WHEN
CHILDREN
ASK ABOUT
SEX

When Children Ask About Sex

A Guide for Parents

Joae Graham Selzer, M.D.

Drawings by Linda Sturges

Beacon Press 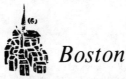 *Boston*

612.6
Sel

Beacon Press books are published under the auspices
of the Unitarian Universalist Association

Simultaneous publication in Canada by Saunders of Toronto, Ltd.

9 8 7 6 5 4 3 2 1

"Spring," by Ruth Whitman, © 1965 by Ruth Whitman.
Reprinted from her volume *The Marriage Wig and Other Poems*
by permission of Harcourt Brace Jovanovich, Inc.

Library of Congress Cataloging in Publication Data

Selzer, Joae Graham, 1926—
    When children ask about sex.
    Bibliography: p. 148
    1. Sex instruction.   2. Children's questions
and answers.   I. Title.   [DNLM: 1. Sex education.
HQ56 S469w]
HQ57.S46   612.6′007   74-4879
ISBN 0-8070-2376-0

Contents

Preface

Children and their parents are now living in rapidly changing times. Established traditions are being questioned and discarded by growing numbers of young people. Adolescents—especially those of college age—are more sexually active than in the past. Girls flock to clinics and doctors' offices for contraceptives. But many others do not protect themselves, and pregnancies and abortions are common. Venereal disease has reached epidemic proportions in this country. Young couples live together without being married. Divorces occur with ever-increasing frequency. Unmarried pregnant girls often decide to keep their babies. Of those who do marry, an alarming number are already pregnant, adding to the stress of adjusting to marriage. A new philosophy, that marriage is outdated and confining, is spreading, and many young people believe they should be able to move in and out of relationships when they feel the need for change. Teen-aged girls beginning to date are told by their boyfriends that virginity is an old-fashioned burden they should rid themselves of as soon as possible.

Many parents are increasingly anxious about the welfare of their growing children in the midst of this upheaval in sexual mores and are unsure about what to tell them. They want very much to be helpful and give them guidance, but they don't want to be met with exasperated rejection by sons and daughters who tell them that their ideas are outmoded and irrelevant.

It is difficult to communicate meaningfully with children about sex today. This book serves as a guide for parents trying to carry out this task. Children still ask questions about sex, although their ways of asking vary with age and their feelings about the person they are talking with. In this book you will find the typical questions asked by preschool, pre-teen, and teen-aged children. The meaning of the questions, not only in terms of what the child wants to know, but of what is going on in his emotional life at the stage of development that gives rise to the question, is discussed. Suggested answers are given and sample discussions between parents and children show how to promote communication and thinking that leads to further conversations within the family and dissuades the child from turning to other unknown and often unreliable sources of information.

The book deals honestly with all kinds of sexual questions and issues and emphasizes the positive aspects of loving sex and marriage. It discusses questions about the new ways of relating sexually and offers guidance through the conflicting maze of today's morality for both children and their parents.

The book gives warnings and reassurances. Parents are asked not to pry, lecture, or interrupt, and not to deride the child's questions or ideas. But no one can handle a discussion perfectly every time. If you feel you made a mess of it, don't be afraid to admit you made a mistake or to apologize and start again. Your sincere wish to understand and be helpful will get through to your child, and that is what is important.

Acknowledgment

The author wishes to express her gratitude to Veronica Tisza, M.D., of the Children's Hospital Medical Center in Boston, Massachusetts, for her helpful thoughts and suggestions.

Part One

Questions the Very Young and Preschool Children Ask

Infant Sexuality

Young children are very interested in their own bodies. The preschool child has a strong desire to learn about himself as well as the world around him. A two or three-year-old learns a great deal by looking and touching, and until about the age of five a young child understands only the simplest verbal explanations.

Babies are self-centered creatures. They are sensitive to their own feelings and needs, but not to those of others. From the very beginning of life their bodies are of the utmost importance to them. The warmth, comfort, and strength of the mother's body as she holds her baby gives it a feeling of security and pleasure, and the sight of mother's face, the sound of her voice, the smell and texture of her skin, the way she carries and holds it become bound up with the simultaneous relieving of unpleasant, distressing feelings of being hungry, chilly, and lonely.

Bathing and being changed are enjoyable for the infant, and rhythmic sensations of being pushed along in a carriage or gently rocked are enjoyable too. Sucking is an intense need in babies and can adequately be gratified by either the breast or the bottle. The important factors are the warmth, relaxation and closeness transmitted to the baby by both its mother and father.

A child's first experience with sexual feelings occurs during the first year while being bathed and changed. The pressure and motion of the washcloth on the genital area brings pleasurable sensations in that very sensitive part of the body which the baby enjoys. When the infant is a little older and better able to control the movements of limbs, s/he may touch the genitals accidentally and then try to touch this part of the body again, simply because it is natural and human to want to re-experience something pleasurable. Baby boys often pull at their penises, but infant girls find it more difficult to touch their genitals because they are more hidden and so we see this activity less in them.

Some parents get upset at this early interest in sexual sensations and worry that it may be somehow abnormal. What the babies are doing is entirely normal, natural, and healthy. *Sex education begins at this point.* It's important to remember that an angry response on your part—bewildering and frightening to the baby—*is* harmful to the emotional development, not the rudimentary masturbation.

Toilet Training and Sexual Feelings

Toilet Training at around eighteen months to two-and-a-half years again focuses both the child's and mother's attention on the child's genitals. If s/he is to remain dry, s/he must become more aware of sensations in this part of the body. S/he must begin to notice when the bladder or bowels are full, and the pressure causes some sexual feelings in neighboring organs. During training, diapers are removed much of the time and the skin of the genitals and buttocks is now exposed to the potty chair or toilet seat and no longer insulated by the diaper, so the child perceives pressures and touch much more acutely. S/he now pays more careful attention to the feeling of urine as it passes through the urethra and this in itself is pleasurable. Little boys must hold the penis as they urinate to control the stream and this feels pleasant to them. New sensations are experienced from the rubbing of toilet paper, especially in little girls, for the urethral opening is next to the highly sensitive clitoris and is also near the vagina.

Often small boys become more aware of the scrotum and testicles during toilet training for as they sit on a cold potty seat, the skin of the scrotum tightens and the two testicles reflexly rise upwards causing a peculiar sensation. If your little boy seems anxious as he sits on the potty chair and resists doing it, you would be wise to keep this in mind and reassure him that everything is all right. Any further explanation such as attempting to tell the toddler about the testicles inside the scrotum is futile, for a child of this age cannot comprehend at all clearly the difference between what is inside the body and what is outside. In spite of your good intentions and correct statements you will end up confusing him.

Young children consistently assert their own fantasies about phenomena they observe or hear about and cling to these erroneous ideas for years. One instance which came to my attention was a very bright eight-year-old who at six had been told simply and clearly by her mother where babies came from and how they were made. The mother believed that her young daughter understood and knew the basic facts and was astonished to hear the girl explain to a friend one day, "You know how babies get made? The mother and the father lie down close together and the sperm go out of his belly button and into her belly button, and they meet and start to grow into a baby."

But one afternoon a year later, at nine, she confidently gave a friend of her mother's a description of where babies come from that was correct. At eight she had not been ready to accept the idea of intercourse and so thought up her own explanation of how the sperm meets the egg; at nine she was able to accept the reality of the concept.

So don't be discouraged that you haven't dealt with your young child's questions adequately if s/he comes out with some completely inaccurate account, very different from the answer you gave earlier. Keep in mind that the inside of the body is very mysterious indeed to children and their emotional needs at various stages of development greatly affect what they perceive and understand. It does no good to argue. When the child asks a question, answer only what s/he is asking in a simple, clear, and honest statement, and that is all.

"Where Do Babies Come From?"

Children usually first begin to ask where babies come from at three or four. In this age of the nuclear family, when young mothers have no aunts, grandmothers, or housekeepers living in the home as ever-available baby sitters, young children are taken about a good deal as their mothers do errands. This can be very educational for the child, especially if the mother answers questions s/he asks. In the supermarket there may be a baby nestled in an adjacent shopping cart; on the trolley a pregnant lady sits down near the child; on the sidewalk ahead an amorous adolescent couple hold hands and occasionally kiss and on the lawn a pair of dogs may be copulating. The young child, with innate curiosity and drive to know and learn, sees, wonders, and at some time asks, "Where do babies come from?"

This universal, basic question makes many parents anxious and tongue-tied because of old, learned feelings of anxiety and possible guilt about sexual matters. They wonder whether the child should now be told about intercourse. But the three- or four-year-old is simply asking about the place where babies come from. S/he has been to enough stores by now and has observed enough packages left at the house by the mailman or delivery man to know that babies aren't bought and delivered in the usual way.

Well, where do babies come from? They come from a mother's uterus. It is as simple as that. And so the answer should be something like this: "A baby comes from a special place inside its mother."

Children under five usually do not pursue the matter further. At five or six they will want to know how the baby got inside the mother, and how it gets out. But at three or four the child is satisfied with this explanation and the matter is usually dropped until a later time when s/he is more aware of what goes on in the world. At five years cause and effect begin to have some meaning for the child.

Of course young children know nothing about tact or appropriate timing. They ask whenever the need arises. The clear, high, four-year-old's voice asks where babies come from in the crowded supermarket as s/he gazes at a sleeping infant in the next shopping cart, or inquires in the trolley car or bus as s/he stares unabashedly at the pregnant lady's abdomen: "Mama, why is that lady's tummy so big?" "There is a baby growing inside her." "Why?" "That is where babies come from."

"How Does the Baby Get Inside the Mother?"

Children are usually not ready to hear about intercourse, sperms, and fertilization until six or seven. If they ask at five how the baby gets inside the mother, you can mention the tiny eggs inside every woman and say that when a woman wants to have a baby, one of those tiny eggs starts to grow into a baby in a special place inside her. Any further explanation only confuses the child at this age. "How does the baby get in?" To a child's mind the only way something can get into the body is through the mouth by eating. So the idea that pregnancy somehow results from swallowing something or kissing is very common in children. A six-year-old girl once told me that you get pregnant when a man kisses you —he has seeds on his lips. Often adults tease children, knowing intuitively about this widespread notion and having remnants of it unconsciously in themselves. They tell children, for example, that if they swallow a melon seed, it will grow into a melon inside them and the leaves will come out of their ears. Most children laugh at this kind of joking, but some worry secretly about it and may develop food phobias.

"How does the baby get in?"

"The mother has a lot of very tiny eggs inside her. They are not the kind of eggs we eat. They are much smaller. When she wants to have a baby, one little egg grows slowly into a baby inside her. It takes a long time."

And if the child wants to know how the baby gets out, you can say, "There is an opening [*or* a little hole] for the baby to come out when it is ready to be born. It is between the mother's legs. The hole gets bigger and the baby comes out."

Because the orifices for the elimination of urine and bowel movements are situated so close to the vagina and because the labia—the fleshy lips covering the vaginal opening—conceal it from view, young children very often believe the baby comes out the same place as urine or bowel movements. This confusion lasts for years and may not become clear until puberty. Nevertheless it's important to explain clearly that there are separate openings. Western society is very concerned about cleanliness, and it is all too easy for a child to form the attitude that bowel movements and urine are dirty and therefore bad, and so the part of the body emitting them must be dirty and bad, too. Since sexual activity occurs in this area, an unfortunate, negative feeling extends to sexuality and may cause inhibitions, anxieties, and guilt which can last throughout life. So it is of great importance that mothers make a consistent effort during toilet training to refrain from expressions of dislike or disgust at the child's waste products, and also that the three orifices be clearly differentiated for the child so that s/he does not believe a baby comes out with bowel movements or urine and associate it with them.

A Positive Attitude Toward Sex Says Much—Nonverbally— To Your Child

It is not only what you tell your child that matters, but your feelings about and attitude toward the body and its sexuality. All kinds of messages are communicated nonverbally to children by adults, and children understand them, even though the adult may not be aware of what s/he is conveying. A facial expression, tone of voice, choice of words, state of muscular tension or relaxation, and a willingness or unwillingness really to pay attention and listen and answer honestly—all tell a child a great deal about the parent's feelings. It is crucial that children feel comfortable about asking questions and learning. If your child senses that you don't want to be confronted with questions about the body, s/he will either repress the desire to learn which may affect how s/he learns new material in school later, or s/he will turn elsewhere for answers and then you have no idea what s/he is hearing and learning.

Should Parents Be Relaxed About Nudity?

Many parents want to believe it's appropriate and helpful to allow their young children to see them nude as one way of answering questions. They feel the human body is a fine, natural thing that need not be covered up or hidden from children; that if it's always kept from their sight, children begin to think there is something bad or shameful about the genitals. A negative attitude about nudity could lead to anxiety, inhibition, and conflict later when the child, then an adult, wants to express sexual feelings and actions in a relationship with a loved person.

This attitude is understandable, but, unfortunately, in practice—at least in our Western culture—difficulties may arise when parents expose their bodies to their young children. The sight of adult genitals is sometimes frightening and exciting to very young children and may cause feelings of inadequacy which affect their basic image of themselves. It is important to remember that to small children we look like giants.

Little boys may feel small and weak in comparison with their big fathers. Much of their swaggering and boasting is a not very successful attempt to feel big, strong, and important. Their exaggerated wishes to be the biggest and strongest in the whole world show how small and vulnerable they really feel inside; otherwise, they wouldn't have to go to such extremes. To be repeatedly reminded by the sight of the father's naked body that they are smaller may emphasize over and over again inner feelings of inferiority and resentment despite reassurances that they will grow up to be as big as daddy.

The sight of adult female genitals may stir up conflict in both small boys and girls. One theory holds that castration fear is aroused in little boys. They think everyone must be made like them, so they conclude that mother once had a penis and worry about what could have happened to it. Many decide it's hidden in mother's pubic hair.

Girls may have anxiety about castration, although it is somewhat different. According to Freud, some already feel castrated and therefore inferior, and the repeated sight of the nude mother keeps stirring up these upsetting ideas.

It's not uncommon for a little girl to become quite preoccupied with her father's penis if she sees him naked often. A mixture of intense feeling may occur. She is excited and tries to get into the bathroom or shower with him because the excitement is pleasurable, but other distressing feelings and thoughts may occur at the same time. She may feel cheated and angry that she does not have this interesting organ.

These conflicts may arise with intensity and cause difficulty in children repeatedly exposed to and stimulated by their parents' nude bodies. In these instances, it seems parents are acting out an unconcious wish to exhibit their bodies and to be seductive, and the child gets the unspoken message and becomes emotionally caught up in it.

One father wanted to know why the sight of his penis would mean any more to his three-year-old son than the sight of his hand or foot. I pointed out that for a number of reasons the genitals are invested with emotion and some measure of conflict in children, and that looking at his father's penis is a very different kind of experience for a three-year-old boy than seeing his father's hand. The penis is special because not everyone has one; father's is much bigger and surrounded by hair; the boy has experienced pleasure from erections and touching the very sensitive skin covering his penis, and he takes great pride in seeing how high or far he can direct his urinary stream.

Let us go back for a moment to the parents who want to foster the attitude that the body is natural, good, and acceptable, and can be viewed without anxiety and shame. I agree, but, caution against a too-eager program of exposure, because it may result in conflict and difficulty rather than calm, easy acceptance.

The unconscious mind is a powerful force which can affect behavior without our being aware of it. A parent who sincerely believes s/he is being natural and non-sexual about being nude in front of the children, may be unwittingly acting on an unconscious wish to be exhibitionistic, seductive, teasing, or superior, and the child perceives it even though the parent doesn't. It is the very rare person in our culture who can be really relaxed and non-sexual while nude in front of others.

Parents shouldn't gasp and run for cover, however, if their child unexpectedly comes into the bedroom or bathroom. This makes the child feel that something is very wrong—that the genitals are shameful and must be kept out of sight at all times. It gives rise to anxiety about the genitals and sexual acts and feelings.

How should one behave, then? I feel the wisest course is to avoid repeated nakedness in front of very young children, but if a child wanders in when you are undressed, be calm and casual about it, go about getting dressed at the usual pace, and be ready to answer questions, for your child will want to know why your genitals are different from his or hers.

A three-year-old girl burst unexpectedly into her parents' bedroom while her mother was nude and preparing to get dressed. The child's eyes widened at the sight of her mother's pubic hair and she exclaimed, "You have hair there!"

"Yes."

"Oh, I don't like it! Why do you have it?"

"All women have hair here."

"Why?"

"When you get to be about eleven or twelve, it just grows."

A three-year-old boy walks into the bathroom while his father is drying himself after a shower. The child is struck by the large size of his father's genitals and the dark hair around them. He observes, "Your penis is too big."

"Yes, it is big. Yours will be big, too, when you are grown up."

"Hair is ugly."

"Grown-ups have hair there."

"Me have big penis too, bigger than yours!"

"When you are grown up, your penis will be big."

This father wisely avoids an argument with his young son and reassures him, allaying his resentment and anxiety.

It is also wise to use accurate terms for the parts of the body. Many parents use babyish or silly words because the correct ones seem too directly sexual and make them uncomfortable; they feel less anxious saying "dingle" or "peewee" or some other word rather than penis. But one of the most important tasks of parenthood is to help children mature, leave babyish ways behind, and feel comfortable about sex. And it is harder to learn something and have to unlearn it later than to learn it correctly in the first place.

One of the most crucial feelings children must sense toward their parents is trust. If you are honest with your child when s/he asks questions, his or her trust will be encouraged. This is basic to any good interpersonal relationship, in childhood and among adults.

A very easy and natural way for children to see nakedness in both sexes without the possible stimulation and anxiety of viewing their parents' bodies is to permit siblings and young friends in the course of everyday living to be together as they dress and undress and bathe. The smaller, hairless genitals are far less conflict-producing and the casual, accepting attitude toward nudity that many parents hope for can be achieved in this way.

In certain primitive societies, nudity and sex play among children are freely allowed and sexual activity—including intercourse—takes place at puberty. This is part of the culture and perfectly acceptable to everyone. But I feel that our society, despite recent extraordinary changes in sexual behavior and attitudes, is not ready for this. If parents feel some change is needed —that behavior which in general is not acceptable should be—they should discuss it with their children after puberty and let them know what they may be facing, and give them the freedom to decide whether they want to be pioneers.

One other important aspect of the question of parental nudity is privacy. Sometimes we think too much about our children's needs, and not enough about our own. We have desires and rights, too. Most people want privacy at times and they should have it. Their children should realize that being alone or apart sometimes is part of living. It is entirely appropriate to set limits in terms of keeping the bedroom door closed at night and the bathroom door closed when bathing or using the toilet. And children's rights and wishes to be alone should be respected as well.

As children grow older, the sight of parents' bodies is not so likely to arouse anxiety and conflict. Parents can be more relaxed and casual about nudity at this time. The admonitions I have outlined are really for parents of very young children whose understanding and security are not yet very great. But again at puberty when the child's sexual feelings and thoughts intensify, modesty in the parent of the opposite sex is once again called for. Early adolescents are very sensitive and tend to assume, because sex is so much on their minds, that everyone is thinking about it too. A father shaving in the nude and thinking about business problems may be accused by his pubertal daughter of being deliberately seductive.

When Do Children First Experience Oedipal Feelings?

Children from four to six years will go through an Oedipal phase of development in which the little boy has yearnings to be the most important man in the world to his mother and the little girl has the same feelings toward her father. They also harbor rivalrous, resentful feelings toward the parent of the same sex, and secretly wish that that parent were out of the picture altogether. Of course these wishes are only part of the totality of the child's feelings, for little girls need and love their mothers and boys adore and imitate their fathers and if through divorce or death the loved and resented parent is actually gone, the child will be severely upset and grieving, and may feel worried that his or her angry feelings caused the terrible loss. Children thrive in the normal, healthy situation where both parents live together and meet the children's needs—where the child can see and experience the reality that his or her rivalrous, hostile wishes don't actually come true, and that in spite of them the parents stick by him or her and love him or her.

Boys and girls at this age will frequently express wishes to marry the parent of the other sex. They should not be teased or laughed at, for they are quite serious and the whole matter is of the utmost importance to them. Neither should they be dealt with seductively, for that may make it harder to get through this stage and leave it behind. Children need parents who are reliable, loving, accepting, and yet help them know and deal with reality.

Psychiatrists treat people constantly whose adult love relationships are unhappy and fraught with conflict because of old, unresolved Oedipal yearnings which a seductive parent often unwittingly fostered. Seductiveness can be expressed in the way a parent talks to a child.

A five-year-old girl yearns to marry her father and replace her mother. Recently her parents have had difficulties in their relationship. Her mother feels neglected by the busy and tired father; her angry and sarcastic comments make him keep away from her even more. One evening, having been detained unexpectedly at work, he arrives home an hour late for dinner.

Father: Hello. I'm sorry I'm late. I didn't expect——
Mother: I didn't think you'd be on time. It seems you just stay away from me as much as you can lately.
Father: (*angry too*) Look, I couldn't help it. Will you please lay off? What are we having for dinner?
Mother: Steak, but it's probably all dried out by now.
Child: Daddy, I'll make you supper!
Father: Well, I'm glad to see someone cares about me around here.
Child: Daddy, let's get married and I'll make supper for you every night!
Father: Okay, honey, I bet you'll be a better wife to me than Mommy!
Mother: (*feeling increasingly neglected*) All right, you two have a nice, happy time together. You probably won't even miss me when I'm gone.

Suddenly the little girl's world is turned upside down. Her normal wish has turned her mother against her. The child is filled with fear and sadness. If this kind of interaction is repeated over and over again, she may be unable to trust her mother, have problems getting along with women as she grows older, and be too tied to a father who extends a promise he can never keep. This may push her in the direction of either not trusting men or choosing men who disappoint her.

When parents are resentful and unhappy, it's very hard for them to pay careful attention to their children's needs. But parents have the great responsibility to listen and answer honestly and helpfully. The situation just described might have been dealt with better in the following way:

Father: Hello. Sorry I'm late. I didn't expect a meeting to be called at the last minute.
Mother: (*annoyed but holding back her feelings*) I guess it couldn't be helped. Sit down, you two, and I'll have dinner on the table in a minute.
Child: (*snuggling up to her father*) Daddy, I want to marry you!

Father: Jenny, I love you, but you know I'm married to Mommy.

Child: Well, Debbie's parents got divorced. They had fights. You and Mommy fight.

Father: Mommy and I get tired and we do get mad at each other sometimes. But I am not going to marry you. Mommy is my wife. You are my little girl.

Child: I want to be your wife!

Father: No, you are my child. I love Mommy and I love you, too, but you cannot be my wife.

Mother: (*pleased to hear that father still has loving feelings toward her, looks and sounds happier*) Jenny, Tom, come to dinner. I think it will still be good.

The child learns that she can compete with her mother and express loving yearnings toward her father without anyone getting angry or leaving her. If her mother had become furious and had walked out, the little girl would have felt abandoned, unloved, guilty, and bad, but when this does not happen, she knows she will be loved and accepted even if she sometimes wishes her mother were out of the way and she had her father to herself.

Here is an illustration with a younger boy. A five-year-old boy watches his parents kiss when his father comes home from work. He feels envious and wants to be the most important male in his mother's life. He wants all of her time and attention. He tries to get between them and tells his mother, "Mommy, Mommy, I'm going to marry you!"

"No, Tommy, I'm married to Daddy. You are my little boy."

"I'm your husband."

"Daddy is my husband. Someday when you are grown up, you will find a nice wife."

"I want you to be my wife!"

"I can't be your wife. You're my little boy and I'm your mother. I love Daddy and I love you."

Should Children Witness Parental Intercourse?

One aspect of family life children should not see because of the psychological damage it can do is parental intercourse. Children characteristically perceive intercourse as an aggressive attack by the father upon the mother, and interpret any sounds associated with it as moans of pain and distress. Some children have revealed to child psychiatrists a fear that their father was killing their mother. This traumatic experience can result in neurosis in the child. A three-year-old girl was found by her young parents in a state of complete panic upon their return from a week's vacation. She had been in the care of loving grandparents who were terribly upset and bewildered by the child's extreme behavior. The little girl refused to get dressed or eat and talked in a babbling monotone. She was taken to the psychiatrist's office wrapped in a blanket. There she repeatedly smashed two toy locomotives together. She was seen in daily sessions because of the severity of her panic, and as she began to speak more intelligibly, she called one train "Grandma" and the other "Grandpa."

At that point, the doctor realized that the child must have seen the grandparents having sexual relations, and when the doctor talked with them, she learned that the child had slept on a cot in their bedroom, for they lived in a small, one-bedroom apartment, and they had made love when they thought she had been asleep. It took several months to work through the child's fear, and much patient reassuring on the part of the psychiatrist and the parents before she emerged as her old smiling, lively self again.

Parents might put a lock on their bedroom door to insure privacy when in bed at night. The ordinary hook kind is easy, practical, and can be placed high on the door. In general during the day children should feel free and welcome anywhere in the house except when a parent or adolescent sibling is using the bathroom, but at night parents have a right to both privacy and rest. Too many young children interrupt their parents' sleep by coming into the bedroom at night and getting into bed between them. Although children like the closeness, they may feel guilty to some degree and this is not helpful. And they need help in learning to tolerate being alone at night.

"Why Don't Girls Have a Penis?"

Let us look now at the kinds of questions typically asked by three-, four-, and five-year-olds as they try to learn about and understand the body.

A three-year-old boy has a new baby sister. He stands next to his mother as she changes her diapers. He is surprised to see that the baby's body is not like his. Because he feels he is the center of the world and everyone's body must be like his, he reasons that his sister must have been born with a penis like his; his anxiety stems from his deduction that something must have happened to it. Does that mean that he could lose his penis, too? He cannot imagine a worse punishment than losing this organ which feels pleasant when he touches it and sometimes gets bigger and stands up and which he can use to make his urinary stream go in any direction he wants. And how could he grow up to be like Daddy without a penis? These worries prompt him to ask, "Where is her penis?" or "Why doesn't Amy have a penis like mine?" or "What happened to her penis?"

Your answers should reassure your small and worried son that nothing will happen to his penis because this is what he really needs to hear.

"Girls don't have a penis."

"Why?"

"They're made differently. Boys are born with a penis. Girls are born with a little place inside them for a baby to grow in when they are grown up."

If he still seems anxious and needs more reassurance, you can say, "You will always have your penis."

Little girls often feel envious when they discover that boys have a penis. They feel they lack something important, for boys obviously derive much pride and pleasure from this appendage. They wonder why they don't have one, too. Some worry that they had one once and somehow lost it. Some secretly fantasize that they possess one, though they know their daydream is not true. It is a rare girl indeed who at some time in her early childhood did not secretly try to urinate standing up as she had seen a brother or playmate do, only to find to her consternation and resentment that urine trickled down into her socks and shoes. Feelings of being inferior and second-rate may stem from this conflict which may trouble a girl all her life.

So it is very important that parents give their daughters the definite feeling that girls' bodies are as complete and good as boys', that girls are equally important and valuable as human beings. Little girls need to know about the uterus, or womb, whichever you prefer to call it. To tell them about the vagina alone is not enough. They need to learn that they possess something uniquely their own, different from the penis but just as important.

Five-year-old Susie watches her younger brother bathing. She wonders why she doesn't have a penis, and worries that her body isn't as good as his. She feels something is missing, something is wrong. She feels uneasy, angry, and sad. She goes to her mother and questions her. Her mother realizes the importance of her little girl's inquiries, and listens carefully.

"Mommy, why don't I have a penis like Danny's?"

"Girls and women don't have a penis."

"Why?"

"We aren't born with a penis. Our bodies are made the way they are on purpose."

"Why?"

"We are made so we can have babies. Boys can't have babies."

"Why?"

"We have a special little place inside us for a baby to grow in. It is called the uterus [*or* womb]. Boys don't have a uterus."

"Where is it? I don't see it. Can you see yours?"

"It is way inside us, in here [*touching her lower abdomen*]. It looks a little like a pear upside down. When we go to the store, we can look at a pear."

"Why is it inside? I want to see it!"

"The uterus is inside so the baby will be warm and safe."

"Will a baby grow in me today?"

"No. It will happen someday when you are a grown up woman."

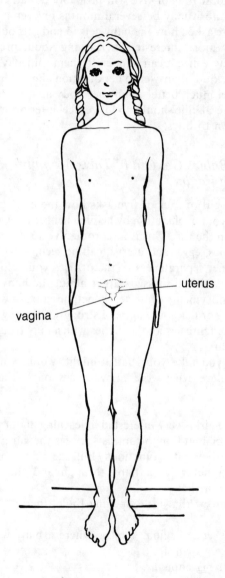

The child at four or five will probably be satisfied with this explanation and it may be several months or even a year or two before you are asked how the baby gets in and gets out. Little girls are naturally more interested in learning about pregnancy and birth, for they realize it can happen to them someday. A little girl who gets this kind of answer to her question about why she lacks a penis will feel much better about her body and, therefore, about herself in general. She should no longer feel inferior or second-rate in comparison to boys.

"How Do Babies Get Out of Their Mommy's Tummy? What Is the Vagina?"

When a girl of four or five asks how the baby gets out, you can support your explanation by helping her see the vaginal orifice when she is in the tub. This is a reproductive structure which, unlike the ovaries, eggs, and uterus, can be seen. Also, by pointing out the distinct separateness of the orifices you help prevent the common confusion discussed earlier about the baby coming out with bowel movements or urine. Sometimes a child wants to have you show him or her your vagina. I strongly advise against this for it may arouse fantasies and anxieties which may trouble the child for many years.

"When you take your bath tonight, would you like to see your little place where the baby comes out? It is called the vagina."

"Yes!"

The little girl is very interested in learning about her anatomy and feels special and important as she sees the various parts and understands their vital functions. But she may worry that her vagina could never let a baby through and she needs to be reassured about that.

"Do you see that little opening [hole] there?"

"Yes."

"That is your vagina. That is where a baby will come out when you are grown up."

"It's not big enough ."

"It will be. You will grow bigger and it will grow bigger too. When the baby is born, the vagina stretches. You know how an elastic stretches; your vagina will stretch like that to let the baby out."

She may ask where urine and bowel movements come out. It is important to comment that the vagina is not the place where urine and bowel movements come out. If she asks where those openings are, you can easily show her by pointing to or touching her anus. The urethra is much more difficult to find and you might just tell her that it is a very small opening or hole in front of her vagina that is hard to see.

You may find the drawings of the infant boy and girl on pages 22 and 23 helpful in explaining the location and function of the orifices. I have not labelled the structures in the pictures because little children take things very literally and would be distracted by lines leading to explanatory words.

The round structure at the top of the genital area is the clitoris. Next is the very small urethra for the excretion of urine. Next is the larger orifice called the vagina although the vagina is actually the entire passageway from the outside of the body up to the bottom of the uterus. At the bottom is the anus.

The drawing of the boy includes the scrotum and the urethra as well as the penis. The word urethra is quite difficult for a young child to master so you could just say it is the little place where urine comes out.

If your child asks what the scrotum is, simply name it. "That is called the scrotum. Boys and men have a scrotum."

Usually young children are satisfied with that. It is not until six or older that they will ask what it is for.

The young girl may ask you about her clitoris, the highly sensitive little organ anterior to the vaginal orifice, whose function is solely to enhance sexual pleasure. Often little girls equate the clitoris with the penis.

"Look at this! This is my little penis."

"That is your clitoris. It is different from a penis."

"What is it for? It feels nice [*laughing*]."

"That's what it's for. To feel nice."

"Do you have one, too?"

"Yes."

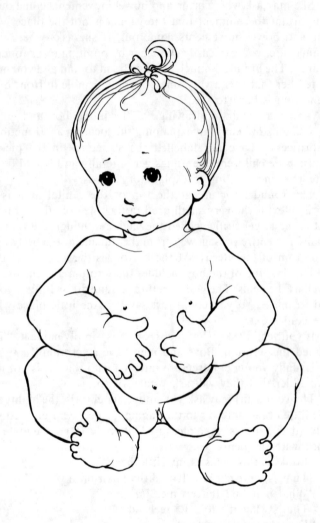

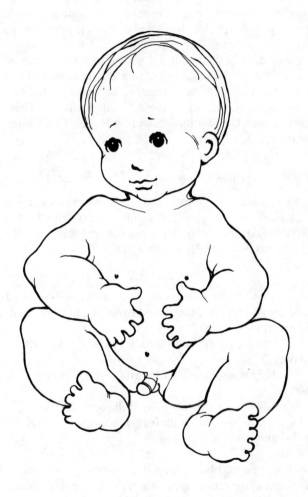

A small boy wonders too how babies get in and get out. If there is an infant girl in your family, you can show him her vagina while changing her, for she is clearly too young to be embarrassed. It is also easy while changing the baby's diapers to show your little boy the infant's anus, again to make the distinction between the orifices and their functions. If you have a son asking about these matters and you do not have an infant daughter, you might ask a friend who does if she would be willing to let you and your son visit while she is bathing or changing the baby so you can point these things out to him. It is amazing how many intelligent adult men are vague and ignorant about female anatomy. They would be more competent and understanding lovers if they knew more about it.

"Why Do Grown-Up Women Have Breasts?"

Boys as well as girls wonder about women's breasts. They look at their own bodies and cannot understand how or why women's breasts are so big. How did they get that way? What are they for? And they wonder whether they will have breasts like that someday.

A three-year-old boy went over to his full-breasted aunt, reached up and touched her breast through her dress, and asked, "Why are these so big?"

She answered, "Grown-up ladies have big breasts."

"Why?"

"If a lady has a baby, her breasts make milk for the baby to drink."

"My Mommy gave our baby milk out of a bottle."

"Some mommies use milk from a bottle and some like to give the baby milk out of their breast."

A four-year-old boy watched his mother nurse his newborn sister. Some of the milk dripped from the nipple. He asked, "What is the baby doing?"

His mother answered, "She is drinking milk from my breast."

"Why?"

"She is hungry and the milk is her food."

The little boy touched his mother's other breast and asked, "Is there milk in this one, too?"

"Yes."

"Why?"

"So there will be enough for the baby."

He was quiet for a moment, and then stuck out his chest and announced in a loud voice, "I have little ones and there's milk in them too!"

"No, boy's breasts don't have milk in them."

"They do too! Mine have milk."

There is no sense in arguing. It is best to calmly, clearly, and briefly tell the child the truth and let the matter drop. Young children are likely to believe what they want to believe and can be very stubborn about it. The boundary line between reality and fantasy is not at all clear, especially in the face of a strong wish.

"Why Don't Boys Have a Uterus and Breasts? What Is the Scrotum and What Is It For?"

Little boys may feel gypped when they learn that they do not possess a uterus and will not ever have a baby growing inside them or produce milk from their breasts. Young children want everything and time and again in their young lives little boys would like to have everything that mother has.

A three-year-old boy with a newborn brother began strutting around the house with his abdomen prominently protruding. When asked why his stomach was sticking out so far he promptly explained, "There's a baby inside me!"

"But boys can't have babies."

"Yes, *I* can."

"Well, you can be a daddy someday."

He also insisted on being called a girl's name. This behavior persisted for six months and disappeared as quickly as it started. This child from four until six was anxious about the possibility of losing his penis. The castration anxiety was expressed almost daily in his comments that a lion or a tiger might bite off his penis. He was fascinated but very tense one day during a visit to the zoo. On the drive back home the family passed a grove of slender, straight trees; he announced that they would soon be chopped down. This phase, like the earlier one, passed spontaneously. His parents treated it casually but reassuringly. They did not argue with him but in an accepting manner let him express his feelings and simply stated from time to time that nothing was going to happen to his penis.

Many little boys have intense castration anxiety, but they soon learn it is not right to talk about it because of the shocked reception their comments arouse. They keep their worries to themselves. This, of course, is unfortunate because they don't receive the understanding and reassurance they need during this phase of development when the concern over getting "hurt" looms large. Sometimes small boys trying to cope with castration anxiety will say that everyone has a penis, including mother, grandmother, aunts, etc. If they can believe that girls and women as well as boys and men have a penis, they don't worry so much about possibly losing theirs.

A three-year-old boy insisted that everyone's body was the same, saying that sister, mother, and grandmother each had a penis. When his mother tried to correct this notion, he was adamant in his denial: "Oh, no, Nana has a penis."

A four-year-old boy announced at dinner one night to the surprise of his family, "Mommy has a penis!"

Little girls sometimes make various attempts to claim that they have a penis, too. They will label the clitoris a little penis, and will give their baby brother's penis a name, thus partly assuming ownership: "That thing is a dingle dangle. Isn't it cute?"

One jealous four-year-old girl teased a three-year-old playmate about his "pee-pee tassel," a name she insisted his penis should be called, but her preoccupation with the teasing revealed her envy. Once she "accidentally" hit him in the crotch. Her aggression diminished markedly when her mother told her about her own genitals, including the uterus and tiny eggs inside her, and how special and important her body was, too.

Little boys are more interested in the penis than in the scrotum and testes, because the penis is in their line of vision and they touch it while urinating. They will ask, however, about the little bag of skin behind the penis and want to know what it is. A parent who does not yet want to go into the man's role in sexuality and the making of babies will answer that it is something all boys and men have, it is a part of their body. The child may be satisfied with that explanation and leave it at that, or may want to know what it is for. The child knows that the penis carries urine out of the body but he cannot figure a use for this other part. I feel one should give a truthful answer rather than be evasive. Even very young children can tell when a parent is not being honest or is try- ing to avoid something. They sense the tension and discomfort in their parent and perceive a change from the customary manner of relating and answering. If the small boy is not satisfied with the statement that this part of his body is called the scrotum and all boys and men have one, and if he really wants to know its pur- pose, I suggest telling him that when he grows up, very tiny seeds called sperms will be made inside the scrotum. These little seeds help start a baby growing. It is often hard on boys to learn that girls can someday have babies inside them and breasts that give milk, and it helps them to learn that they have something impor- tant to do in making a baby.

Both boys and girls are curious about the navel and at some point they all ask what it is for. You might say that when they were babies inside their mother, they got food through a tube that went from the mother's uterus to their own tummies. When they were born and began to take food in through their mouths, they didn't need the tube anymore. It dried up and fell off when they were about a week old. What remains on their tummy is the navel.

Young Children and Masturbation

Young children's interest in their bodies and the pleasure they experience in touching their genitals give rise to some mastur- bation which is entirely normal and pleasing to the child. It is human and natural to want to repeat an experience one finds enjoyable. Children, having learned quite accidentally from being washed or carrying out toileting activities that touching the genitals brings definite pleasure, will do it again. Children tend to masturbate in bed at night because it feels good and compensates for the separation from the rest of the family and the loneliness they often feel at that time. Some children masturbate when anxious, to release uncomfortable tension. Also little boys may clutch their penis when nervous. The important thing to remember is that masturbation is pleasant, completely harmless, and the old wives' tales about its deleterious results are simply not true. Masturbation can be harmful only when parents react with anger and punishment, making the child feel that s/he is bad or that the genitals are dirty. Parents' negative reaction to masturbation can result in a child's lowered self-esteem and problems in accepting and feeling comfortable with sexuality when s/he is older.

Part Two

Questions Pre-Teens Ask

Overview of the Pre-teen Years

The span of years between six and ten has been called *latency,* a word coined by Freud who believed that interest in sexuality was latent in children during this stage of their emotional development. We now know that interest in sex is not entirely latent in this period. During these years children emerge from earlier preoccupations with their body and are more interested in learning about the world around them. Their attention is focused more outward than inward. School is a very important part of their lives and the information they learn and the new adults they relate to outside the family all greatly expand their horizons. Typically the pre-teen child is busy and active. Learning the details of life in the world takes up much of his or her energy and time.

Questions about the body and sexuality do arise, and the child is now ready for more detailed information. S/he wants to learn more about the body, pregnancy, and birth. Boys want to know the man's role in these vital processes. Girls are interested in finding out more about the inside of the body, for they know that babies will grow inside them, and many have heard something about menstruation. They also know that their breasts will grow and someday produce milk. And they are curious about what it is like to give birth.

The pre-teen child is constantly engaged in the difficult task of mediating between inner urges and drives and the demands of the external world. For instance, s/he may feel like talking out in class or getting up and walking around to relieve tension, but, on the other hand, s/he also wants to win the teacher's approval and good will through acceptable behavior. S/he must experience over and over again having to forego childish gratification for the deeper, more lasting, and meaningful satisfaction of behaving in a more mature way. This ever-present struggle makes the pre-teen child feel unsure and fear that his or her equilibrium will be upset. The conscience is also being formed; the child integrates the standards of parents and those teachers and other adults whom s/he likes and respects. These internalized principles and prohibitions have a profound influence upon attitudes and behavior.

In the child of six or seven the conscience is new and harsh and this accounts for many of the child's contradictory actions; s/he alternates between being obedient and rebellious. In the child of eight to ten the conscience, or superego, is less strict and the child copes with reality more easily and with less conflict. The child of six or seven is still concerned with earlier issues and makes jokes about anal matters, while eight- to ten-year-olds are usually beyond this. Entering the pre-teen age, children gradually resolve Oedipal issues. They give up their earlier yearnings as they realize and accept the reality that their wishes are not going to come true. The longings are never given up entirely, but become repressed and largely disappear from conscious thinking. In pre-teen years the child identifies with the parent of the same sex.

Many pre-teen children are in a conflict over masturbation. They know that touching or rubbing the genitals is pleasurable, but they may have been conditioned to feel that it is something they should not do. Other children masturbate quite regularly and frequently, and some only occasionally. Of course, masturbation is an entirely normal and natural activity—part of the child's development. Most often it occurs under the blanket before going to sleep at night. An important factor is your attitude about it; if you are accepting and reassuring, your child will not feel fearful and "bad." We have all heard the old stories of softening of the brain and other hideous conditions supposedly caused by masturbation—these stories have no basis in fact. Masturbation increases greatly at puberty when sex hormones are produced and circulate in the bloodstream, intensifying sexual feelings.

The phase of development from about nine or ten until twelve or thirteen is called preadolescence. During this period the child's physical strength and activity increase. The child is more mobile socially and quite engrossed in the interests and activities of the peer group.

During the preadolescent stage the children's interest in their bodies and sexuality will be greater because of physical changes they experience and observe. These changes cause a variety of feelings—bewilderment, anxiety, and pride. The girl notices the growth of her nipples and breasts and the appearance of hair, sparse at first, under her arms and over the pubic area. If she is anxious about these changes, she will make remarks about not liking them. At this time parents should reassure her that what is going on is a normal part of growing up. The boy's voice, on the other hand, begins to deepen and he also has new hair growing in the axillary and genital areas. These changes take place in boys usually about two years later than in girls. The penis will increase in length. In both boys and girls there will be a spurt in height and weight gain.

Puberty or adolescence actually begins when the girl first menstruates and the boy first ejaculates semen, either during sleep as a wet dream or nocturnal emission, or while masturbating. It is important for preadolescent girls to understand fully what menstruation is; otherwise they may be extremely frightened and think they are ill or injured. It is also important for boys to be prepared for ejaculation. Boys can be very anxious and upset if they do not understand that what is happening to them is perfectly natural.

As these changes take place, the children's interest in their bodies is strongly reactivated. External events in the child's life arouse interest in sexuality. Marriage, pregnancy, and birth stir up questions and fantasies. With the change in sexual mores, children learn of young adults living together without being married, of young women becoming pregnant and perhaps keeping babies without a husband to help. Children hear about adoption and wonder where those babies come from and why they are being adopted. They hear about abortion and wonder what it means.

Sex-education classes in the schools, if carefully thought out and taught, can be very helpful in giving children the information they need to understand much of sexuality and to use that understanding wisely. However, parents should be prepared for questions when their children come home from the classes. Children may be confused on some points or may want to understand more fully something briefly touched upon. I have found that many films shown to fifth- and sixth-grade children discuss facts about the testes and ovaries, breasts, and skin (such as the formation of acne) that most parents, despite adequate education in other areas, are not thoroughly acquainted with. It can be very helpful to parents and children if schools invite parents to see the materials and films. Elementary schools I have worked with in sex education in Brookline and Newton, Massachusetts, offer this option to parents. Sometimes parents are invited to view films on an evening preceding a showing to the children; or parents and children are invited to attend together—and early in the evening so that fathers can take part. I feel that sex education for pre-teens will be more successful if parents support and take part in the school's effort.

If you conscientiously listen to your child's questions in general and give thoughtful and truthful answers, your child will be much more inclined to go to you with questions about sexuality and not turn to peers or others as lacking in understanding and perspective as s/he is.

Questions Pre-teens Ask About Sex

My discussions with parents of elementary school-age children focused on the specific questions their children asked them about sex.

A six-year-old girl asked her pregnant mother several questions about babies, her curiosity aroused by her mother's changing shape. When she asked, "Mommy, why is your tummy getting so big? You'd better go on a diet!" her mother answered that she wasn't getting bigger because of overeating, but because a baby was growing inside her in a special place called the uterus.

The child was intensely interested in this news and wanted to know when the baby would come out, and how it got in there. Would it be a boy or a girl? How would it come out? Would the mother have to be cut open? Would it hurt when the baby was born?

The mother found most of these questions easy to answer. She told her daughter the due date, but added that often babies are born a few days before or after the due day. She said she didn't know whether it would be a boy or a girl because she couldn't see inside; they would just have to wait until it was born to see which it was. The baby would come out of an opening between her legs called the vagina that would stretch so the baby could pass through.

The child was told that her mother would not have to be cut open to let the baby out, an acceptable answer because the mother had been through an uncomplicated delivery with her first child and there was no reason to anticipate a Caesarean section. But in the age of TV, when children learn all kinds of facts their parents were not exposed to until they were much older, parents must be prepared to answer questions that were not asked by pre-teens a generation ago. Children nowadays have heard of a Caesarean section and want to know what it is and why it happens.

"Why Are Some Mothers Cut Open to Have Babies?"

A mother might answer this question as follows: "A Caesarean section is done when the baby needs to be born quickly. Inside the uterus is something called the afterbirth which has many blood vessels in it. The blood vessels come from the heart and are like the branches of a tree that carry blood to all parts of the body. In order to stay alive every part of our body needs oxygen from the air we breathe and nutrients from the food we eat. These things get circulated inside us through branching tubes called blood vessels. The afterbirth has a lot of blood vessels in it to carry oxygen and food to the baby, because the baby inside the uterus cannot breathe and eat as we do. Usually the afterbirth comes away from the inside of the uterus and comes out after the baby is born—that is why it is called the afterbirth. But once in a great while it starts to come away from the uterus too soon, before the baby is born, and bleeding starts. The doctor takes the baby out quickly so it won't die. S/he gives the mother some ether so she will fall sound asleep and not feel any pain. Then the doctor carefully cuts the skin of the mother's tummy so s/he can get to the uterus. Then s/he makes a cut in the uterus and reaches in with his or her hand and lifts the baby right out."

You may also tell your child, "Sometimes a woman's bones are too close together inside to let the baby through at birth. The doctor has a way of measuring the space between bones. If the space is too small, the doctor plans way ahead of time to bring the baby out by section."

If a mother has had one baby by section, she will have others the same way, for the place where the uterus was opened does not heal as strongly as it was before (scar tissue is not as strong as muscle) and there is a chance that the uterus could open up by accident when it is pushing the baby out (rupture of the uterine scar during labor could occur).

Sometimes a child hears the term Caesarean section and wants to know how it got that odd name. It is named after Julius Caesar, who is said to have been delivered by this method.

"Does It Hurt to Have a Baby?"

Girls especially want to know if it hurts to have a baby. Again, it is best to be truthful in a reassuring way. The child can be told that the uterus is a big muscle that can push the baby out when it is time for it to be born. The pushing of the uterus does hurt some, but the nurse gives the mother medicine so it won't hurt as much. Some mothers prefer no medicine because they have done special exercises to prepare them for the baby's birth. The mother is so excited and happy to see the baby that has been growing in her for such a long time that she soon forgets the pain.

Younger children do not need to hear about possible complications with childbirth, but if they have heard of some problems and ask about them, it is best to answer honestly and reassuringly. Children do not have the perspective adults have. A six- or seven-year-old may hear of a baby born dead or deformed, or a woman being "cut open" to have her baby. These are very frightening ideas to the child. We know these things happen rarely, but children do not, and they very much need to be reassured.

"How Does a Baby Get Inside a Mother's Tummy?"

The question the six-year-old's mother found most difficult was how the baby got inside her. She said that a little egg inside her tummy grew into a baby. Two problems arise with such an answer. First, the child thinks the stomach where food goes and the uterus where the baby grows are the same place. Second, a girl may develop an aversion to eating eggs, fearing that a baby will start to grow inside her, and she knows she isn't ready for anything like that.

A better answer would be: "All girls and women have many, very tiny eggs inside them. They're not like the eggs we eat or see in a bird's nest, but are so small that if you took a pencil and made a dot, they are even smaller than that. Though very tiny, the eggs are also very important. When a woman wants to have a baby, one of those little eggs starts to grow into a baby inside a special place called the uterus. The uterus is inside the mother, and looks like a pear upside down. It is not the same as the stomach where the food you eat goes. The baby grows for a long time—nine months—the time it takes for a whole school year to go by before it is ready to be born."

"How Does a Baby Breathe and Eat Inside Its Mother's Tummy?"

The previous question probably would lead to queries about how the baby breathes and eats inside the uterus. It could be explained like this: "The baby inside the uterus does not breathe and eat and drink as we do. It gets air and food from its mother's blood through a long white tube called the umbilical cord. After the baby is born, it breathes and drinks milk, so it doesn't need the cord anymore. The doctor cuts the cord after the baby is born. This doesn't hurt the baby at all, because the cord has no nerves in it. Nerves inside us are what makes us feel things like pain, and warmth and cold. After a few days the piece of cord dries up and just falls off the baby's tummy. What is left is called the navel."

"How Does an Egg Start Growing Inside a Mother's Tummy? What Is Intercourse?"

A six-year-old is usually not able to understand details about intercourse, but of course, there are precocious exceptions. When a child is seven or eight, you can tell him or her that a sperm from the father's body joins with the tiny egg inside the mother to start the baby's growth. Of course, the child then wants to know how the sperm gets inside the mother, where it comes from, and just what it is. People feel more uneasy and embarrassed about telling children about intercourse than about anything else. This is partly due to old culturally conditioned anxieties, inhibitions, and worries our elders taught us, that these things are "bad," dirty, or sinful, and partly from fear that one's personal sexual life will be revealed to the child. Both are untrue; sex is a healthy, natural part of life; and one's private sex life with one's husband or wife is not something the child need hear about.

Questions about intercourse should be answered adequately and truthfully by telling children how a man's body is made to fit with a woman's body so that sperm have a way of getting to the egg. The reason why mammalian bodies evolved with the female's reproductive organs inside and the male's outside was to insure a way of getting the sperm to the egg and keeping the developing baby warm and safe. One function of the penis is to deposit sperm at the mouth of the uterus (cervix) where it can meet an egg.

When the body is thought of in this biological way, it is much easier to answer questions about sex because it is all so logical. Intercourse is a way of getting the sperm to the egg. The child asks how the sperm gets to the egg inside the mother.

"The mother and father lie close together and feel loving toward each other. The father's penis gets hard and fits into a special opening between the mother's legs called the vagina. The sperms come out of his penis and swim up into the uterus and find the egg. One sperm swims right inside the egg and then the egg divides into two halves, and then four parts, and more and pretty soon begins to grow into a tiny baby."

Before they are adolescents and begin to have adult sexual feelings, children cannot grasp the notion of pleasure in intercourse. It is perhaps just as well not to try to go into that when

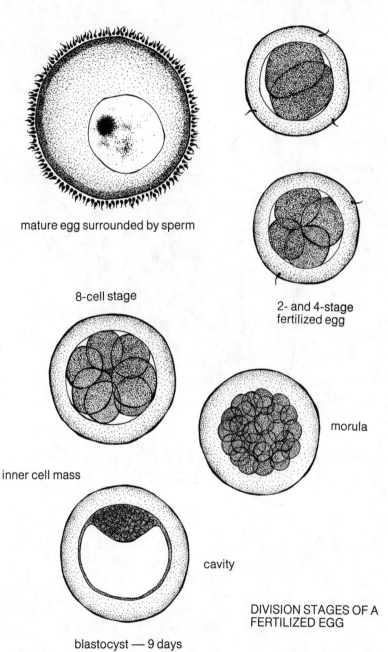

mature egg surrounded by sperm

8-cell stage

2- and 4-stage
fertilized egg

inner cell mass

morula

cavity

DIVISION STAGES OF A
FERTILIZED EGG

blastocyst — 9 days

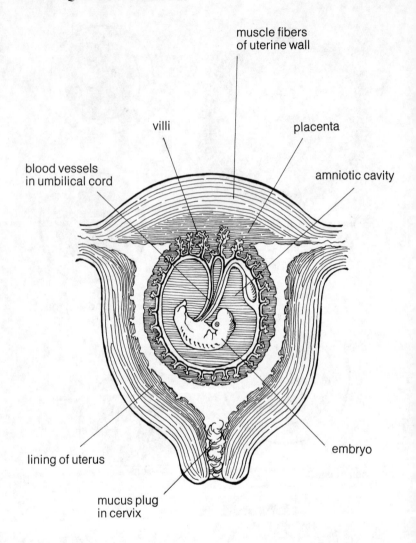

THE PREGNANT UTERUS IN THE THIRD MONTH

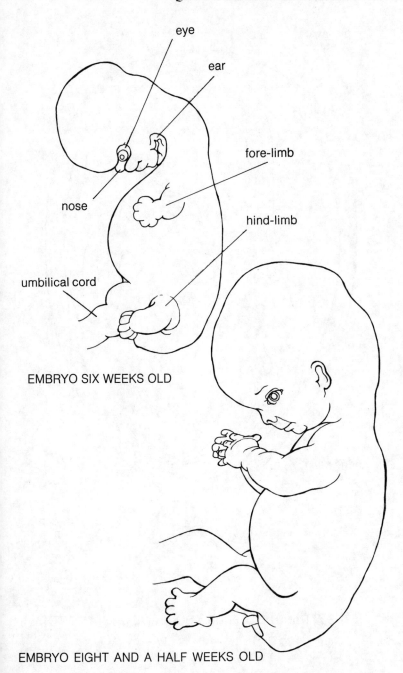

EMBRYO SIX WEEKS OLD

EMBRYO EIGHT AND A HALF WEEKS OLD

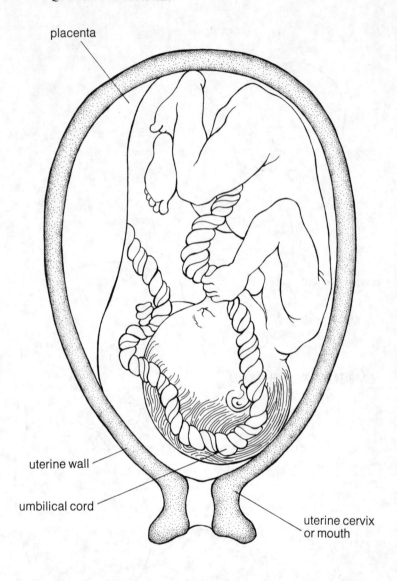

FETUS WITHIN THE UTERUS, ABOUT FIVE OR SIX MONTHS

they are young. Sometimes they will ask about it, because they worry that the penis might hurt and want to be reassured, or because they have experienced pleasurable genital feelings during masturbation or bathing. One mother reported that her nine-year-old daugher asked, "Does intercourse feel good?" When the mother said it did, the child was dubious; at nine she could not imagine the pleasure of making love.

One six-year-old girl wondered how the baby gets bigger inside the mother, knowing it did not eat as she did. The mother said that the baby gets its food from a woman's body, and that satisfied the child, but another child might want more details. One has to take care when explaining anything concerning blood to children, and blood is very much involved in describing how food and air get to the baby growing inside the uterus, menstruation, or erections. It is blood rushing into the spaces in the tissues of the penis that makes it erect. Children worry about blood, associating it with injury, and they should be told that blood is very important and necessary, that we could not live without the food and oxygen it carries to all parts of our bodies, pumped at all times by our heart. When they understand that, they are ready to hear about blood's role in sexual processes and not feel threatened.

An example of misconceptions in children's minds is a six-year-old boy's statement, after hearing about sperms from an older brother, that tadpoles crawl up inside the lady to make a baby. Happily, if children feel free enough about sex to verbalize their thoughts, parents can help correct such misconceptions.

A seven-year-old boy asked about erections, curious about why his penis sometimes stiffened and then went down. His mother said in our discussion group that she hadn't been sure precisely what to answer, but told him that this happened naturally and was perfectly all right. She also suggested that he talk with his father about it if he wanted to. I felt this was an adequate answer for a child of seven, while an older child could hear in more detail about what actually causes an erection when the penis is touched and stimulated. One could say casually to the little boy that that's the way penises are, they do that and it's fine, for the child's anxiety that something might be wrong, as well as curiosity, prompts the question, and he is hoping his parent will allay his fear.

"When Am I Going to Grow Up?"

An eight-year-old boy asked when he was going to grow up. He had noticed some bodily changes in his pubescent brother and, having only a hazy idea of when these things occur, thought they might happen to him at any time. Children need help in getting perspective on not only what occurs but when. And they should realize that human beings are a various lot, some growing very tall and others short, some maturing earlier than others—that we are much more interesting with our differences than we would be if we were all exactly alike.

Children are most absorbed in what is happening and what is going to happen to them, but they are also interested in the bodies of their siblings and friends and they do a lot of comparing. A nine-year-old boy came home from school and asked his mother why girls' breasts got bigger, having noticed this development in one of the girls in his class. Girls watch others to see how their bodies are changing and a lot of unspoken competition occurs concerning breast development and the onset of menses. Boys compare height and penis size and worry if they are smaller than their contemporaries in either category. One mother wisely told her son that although the men in their family tended to be short, manliness was measured by many other factors than just height. And she outlined some of those qualities she felt were important.

A child of six or seven asking why girls' breasts get big may be told simply that women's breasts make milk for a baby to drink, while an older child can hear about cells dividing and glandular tissue developing and increasing within the breasts which someday will produce milk when it is needed.

One mother reported that her nine-year-old son had become involved with a group of somewhat older boys who were looking with great excitement (and probably anxiety, too) at copies of *Playboy* magazine in secret. She asked if he was curious about the pictures he had been seeing and he said he was, but hadn't dared ask questions because the other boys would think he was dumb. So the mother and son bought a copy of the magazine and looked through it together, the boy asking about why the women were undressed, why their breasts were so big, why they had hair where their legs came together, and why the bigger boys laughed and got excited when they looked at the pictures.

His mother told him that teen-aged boys and men enjoy looking at pictures of pretty, naked women; that women's breasts are big because they make milk when a baby is born; and that both boys and girls, when almost teenagers, grow hair under their arms and where their legs meet. She told him that the bigger boys aren't sure of themselves yet and sometimes laugh because they feel nervous or they want to look as though they know a lot when they really don't.

She added that people's bodies are different—most women don't look like those in *Playboy*. Some women have smaller breasts than others, just as some are tall and some are short. And all breasts, regardless of size, produce milk. When explaining this to a boy, one could casually comment that boy's penises differ in size, too; some are a little bigger than others—the way some people have bigger ears, noses, or hands and feet. All these sizes are normal. This discussion—an excellent example of informal sex education—was very helpful to the child and after that he was no longer interested (at least for a few years, perhaps) in looking at *Playboy*.

Both boys and girls become very interested in the changes taking place in their bodies as they enter puberty. The changes occur as early as nine years in girls, although usually the budding of breasts and appearance of axillary and pubic hair occur from ages ten to twelve or even thirteen. Boys on the average begin bodily changes two years later than girls. Both sexes experience a spurt in height and weight during puberty. At this point we will review some of the typical questions girls anticipating the onset of menses ask, and what they mean.

"When Will I Menstruate, and What Happens to Me?"

This first group of questions was compiled by an eleven-year-old girl and her best girlfriend and brought by her mother to our parent-discussion group.

"Does it hurt when you put in a Tampax?"
"Will a Tampax affect your daily activities?"
"Can you urinate when you're menstruating?"

These anxious queries reveal a fear of pain, of being hampered, and of something going wrong when menstruation occurs. The girls need confidence that they will be free to do everything they ordinarily do during these times, that other bodily functions are not affected. Inserting a tampon can be uncomfortable the first time, and girls should be free to choose between tampons and pads and experiment with both. Smaller tampons now on the market are easier for young adolescent girls to use.

"When does your period start?"
"How long does a period last?"
"Once you begin to menstruate, do you always have to wear a tampon or pads?"
"Are the pads noticeable?"
"Should you take out the Tampax when you take a bath?"

These questions indicate a real wish to be prepared so that they can cope when bleeding begins. Some girls worry that once it starts, they will bleed forever and are relieved when they learn of the cyclical nature of menstruation. They anxiously wonder whether boys can tell they are menstruating and worry that they will be teased. They need to be reassured that no one can tell they are having their period as long as they change the pad or tampon frequently. They will soon learn how often to change tampons as they experience their periods and find out for themselves what they are like. Again, they should be aware of the normal variations—that some girls flow more heavily than others and need to change the pad or tampon more often; that some girls' periods last a week, and others' three or four days.

Children at this age are confused about the inside of their bodies. They know that urine, bowel movements and menstrual blood all come from somewhere inside, but they are not at all clear about the sources. They need to learn about the urinary bladder, uterus, and bowel. Old ideas about menstruation being "dirty" because it is often associated in their minds with urine and bowel movements come to the fore at puberty. Girls should be told that menstrual blood is clean and learn what the purpose of menstruation is.

Another group of preadolescent girls asked these questions about menstruation in a sex-education class in the fifth grade:

"Will every girl menstruate?"
"Do you have to menstruate before you have a baby?"

Because of old ideas stemming from early childhood that bleeding signifies injury and something wrong with the body, some girls want to avoid the process of menstruating. They secretly hope that they will be able to have a baby someday without going through the monthly bleeding.

An eight-year-old girl learned of menstruation from listening to a conversation between her older sister and her sister's friend, who were discussing their coming menses. She asked her mother about it and was told the monthly bleeding from the uterus inside was to get ready for a baby to grow someday. She grimaced and said emphatically, "That's not ever going to happen to me!"

By the time girls are ten or eleven they are more accepting of this important event, but still anxious. There is a great deal they do not understand that needs to be clarified.

"Does intercourse cause you to menstruate?"
"Does it hurt to menstruate?"

You can see how they still associate bleeding with injury and pain, and how they need reassurance that the bleeding is a normal, usually entirely painless event—although some girls and women have cramps in their lower abdomen the first day or two of their period which should not interfere with their usual activities. One twelve-year-old girl whose periods had not yet begun told her mother as she placed her hands over her pelvis, "Mom, I've been feeling heavy here."

She was not distressed, but seemed pleased as her mother explained that her body was making itself ready for menstruation and this meant that she was growing up. If a mother accepts her own menstruation calmly, her daughter will be much more likely to take the onset of her menses in stride and to feel pleased at this evidence of developing womanliness.

Girls naturally worry about getting their period in school. They wonder what they should do then: "What do you do if you start in school?"

It is rare for a girl who has not yet begun menstruating to be willing to take a belt and pad with her to school just in case she begins. In some it is a denial of the inevitable, in others a fear that a classmate will see the pad in her pocketbook or locker and tease her or tell others. One fifth-grade girl told me that a boy saw a Kotex in a girl's pocketbook partly open on her desk, and that he took it and held it up for everyone to see. Whether this really happened or is one of those anxious stories that makes the rounds at this age, I don't know, but it shows the girls' worry that something very personal will be revealed in public. They especially fear boys' ridicule and wish they had to experience menstruation, too.

"Do boys have anything like menstruation?"
"Do boys have periods too?"

The anxiety about boys' teasing may stem from old experiences in early childhood when brothers or playmates may have teased them about their lack of a penis, which at that time made them feel inferior and envious. Now the boys' derision stirs up those old distressing feelings, for the boys are pointing out that girls' bodies are different from theirs. If girls are developing psychologically along normal lines, they will take this in stride; they are proud of their growing breasts and of their uterus with its ability to carry a baby, and they are willing to tolerate periods because those gratifications outweigh the discomforts of menstruating.

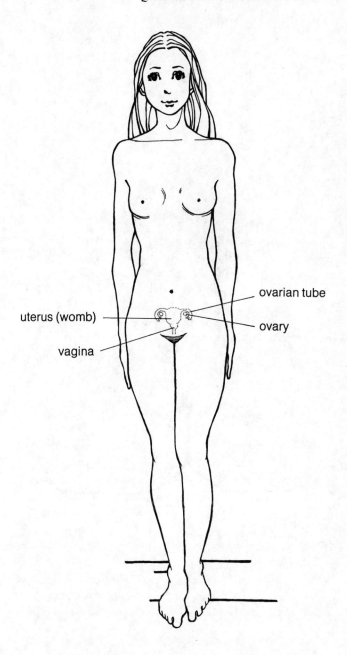

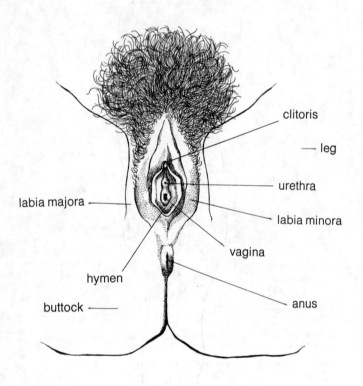

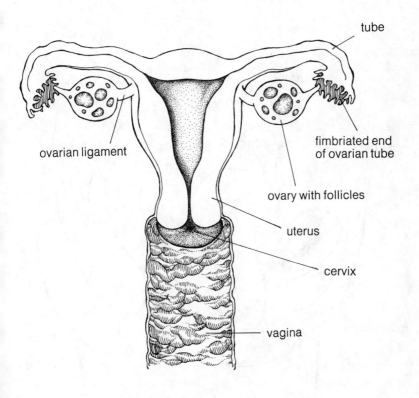

FRONTAL CROSS SECTION OF VAGINA, UTERUS,
UTERINE TUBES AND OVARIES

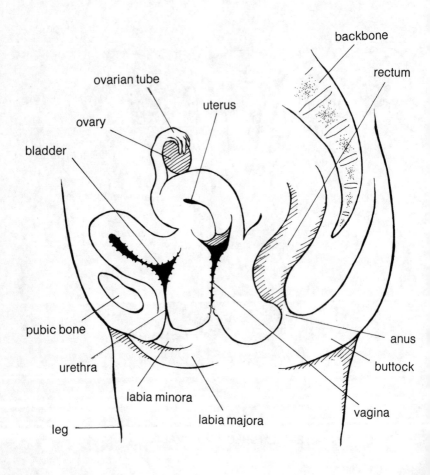

Preparing for Menstruation

Our discussion group focused on how to prepare a girl for menstruation. By age nine girls should be learning about it, for recent studies show that girls are menstruating two years earlier than their mothers did on the average, so that many girls of eleven and even ten are having their first periods and need to be ready for this very important event. It has great psychological impact, and the way they cope with it emotionally affects their entire feeling about being women.

I like to begin by telling a girl about the uterus, tubes, ovaries, and vagina. If you can draw passably well, a sketch helps. The uterus is the size of a girl's or woman's fist, so you can ask her to make a fist and tell her the uterus inside her is shaped like an upside-down pear. They should learn that many thousands of very tiny eggs—so small they can only be seen through a microscope—are in their ovaries, and that about two years after they begin having their periods, one of those tiny eggs will ripen, grow larger and leave the ovary, and enter the tube near the ovary. One month one ovary produces a ripe egg or ovum and the next month the other one produces it. The egg passes down the tube, taking a few days to make its journey, and into the uterus.

I tell them that the uterus is the special place where a baby will grow someday. The baby begins to develop when a sperm joins with the egg. Even though girls don't marry and begin to have babies at eleven, twelve, or thirteen, the uterus doesn't know that and each month gets ready in case a baby begins to grow in it. The lining of the uterus builds up and becomes thicker by developing more tiny blood vessels that bring more blood to it so a kind of soft bed or cushion is made ready for the baby. But when no sperm joins the egg, this built-up lining is no longer needed; the tiny egg breaks up and passes out of the body unnoticed, and the extra lining comes away from the inside of the uterus and passes out of the vagina as menstrual blood. This takes anywhere from three to four days to a week. It is necessary to wear something to soak up the small amount of blood so that it doesn't get on one's clothes, and this is why pads were made. The pad is supported by a belt around the waist with tabs in front and back that have pins or little hooks that attach to the two ends of the pad worn between the legs. Some pads come with tabs that stick to the underpants and make belts unnecessary. The outlines of the pad don't show in ordinary clothes. Every three or four hours the pad should be changed as blood accumulates.

The girl needs to know about how to change the pad—especially in school—and girls' bathrooms in schools should be equipped with covered cans and small paper bags for disposal. The girls should know whom to go to if they need pads or help. If there are no paper bags, the girl should know that she can fold the discarded pad, wrap it well in toilet paper and put it in the covered can, or if there is none, in the wastebasket. She needs to know that nothing is wrong if a little blood gets on her underpants—she can wash them out when she gets home—and such a small amount of blood will not go through her clothes.

Girls learn quickly about their periods as they experience them and become adept at dealing with them. They take note of their feelings and can usually tell when a period is approaching. Monthly periods give them a feeling of cyclic regularity that they can count on and this helps them feel more settled. Often the scattered, hyperactive, seemingly disorganized behavior of the preadolescent girl calms down remarkably once her menses have begun.

Girls at this age are also concerned about breast development and do a lot of covert comparing, observing their friends and classmates to see whose breasts are developing faster or growing larger than the others. If she is slow in this regard, the girl may worry that she will never have breasts large enough to please her: "I am starting to develop but my nipples are not coming out. Will they ever come out?"

She needs to be told that breasts, like other parts of the body, vary a great deal in size and somewhat in shape in different people. Girls know very well in preadolescence what breasts are for. Now they are more interested in more details about the breasts' functioning and may ask how milk is made inside the breast.

"Where does the milk come from inside the breasts?"
"Does milk only come when you have a baby?"
"Do I have milk in my breasts now?"
"What happens to the milk when the baby gets older?"

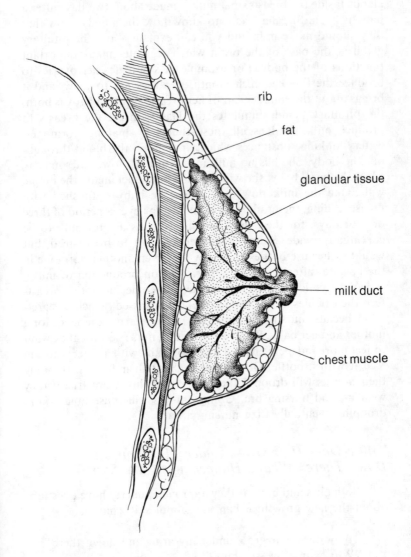

You can tell your daughter that the milk is made by special glands inside the breasts, that milk is made about two days after a baby is born. She may want to know how the glands know that they should make milk and you can explain about the pituitary gland at the base of the brain which regulates many important functions of the body. For example, it stimulates her ovaries to produce the tiny egg each month, it causes her to grow, and it brings about the enlargement of her breasts. When a baby is born, the pituitary gland stimulates the glands inside the breasts to produce milk. It does all these things by making hormones, watery-looking substances which circulate in the blood throughout the body. She has no milk in her breasts now, but someday when she has a baby, she will, and the baby sucking on the nipple will make the milk flow out. When the baby is finished with breast-feeding, the production of milk stops over a period of three or four days, for the baby's sucking is necessary for milk to be continually made. Some women choose not to breast-feed, but would rather use bottles, and they are given another hormone in the hospital after the baby is born to stop production of milk.

Your child may ask why some women decide not to breast-feed their babies. Some women feel embarrassed, which is regrettable, because nursing can be a very happy, warm experience for a mother and her baby. Some women don't nurse because they want to feel more independent and leave the baby with a sitter who can feed it with a bottle. Others worry about their figures, thinking their breasts will droop if they nurse, but this is not true if they wear a good nursing bra. Going bra-less will cause much more drooping eventually than nursing a baby.

"Why Does Hair Grow Under My Arms and Down There? What's Happening to My Skin?"

Both girls and boys as they approach puberty have questions about the new growth of hair and about skin changes.

"Why does hair grow under my arms and down there?"
"Why is my face so shiny?"
"Is this a blackhead?"

The most understandable way of explaining hair growth is to remind them of early man whose hair covered his body to keep it warm and to act as a cushion against attack. Now a few vestiges remain, covering two of the most vital areas of the body, the head and the sex organs. As far as we know, hair on these two areas serves an ancient protective function, but why we retain hair growth under the arms (called axillary hair) is not as well understood. Now hair on the head is considered an ornament, and children know from TV commercials, magazine advertisements, and going to the corner drugstore how much emphasis is put on beautifying the hair by both men and women.

Preadolescent children may have heard the word "blackhead" from their siblings and peers. Noticing the onset of an oily shine on their faces, they spend some anxious moments alone in the bathroom peering in the mirror at this age, eager yet anxious about bodily changes that signify they are growing up, worrying that somehow their budding sexuality may be dirty and bad. This unfortunate notion sometimes stems from toilet-training days, if a parent showed aversion or disgust at the child's urine or bowel movements, and sometimes from parental prohibitions regarding masturbation. Often negative attitudes toward sexuality have been picked up by children who have heard parents make condemning or rejecting statements about sex. They are concerned that oily skin, perspiration, and menstrual blood are dirty and sometimes become overly upset about them, for in the unconscious mind to be dirty is the same as being bad, and if you are bad, there is the risk of loss of love.

Understanding these conflicts and feelings is helpful in reassuring the pubescent child. Parents can remind children that their bodily changes are normal, that the oil and sweat the skin produces are clean substances. Blackheads form with their dark coloration because dust particles fall on the skin and cling to the oily surface. Again, both boys and girls should be told that menstrual blood is clean. If an odor develops on the pad, it is caused by the action of bacteria that live on the outer skin surfaces.

Children find it helpful to have some notion of what is going on in the functioning of their skin at this age. Oil glands produce oil to prevent the skin from drying and they empty into the hair follicles. At puberty the oil glands pour out more oil than before; hair on the head and facial skin become oily and need to be washed more frequently. The amount of oiliness varies from one person to another. Excess oil, old sloughed-off skin cells, and dust particles in the air all tend to plug the openings of the hair follicles so that blackheads may form. If the oiliness is quite severe and the child has an inherited predisposition to acne, pustules, commonly called pimples or whiteheads, may develop. The pus material in these eruptions consists of dead bacteria and broken down white-blood cells, for the body fights infections by mobilizing its white cells, which engulf and destroy the bacteria.

It is very tempting to squeeze these whiteheads, but the pressure on the skin can push the infection out to a wider area, making things worse. Children should be encouraged to wash their faces gently two or three times a day with a clean washcloth, tepid water, and mild soap. Frequent shampooing is not harmful; again, it should be with tepid water and oily shampoos should be avoided. The child needs to be reminded to wash combs and brushes when shampooing to avoid introducing bateria into clean hair. Often children think that very hot water will get hair and skin cleanest. They should be cautioned against this, because hot water stimulates the oil glands.

The sweat glands' openings onto the skin surfaces are called pores. The child perspires more than in the past, during exertion and when anxious or tense, and for the first time the sweat has an unpleasant odor. Learning about the use of deodorants is helpful. I'm not too keen about new spray deodorants because particles can be inhaled into the lungs, and I recommend the traditional cream, or roll-on types.

"What Is in a Man's Balls? What Are They For?"

Boys are very interested in the changes in their bodies, and take careful note of what is happening. The preadolescent boy notices the growth of pubic hair, the increasing size of his penis, and the appearance of oily skin and perspiration. He begins to wonder again about erections and about the purpose of the testes.

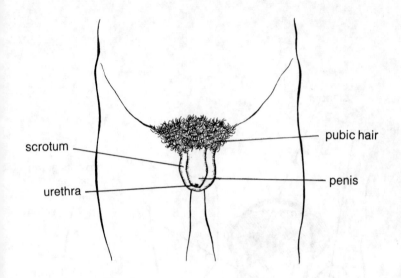

scrotum

urethra

pubic hair

penis

FRONT VIEW OF UNCIRCUMCISED PENIS

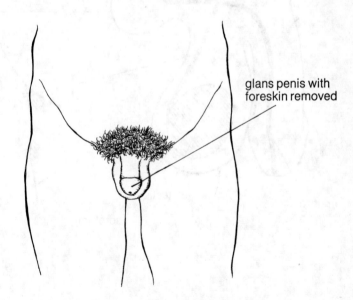

glans penis with
foreskin removed

FRONT VIEW OF CIRCUMCISED PENIS

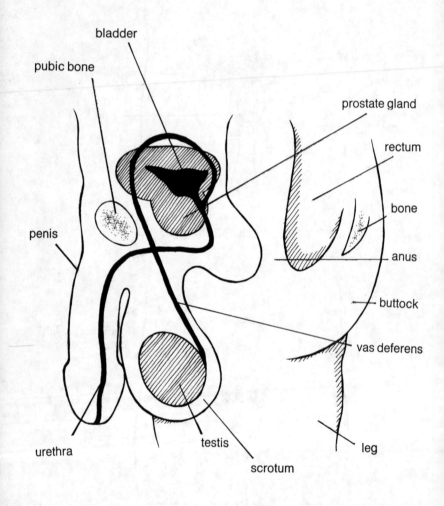

pubic bone

bladder

prostate gland

rectum

bone

penis

anus

buttock

vas deferens

leg

urethra

testis

scrotum

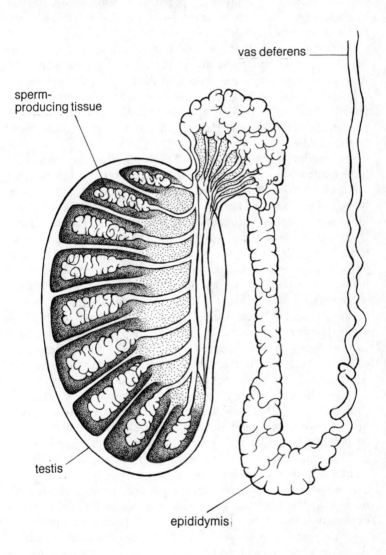

One question brought up in my parent-discussion group, relayed by the parent, was from a ten-year-old boy: "What is inside my balls? What are they for?"

Most parents without a medical background find it very difficult to answer questions about the interior of the penis and testicles because they were never told themselves and have only a vague notion about it. They know that sperms are made in the testes but are not sure how, and most people have no idea of the physiology of an erection. Here is one way to explain these things to the child.

Sometime between the ages of twelve to fifteen, sperms begin to be made within a boy's testes. Special cells turn into sperms and millions are made. They are extremely small and can only be seen through a microscope. If you could look at some, they would seem like young tadpoles with an oval head and a long tail that lashes from side to side so it can propel itself. The sperms move up small tubes within the testes to a larger tube called the vas. This tube joins with the tube inside the body that carries urine through the penis. When the boy is dreaming some night, or masturbating, some milky-looking fluid will come out of the opening at the end of his penis. The sperms are in this liquid, called semen. It is perfectly normal and ordinary for this to happen to him from time to time when he gets older. When it happens during sleep, it is called a wet dream (nocturnal emission). Some morning he may wake up and find a wet spot on the sheet and he will know why it is there. His body will make sperms continuously all his life, so he shouldn't worry that he is losing some when semen comes out of his penis—millions more are being made all the time in his testes. Although the sperms are so very tiny, they are extremely important, for it is when a sperm joins with an egg cell inside the woman's body that a new life begins.

Boys in their pre-teens may experience anxiety about erections if they do not understand what is going on. Not only does an explanation help a boy of this age, but it prepares him for very frequent erections in adolescence. If he knows erections are entirely natural and normal and happen to all boys, he will not be worried but take this in stride.

The interior of the penis is made up of three compartments filled with tissue that has many small spaces within it. When a boy or man becomes sexually excited either from physical stimulation of the penis or by erotic fantasies, the spongy tissue within these three elongated and parallel compartments becomes filled with blood, causing the penis to increase in size and become erect. When the excitement subsides, the blood empties out again into the pelvic blood vessels and the penis assumes a flaccid state. Many children wonder if there is a bone in the penis. Sometimes they get this idea from pictures of animal skeletal structures and observing a bony structure within the tail. You can tell them that there is no bone inside the penis, but you can understand their question, because an erect penis is hard.

This brings up the importance of not laughing at children's questions even if they seem amusing. They are quite serious about them, and often worry about seeming babyish or stupid. If their questions are met with derision in the form of scorn or amusement, they will not ask again.

"Can a Sperm Get Into a Woman If She Isn't Married?"

Preadolescent children become more interested in teen-aged behavior as they approach this important phase in their development. These two questions were asked by ten- and eleven-year-old boys and girls:

"Why do some teenagers have babies when they're not married?"

"Can a sperm get into a woman if she isn't married?"

Older pre-teens realize that sometimes pregnancies occur when young people aren't married, and that a baby can begin to grow inside a woman when it is neither wanted nor planned. This perplexes them and makes girls, especially, feel anxious, for when they were younger their parents told them that when a man and woman love each other and want to have a baby, they have intercourse and the sperm meets the egg. In a few years in school and somewhat out in the community—in watching television, listening to conversations, beginning to read newspapers and magazines —they have learned a great deal and know that pregnancy is not always the happy and planned event they once thought it was.

Girls worry that somehow sperms, too small to be seen, can get into them and make them pregnant, and they want to know how to keep the sperms out. They know by this age that an unmarried, pregnant teenager causes unhappiness and conflict in her family, and preadolescents are still children very much in need of the security of their parents' love and acceptance.

Although the questions now are more complex, the best way to answer is honestly, clearly, and simply. You can say that some teenagers don't think before they do things, but feel a strong urge and act on it. A boy and girl may like each other a lot and enjoy kissing each other. When teenagers kiss and pet, they get excited; the boy has a strong urge to put his penis into the girl's vagina, and the girl has a strong desire to let him do it. If they forget to think about what it can lead to and go ahead with intercourse, there is no way to get the millions of sperms out of the girl's uterus. If one meets an egg cell and joins with it, the girl becomes pregnant.

This will probably lead to questions about what the boy and girl do then. They should be told about the conflict and unhappiness that follow, for to omit it is unrealistic. They should learn about alternatives open to the couple and the pros and cons associated with them, for this prepares them to deal with situations they may face in the future. We find that teenagers who are well informed get into less difficulty than those who have been kept ignorant. The problem for parents here is how to tell preadolescent children about these matters in a way they can understand so that what is said will be meaningful and helpful.

When my children or child patients ask me these questions, I tell them, "It is very difficult when an unmarried girl learns that she is pregnant. For thousands of years people have known that children need a father and mother and to be part of a family to be happy, so people have felt for a long time that it is unwise for a woman to get pregnant and have a baby when she is not married. Nowadays people don't get as upset about this, but still parents are unhappy and worried when it does happen and this makes the girl sad, too.

"There are several alternatives in this situation. The boy and girl can marry and have the baby. But often teenagers are not ready for the responsibilities of marriage and of being parents, and their marriages very often end in divorce. The girl can have the baby and arrange for it to be adopted. There are married people who cannot have a baby of their own who are happy to adopt a baby. Sometimes a girl decides to keep her baby even if she isn't married, but it's not easy with no husband to help her. And sometimes a woman decides to have an operation in the hospital called an abortion. An abortion is taking this still tiny fetus, which doesn't even look like a real baby yet, out of the uterus so it cannot develop into a baby."

"Why Do Some Parents Adopt Babies Instead of Having Them?"

In describing the reasons for adoption, I tell the child, "There are some men whose testes make very few sperms so that the egg inside the woman cannot be joined by a sperm and a baby does not start growing. The joining of the egg and sperm is called fertilization. Sometimes a woman does not make eggs, and no one knows why. When fertilization does not happen for a year or more and the wife does not become pregnant, a couple may decide to adopt a baby. They go to an adoption agency. The babies come mostly from unmarried women who believe their baby will have a happier life in a family with a father. Sometimes a married couple who have several children and very little income feel it will be impossible to take good care of another baby, and they will give the newborn baby up for adoption. This does not happen very often in this country, but in other countries and in earlier times, giving a baby up for adoption by rich parents was one way poor parents could be sure their baby had a chance for a healthy, happy life."

I feel that very young children should initially hear of pregnancy as a wanted and planned event, occuring in a loving context, for this promotes a positive attitude about sexuality and having babies. There is plenty of time later for children to learn about unwanted pregnancies. To tell them when they are very young may only bring confusion and anxiety about sexual matters. When they are preadolescent, questions about divorce, illegitimacy, abortion, and premarital sex arise as children begin to hear and read about them.

You have a responsibility to try to instill in your children your values and attitudes concerning these issues. Preadolescents should know about the risks of premarital sex. A good way to begin this kind of discussion is to ask the child what s/he thinks about it. Children don't like long lectures; like everyone else, they appreciate the chance to express their own opinions. This is a good way to learn how your child thinks and what his or her ideas are. Ask what s/he thinks life would be like for a baby or a young child without a father. How could an unmarried mother earn money to live on and still spend time with the child? Of course, many of you are working and/or divorced mothers and you can talk to children about the difference between having a father who doesn't live with the family but whom the child knows and sees, and essentially having no father at all. You can discuss the differences for mother and child between a mother's working because she wants to or has to, and working part time or full time. This kind of conversation gets the child thinking about responsible behavior and helps answer questions in an interesting and useful way.

"How Can a Woman Keep from Having a Baby?"

Some preadolescents ask about contraception because they may have heard about it or, as the earlier question revealed, they simply wonder how sperms can be stopped from reaching the egg if a girl or woman does not want to have a baby. There is always latent interest in girls about having a baby. It starts in very early childhood with their interest in mothering dolls and baby animals and often becomes intense again in pre- or early adolescence if they are around animals. But this wish conflicts with the desire to be free of another person, to be independent and able to pursue educational and career choices. They sense an inner urge to produce a baby and want to defend against it. Again, I feel children should be fully informed, especially about basic methods of contraception.

You can say, "Sometimes a man and woman want very much to be as close as they can be and the man has an urge to put his penis into the woman's vagina because it feels good to them both.

But they don't want the woman to become pregnant—either because they're not married, or if they are, because they don't want a baby yet. Some young people will decide not to have intercourse, and some will decide to go ahead with it. In that case, they would be wise to do something to keep the sperms out of the vagina and uterus. There are several ways to do this. One is for the man to put a little rubber covering over his penis. This is called a condom. When the semen comes out of his penis it stays in the condom and is kept from getting into the woman's vagina.

"Another way is the use of a diaphragm, a round rubber cap the woman puts into her vagina and pushes against the bottom part of the uterus so that the opening of the uterus is covered and sperms cannot get past it.

"Another way is to have the doctor put a special small loop of plastic into the uterus. It is kept in constantly and doesn't hurt. It stops a baby from growing in the uterus.

"Still another way, not as sure a method as the others, is for the woman to put some special ointment that kills the sperms into her vagina before she has intercourse.

"Then there is the Pill, a special medicine made of hormones. The woman swallows one pill every day and it stops an egg from ripening each month, so when sperms get into the uterus they cannot find an egg to fertilize and she cannnot become pregnant."

The children may wonder what happens to an egg when it is not fertilized, and what happens to those millions of sperms that do not find and join with an egg. The egg breaks down and passes out of the body unnoticed; the sperms also disintegrate and are absorbed by the woman's body.

"How Do the Sperm and Egg Turn Into a Baby?"

Fifth- and sixth-graders asked these questions:

"How do the sperm and egg turn into a baby?"
"What decides whether the baby will be a boy or a girl?"
"How can you tell when the baby is going to be born?"
"How do you get twins or triplets?"
"How do twins and triplets come out when they are ready to be born?"

The first question deals with embryology and it is difficult to give a simple answer. By fifth grade, children probably have learned about cell division. The fertilized egg divides repeatedly and soon becomes a tiny hollow ball or sphere. Then it changes in shape and continues growing and begins to look something like a little shrimp with big eyes. The heart begins to beat and circulate blood. Cells divide into three types that will form nerve, muscle, and skin tissue. Buds for the arms and legs appear. This very important forming of the parts of the body, inner and outer, takes place during the first few weeks of pregnancy. After that the baby simply continues growing and near birth hair grows on the head, and nails on the fingers and toes.

Half of a man's sperms carry a Y chromosome and half an X chromosome. Chromosomes are structures inside each cell of the body that determine inherited characteristics like height, curly or straight hair, and hair and eye color. If an X sperm joins with the egg, the baby will be a girl; a Y sperm produces a boy.

There are two kinds of twins—identical and non-identical, or fraternal, twins. Identical twins are the result of the fertilized egg dividing an extra time immediately following conception, and no one knows why this occasionally happens. Because both babies develop from the same sperm and egg and therefore have the same chromosomes, they will look exactly alike and have to be the same sex. Fraternal twins occur because there happen to be two ripe eggs ready to be fertilized instead of just one. One sperm joins with one egg and another finds the second egg, and two babies form. They may be two boys, two girls, or a boy and a girl, and they are no more alike than brothers and sisters except that they are the same age. They may look quite different because they carry different chromosomes, not being formed by the same sperm and egg. One birth in every seventy is twins. Triplets are made when three eggs are fertilized by three different sperms. This is much more rare.

Twins and triplets are born one at a time, and some are breech, or feetfirst, births, for two or more babies fit more easily into the uterus if the biggest part of the baby, the head, of one is high up in the uterus, and another's head is lower down. Most babies are born headfirst.

Of course, mothers can easily answer the question about how you can tell when the baby is going to be born, but it is best not to emphasize the painful aspects of labor and delivery, to avoid frightening children, especially girls. They may ask if it hurts, for a preadolescent girl cannot imagine how a baby could come out of her small vagina, which she imagines is always the size of her small orifice, without causing immense pain and tearing. You should be honest about the fact that it does hurt but not constantly, and that the doctor will give the mother medicine to ease the pain, if the mother wants it. You might explain about the stretching of the vagina to let the baby out. A good comparison she will readily understand is with an elastic band that can stretch bigger and go back to its original size again. I do not tell children of this age about the incision enlarging the vagina at delivery to prevent tearing (episiotomy) because this is too scary and they have plenty of time in the years ahead to learn about it, when they won't be so alarmed.

I have been impressed by the number of preadolescent children asking about things going wrong during pregnancy and birth. By this age they have heard about babies born dead, or with some kind of deformity, and they are anxious about it. Again, their characteristic queries reveal not only a wish to learn and understand, but a hope that they can control what happens to them in the future.

"Will smoking cigarettes affect the baby?"
"Will alcohol hurt the baby?"
"What is a premature baby?"
"Will the baby die if the mother doesn't eat?"

These questions are asked quite urgently, mostly by girls, for at ten they cannot be confident that their bodies will ever produce a normal, live child.

"Does the process of birth harm the baby?"
"Can you have another baby after a Caesarean section?"
"Why sometimes doesn't the baby stay inside the mother long enough?"

"Can a baby live if it is born early?"

"Why does the baby die sometimes?"

"Why are some babies put into incubators?"

"Why are some babies born dead?"

"If one Siamese twin dies, will the other die too?"

"What causes a baby to be mentally retarded?"

"What causes some babies' heads to be too big?"

"What happens to make a baby be born without arms or legs?"

"What is a blue baby?

"Why do some babies die before they are born?"

These are difficult questions to answer if one is not a physician or a nurse. Birth is hard on the baby, but is not harmful. Women who have delivered by Caesarean section can have more babies. It is not known why some babies are born prematurely, though we do know that cigarette smoking and poor nutrition during pregnancy results in prematurity in some cases. A baby can live after six months of pregnancy if it is given expert medical care and its lungs function normally. The baby can die before it is born from bleeding when the placenta or afterbirth separates from the wall of the uterus too soon or from a serious illness or accident. Premature babies are put into incubators to help keep their body temperature normal and sometimes to provide them with extra oxygen if their lungs are having difficulty functioning at first. If one Siamese twin dies after birth and surgery is performed immediately, the other could be saved. It is not known why some babies are born mentally retarded, but there are a number of diseases which can cause it. In rare instances babies are born with a defect in the brain that causes their heads to grow too big; this is called hydrocephalus and if it remains untreated, their brains are damaged by the increasing pressure of the cerebrospinal fluid which is constantly manufactured but in these unfortunate babies is not reabsorbed, so that it piles up and puts too much pressure on the soft brain; luckily nowadays there are operations which drain off the fluid and spare the brain from damage.

The children have heard and probably seen pictures of thalidomide babies which interest but alarm them; they want to be sure that the baby they have someday will not be like those children. They can be told that the drug which caused the defects is no longer being made and that there is little danger that their baby in the future will be so afflicted, although extremely rare cases occur for some unknown reason. A blue baby is one whose heart has an opening between the two sides; blood from the lungs carrying oxygen mixes with blood without oxygen returning from the rest of the body to the heart, so that the blood being pumped by the heart out to the rest of the body does not carry enough oxygen and makes the skin look bluish. The defect can be corrected by surgery.

There is a great deal to think about and be aware of as one's children come with questions of all kinds about sexuality and the body. I have tried to deal with the typical questions that arise, but no doubt children with their curious, inquiring, and active minds will think of many others. Parents should not be reluctant to say that they don't know the answer if they don't, for a child has a great respect for honesty and can learn much from a mother or father who figures out how to find an answer by looking in books in the home or library or consulting the family physician.

I would like to end this section on pre-teens with a poem written by a woman poet, now a mother of growing children, who remembers and beautifully expresses the distortions, anxieties and fantasies of a girl just entering adolescence:

Spring

When I was
thirteen I
believed that
the mailman
had sperm on
his hands and
if he touched
me I would
be pregnant
if he brushed
against me
in the hall

from my pores would sprout twigs branches leaves
buds blossoming unfurling I'd be an apple
tree in my white wedding dress swelling
the room until flowers exploded into the street
and rose up filling the sky blowsy with
        fruit to come

Ruth Whitman
The Marriage Wig and other poems

Part Three

Questions Adolescents Ask

Overview of Adolescence

Adolescence officially begins with the onset of menses in the girl and the first seminal emission in the boy. Girls enter puberty about two years before boys, but the age for the individual child varies greatly. Some girls have their first period at ten or even nine, and some at fifteen or sixteen, with most beginning from eleven to thirteen. Girls now start menstruating two years earlier than their mothers did on the average. Boys experience the first ejaculation of semen at thirteen or fourteen.

This is a time of enormous physical and emotional change and growth. The child changes into an adult—often in uneven spurts and leaps, leaving the amazed parent wondering what has happened so quickly. Then there are stretches when parents feel a certain phase is going on terribly long and they worry that the child will never get through with it. Teenagers swing from being dependent children to rebellious youths, trying desperately to be independent and self-sufficient. Their erratic, often unpredictable behavior causes much upheaval and consternation in others and in themselves. It is an exiting but trying time for the family, but at least it is never boring!

At adolescence, hormones stimulated by the pituitary gland at the base of the brain circulate in the bloodstream and affect important endocrine glands which in turn pour out their own secretions within the body. The production of sex hormones—estrogen and progesterone in the girl's ovaries and testosterone in the boy's testes, as well as androgens secreted by the adrenal glands—have a very great impact on the child, both physically and emotionally. The resulting secondary sex characteristics, the physical changes that occur in the body during early adolescence, are described in the next pages.

Girls, who often gain weight at about eleven, experience a continued weight gain but a growth spurt at the same time so they look slimmer despite weighing more. Some girls, (and boys, too) gain at this age to the point of chubbiness and need help in learning about low-calorie foods, for they are self-conscious and unhappy about their appearance and the problem should not be ignored. By twelve the breasts are growing toward their adult form and the nipples and surrounding skin (called the areolae) are becoming darker. Hair continues to grow under the arms and over the mons pubis in greater abundance. Perspiration with its characteristic odor occurs in the axillae and both girls and boys need to learn about deodorants. They may resist them at first, perhaps as an expression of their anxiety about growing up and their wish to remain children, but if you tell them about deodorants and put one or two kinds in the medicine closet, they will try them out when alone.

Menarche, the first menstrual period, has a great psychological impact on the girl, and it is crucial that she be prepared well in advance for this event. (See pages 53-54.) If she knows the bleeding is a perfectly normal and natural occurence and if she understands where the blood comes from and why, she will be able to take it in stride. Many girls anticipate their first period eagerly, and feel pride and a sense of becoming a woman when it finally arrives. But girls who are not prepared—either because they are not aware of it or because they have heard vague and conflicting stories—are frightened by the sight of blood on their underpants. They believe something is wrong with them, that they have been injured or have some disease, and they are not easily reassured. Unfortunately, even though they may learn of the purpose of menstruation, their anxious and negative feelings may persist, though to a lesser degree, and affect their attitudes about being women and about sexuality.

Girls entering puberty younger than twelve have more difficulty adjusting to their periods than those who menstruate at twelve or thirteen, simply because they are less mature, experienced, and knowledgeable. Some of the ten- and eleven-year-olds refuse to go to school or dancing class when menstruating, or to take gym. They fear their classmates will know that they are having their period and that they will be teased. Some worry that they can't manage the pads on their own, and are too embarrassed to ask the teacher or nurse. It is very important for schools to be set up so that girls can be helped to cope with their periods during school hours, as was discussed in detail in the previous section on pre-teens.

Boys also gain weight at eleven or twelve, and some are very upset about looking too bosomy because of the fat deposits in their breasts. If your son is going through this stage, try to sympathize with his reluctance to appear in public in a bathing suit. Of course, he is afraid that his friends will tease him about looking like a girl. He needs to be reassured that this is a normal stage in his growth, that he will grow in height and increase his muscular strength; the fat that shows now will not show later.

At twelve, both penis and scrotum grow larger and hair begins to appear at the base of the penis and under the arms, though many boys do not experience hair growth in these areas until thirteen. Erections occur more frequently and boys should be prepared and know that they are entirely normal. At thirteen erections occur often, stimulated by sexual fantasies and feelings, and may cause considerable embarrassment when they occur unexpectedly. Masturbation is common at this age, and the boy's voice begins to break and become deeper and his vocal cords grow under the hormonal stimulation.

Boys grow taller rapidly at fourteen and muscular growth is evident. Hair continues to grow around the penis, under the arms, and now makes its appearance on the forearms and legs and at the corners of the upper lip and in the sideburn areas. Most boys are masturbating and they all have seminal emissions in their sleep. About half ejaculate semen at thirteen, and by the end of the fourteenth year, they all experience ejaculation.

It is important for boys to be prepared for seminal emissions, but all too often they are not. Fathers on the whole seem to have more difficulty talking about sexual feelings, and tend to leave sex education to the mother, who obviously finds it easier to talk with her daughters than her sons. Mothers are more vague and uncertain about what boys go through, so sometimes hesitate to talk about sex with them; they should remember that it is perfectly all right to be honest and say they aren't sure about the answer to a question, but will consult books or an expert. Teenagers respect honesty and they are so filled with uncertainty and questioning themselves, they are relieved to find out they aren't the only ones who don't know everything. They often try to cover up their lack of knowledge by acting as though they know all the answers, for they are plagued with fears of being stupid and inadequate. Several times, in discussing sexuality with a class of high-school students, I have been told at the start that they know everything and have no questions! This soon changes as I bring up some aspect of sex and ask them what they think.

Emotional Conflicts

Emotionally, adolescence is a time of conflict and growth. The adolescent has some vital tasks ahead: to relate to other people with a genuine concern for their needs and feelings instead of the primarily narcissistic interest typical of the younger child; to achieve a sense of his or her own identity, choose a vocation, and adjust to a very complex and changing society. S/he must largely break away from his or her parents and a dependent position in the family and become a self-supporting adult. This difficult process takes years and is characteristically uneven, and at times stormy, for old childish yearnings persist and must be struggled against, and often the adult world is perceived as threatening and scary.

Parents have much influence on the teenager's struggles and their attitudes and responses to the child's behavior and ideas can ease or worsen conflicts. If parents really try to be accepting and understanding; take time to listen, reassure, and guide without being autocratic; refrain from teasing and at the same time conduct their own lives as responsibly and maturely as they can, children have a much better opportunity of getting through this trying stage of life successfully. This is a tall order indeed, and understanding what the adolescent's conflicts are helps.

Consciously the teenager is very concerned about self-esteem, confidence, and appearance. At this stage old conflicts from earlier phases get stirred up, and make adolescence more difficult. Little boys feel small compared to their fathers and these old ideas may emerge again in adolescents and plague them; they may withdraw some or compensate through athletic or intellectual achievements and be overly upset if they don't reach their goals. Little girls also feel small in relation to their mothers, but boys are more conflicted about it because our society equates height and strength with manliness. Messages from the culture come through insistently and early that men should be strong, and women beautiful and slender. All adolescents therefore worry, some quite openly and others secretly, they they are ugly and inferior. Because they fear rejection, some drive others away by being rude, sullen, or snobbish; they do the rejecting first to avoid being rebuffed themselves. Some try to win esteem in their peer group by being a wise guy or a clown. Many work hard to excel at something that has meaning for them—an academic subject, sports, art, dancing, or music—to bolster their own self-esteem and win admiration from the group.

The feeling of inferiority makes them extremely sensitive to teasing and criticism. Their feelings are easily hurt. Their unhappiness makes them impatient to have the desired experience or object—whatever it may be at the time—right away, so they become demanding, impulsive, and intolerant. They try to counteract feelings of inferiority by being hypercritical of others and acting like know-it-alls. Inside they may feel weak and helpless and may try to strengthen their egos by identifying with a close friend, having a crush on someone of the same sex who is a few years older, or through hero worship.

Sexual Energy

One of the most difficult problems for teenagers is the new push of sexual energy. Masturbation arises as a repetition of an activity that had been pleasurable when the adolescent was a young child. Some children repress the urge to masturbate because of feared parental disapproval, but at puberty sexual feelings intensify and soon override the self-imposed prohibition. Others masturbate throughout their childhood but much more during adolescence when sexual excitement is so easily and frequently experienced.

Boys masturbate usually by rubbing their penis with their cupped hand. Girls masturbate by stroking the clitoris with one or two fingers; often the vagina is neglected during autoerotic activity until late adolescence, although not in all girls. Girls are curious about the vagina and will explore it with a finger, and some insert objects into it. At the moment phallic-shaped vibrators are in favor with a few older adolescent girls, but are used still more by young adult women as a substitute for a sexual partner.

The first orgasm is a frightening experience for many boys and girls because they don't know what's happening to them. A few fortunate boys have been prepared for seminal emissions and know that the experience is an exciting and natural one. But very few parents prepare their daughters for what orgasm is like, or even tell them it will occur. Girls are baffled and so anxious and often guilty about orgasm that they don't talk about it to anyone. Unfortunately adolescents tend to think their feelings and anxieties are peculiar only to them—that no one else would feel this way, inhibiting them from sharing experiences and worries and getting much-needed reassurance.

You might tell your child that touching or rubbing the sexual parts of the body feels exciting and if continued the excitement grows stronger and eventually results in a climax called an orgasm. In boys, muscles at the base of the penis contract several times and semen comes out of the urethra. In girls, muscles in the walls of the vagina contract. The experience for both boys and girls lasts a few moments and is intensely pleasurable. Afterwards, there is a feeling of relief and relaxation. Orgasm can be a little scary the first time, but is perfectly natural and normal. You might add that when people get older it can happen to them and their partner during intercourse.

The Search for Identity

The vital search for personal identity is revealed in typical questions adolescents ask themselves about who they are, why they are living, and what they will become. A thirteen-year-old girl wrote in an essay entitled "My Philosophy": "I go to my favorite place and think very hard. I block out the outside world. I think as hard as I can and I ask myself, what am I going to do with my life?"

There is a feeling of being special and unique, of being destined to do something important and meaningful which gives the adolescent exuberance and hope and helps balance painful feelings of inadequacy. A fourteen-year-old boy wrote: "The world of outdoors, animals, medical service, health and freedom are my hobbies and my subjects because I think I was meant for them."

And another thirteen-year-old girl wrote in a poem entitled "If I Were":

> If I were a tree
> I'd stand straight and tall
> Fingers touching the sky
> Swaying in the wind
>
> If I were a star
> My gleam would light the darkness
> I'd shout across the sky
> And wait to be wished upon
>
> If I were a wave
> My crash would break the silence of the sea
> My height would frighten all around
>
> If I am me
> I'll grow tall and proud
> And be what I want to be

The adolescent vacillates between old childish wishes to receive from others and maturing wishes to be giving, causing him or her to be selfish one moment and generous and altruistic the next. S/he daydreams of helping others, of making the world a better place, of being a hero. People are often more generous and helpful during adolescence than at any other period in their lives.

Strong sexual drives begin to override old prepubertal fears and dislikes of the opposite sex and both girls and boys become quite preoccupied with their looks. They spend hours in the bathroom looking at their faces and experimenting with their hair.

They think about clothes and want to dress like their peers so they will be accepted. Pulling away from parents makes it imperative that they feel part of another group—the peer group.

Teenagers tend to idealize a boyfriend or girlfriend and feel unworthy themselves. These reactions are derivatives of old feelings toward parents during early childhood. Teenagers seem fickle, but becoming involved with a number of people teaches them about others and helps them in their own quest for identity.

Often adolescent behavior at home is annoying and perplexing to parents. Teenagers can be patient and helpful with their peers, only to turn and suddenly be rude and surly with their parents. There are valid reasons for these paradoxical actions. Boys need to defend against old Oedipal yearnings toward their mothers which were paramount when they were four and five years old. In adolescence these wishes threaten to erupt again. So the boy may act withdrawn around his mother or be rude and antagonistic in order to keep distance between them. He won't listen to his father's advice because again he feels too much like a little boy; he must forge his own way, make his own decisions, if he is to become an independent adult. This is very hard on parents, who see the youth making errors in judgment and heading in regrettable directions, but if teenagers are to evolve into individuals with their own standards and philosophy, they must experience life and inevitably they will make mistakes.

Adolescent girls fight with their mothers, to avoid becoming carbon copies. They also fight with their fathers to defend themselves against their old Oedipal impulses. They fight to keep a distance from the father, yet the fighting gets him to pay attention. Some girls are so conflicted about their wish to be close to father and their need to keep distance that they unconsciously make themselves unattractive. So parents feel pulled and pushed by their teen-aged children, and this stage, although it has its fascinating and happy aspects, is far from easy.

Teenagers tend to be self-centered because they are involved in their own feelings. Their struggles take up so much of their energy, attention and time they don't notice things parents feel they should be aware of, so mothers get upset about messy bedrooms and clothes left in a heap. Teenagers aren't being deliberately thoughtless or selfish; they have other concerns that to them are much more pressing and important. Often the messiness and reluctance to take baths is an expression of an earlier anal phase when there is a natural wish to mess and be dirty; this will pass. Other teenagers defend against the wish to be dirty by becoming overly neat and clean to the point of fastidiousness. Some teen-aged girls become overly modest as they defend against the urge to exhibit their bodies in a sexual way.

All these conflicts occur in the larger context of the necessary adjustment to a complex and changing society. One factor that contributes to the complexity in this country is that so many different groups with their own mores and traditions have settled here side by side. Another is the lessening faith in traditional religions so the old rules and beliefs have weakened and become much less useful to young people. The burgeoning interest in Eastern religions and the so-called Jesus freaks are attempts to sort out what is important, to find some guidelines and ideals which they have not found elsewhere and differ from their parents' ways of doing things. We all feel insignificant as we compare ourselves to the vast reaches of space and we're anxious about the possibility of devastating nuclear war over which the individual feels s/he has no control. Young people also face a myriad of career choices and one of the most difficult things about deciding upon a vocation is the necessary giving up of so many other possibilities. How much simpler it was in times past when a boy learned a skill from his father, when his identity was clear and definite, and when angry gods could be appeased by sacrifice or prayer. It is an enormous task for today's adolescents to rebel against parental restrictions and fashion for themselves a personal code of behavior when they are bombarded with such a bewildering and complicated number of forces, temptations, and choices from the outside while they struggle with their own inner urges and anxieties. A period of sexual and social revolution is not an easy time for adolescents, nor for their parents who are also trying to make sense out of all that is going on and trying to be helpful to their children.

As a result, parents today are being confronted with much more complicated and difficult questions than in the past. What some of these questions and problems are and how they might be answered constitute the remainder of this book.

Questions Teenagers Ask About Sex

Young teenagers will still ask questions, although not as freely and openly as they did when they were much younger. As they get into adolescence, they begin to defend themselves against their inner feeling of inadequacy by acting as though they know everything. But their anxieties often override this idea, and they ask questions not only because they want information and understanding, but because they hope the answers will diminish their anxiety. Again, your answers should be clear, reassuring and need only address the question asked. If there are more questions in the youth's mind, they will emerge later, especially if parents answer calmly and truthfully, and do not give the child the feeling that it is wrong or bad to ask about sex.

Another factor leading to questions at this age is that young adolescents hear from peers all kinds of new words they do not understand. These words are said with anxious laughter and smirking which arouses the other's curiosity. What could these words which they don't hear at home mean?

Because adolescents' questions are so numerous and varied, I will only try to give examples of typical questions and discuss the major issues they want to understand and know more about. Their questions arise from the changes in their bodies, from first experiences with dating, from their thoughts and anxieties about growing up and their future role as adults, and from new social and sexual patterns.

"What Do You Do On a Date?"

Although adolescents these days socialize in informal, friendly groups of boys and girls much of the time, dating is still very much an institution in our culture, and young adolescents think a lot about it. Early adolescent boys and girls are thinking a lot about dating. They wonder just what a date is, and how you behave on a date. It's a new, exciting, but scary experience, different from any they have had before. They worry that they won't know how to act or that they will say or do the wrong thing, feel foolish and stupid, and perhaps be laughed at by their peers.

"What is a date?"

"What do you do on a date? Where do you go?"

"What does a girl expect from a boy when they are out on a date?" (And vice versa.)

"If a boy wants to kiss you on a date, what do you do?"

"What is going parking?"

"Why do girls have to wait till a boy calls them for a date?

"Why can't girls call boys if they want to?"

"What should a girl do if her best friend's boyfriend asks her to go on a date?"

"If a boy is not very tall yet, or if he thinks he isn't handsome, should he ask a girl he likes for a date or will she always say no?"

"What is going steady?"

"What is making out?"

"What is petting?"

"Is it dangerous to go on a date in a car?"

"What do you talk about on a date?"

"How long should you stay out on a date?"

Despite changing customs, questions about how to relate to adolescents of the opposite sex in a close context have been asked by adolescents for generations. They want to try this new experience, so attractive and absorbing for their somewhat older friends, schoolmates, and siblings. They are eager to feel more grown up and independent, but they are anxious that they won't know how to behave or won't be able to think of something interesting to say or won't be able to handle the situation. It's their first time away from the familiar settings of home, school, and camp with someone of the opposite sex. Because they worry that they are ugly, inadequate, and not very bright, they fear no boy or girl will think them attractive. It's usually easier for them to begin their dating experience with a familiar group, and then go on to single dates.

With dating, we are now getting into areas with questions which are not simply answered, where your personal attitudes and standards as parents play an important part. It is helpful to know that "making out" means kissing or petting nowadays, for many parents assume it means having intercourse as it did in some parts of the country twenty or twenty-five years ago. In general, as well as giving your children information they want, it is wise to emphasize impulse control—stopping to think—in addition to consideration of the other person's feelings. I personally would answer the questions about parking, making out, and petting in the following ways.

Going parking is when a couple drive to a quiet, dark place where there aren't many other cars going by. It really is searching for privacy, a place to be together without being disturbed. The boy wants to stop in such a place because he hopes that the girl will let him hold and kiss her. (The girl, of course, may be eager for the experience, too.) He may want to touch her body where it feels exciting, like her breasts or her vagina. This is called making out or petting. It's enjoyable and exciting for both, but sexual feelings may become strong, and it may be hard to hold back from "going all the way."

Having intercourse (some people just say "having sex") before you are really ready for it emotionally can cause a lot of unhappiness, especially for a girl. If one hasn't learned about contraception, pregnancy can result, and sometimes a disease transmitted from one person to another through intercourse can develop. This is called venereal disease and it is serious and must be treated by a doctor with certain medicines if the person is to avoid becoming very ill.

There is such a thing, unfortunately, as the double standard. This is the attitude that boys can be more free about sex, while girls are supposed to be modest and more restrained. This is unfair, and even though times are changing and women are moving toward equality with men, this old idea persists. It is especially hard for girls, who are sometimes pressured by boys to pet and even have intercourse; they also feel pressured by their parents not to do these things, and may themselves feel it is not wise. They are torn in two directions, one toward intercourse because of pleasurable excitement when they feel close to a boy, and one away from it because they don't believe it's right for them.

Again, because of the double standard a lot of people unfortunately look down on a very young girl who has permitted intercourse, or "gone all the way," if it gets to be known. This is not true nowadays for girls of college age, but it is still true for a girl of junior-high and high-school age. She is not thought of as "a nice girl" by a lot of people. It shouldn't be this way. A girl who is emotionally ready and knows about contraceptives should be able to choose whether she will have intercourse with a boy she likes very much or not, and it should be her and the boy's business and no one else's.

The Importance of Self-Esteem

I have found that self-esteem is extremely important in determining how people behave with others. If your boy or girl appears to think pretty well of him- or herself without being conceited (a defense against feelings of inferiority) and to be fairly confident, the chances are he or she will do well with other people in general. An adolescent boy who believes he is a worthwhile person will conduct himself in ways that bear out that reality. He will be law-abiding, dependable and, at times, at least, thoughtful and helpful. He will tend to be attracted to friends and girls who are pretty much like him. He will not need to brag, be tempted to steal, or take hard drugs, because he does not feel deprived and worthless. He will not mistreat his peers, because he will not be angry and constantly self-preoccupied. Although he often feels inexperienced, anxious, and inadequate, these are not deep-rooted feelings but temporary reactions to situations he has not yet learned to handle with ease. He will not feel the need to manipulate or pressure girls into having sexual relations so he can feel masculine and win the admiration of other boys. He can be patient and will have a positive attitude that good things will come to him in time; he will not be impulse-ridden despite the strong pressure of inner urges. He thinks well enough of himself to choose companions and girlfriends who are well regarded, for their behavior, as well as his own, reflects what he thinks of himself.

Girls with a good measure of self-esteem do not become promiscuous. They do not feel that sexual satisfaction is the only way to keep a boy as a friend. They do not choose a boyfriend or girlfriend who acts out in antisocial ways, not only because this would reflect poorly upon them but also because they wouldn't enjoy delinquent activities. Girls with low self-esteem often find themselves a boyfriend who is delinquent or into hard drugs or a lot of drinking because they feel this is the only kind of person they deserve or could get to be interested in them. Their poor choices advertise their poor opinions of themselves.

"What Do You Think About Premarital Sex?"

Adolescence does not exist in animals, including the primates. It is a purely human phenomenon. Animals go directly from childhood to adulthood when they become sexually mature and able to mate. We are the only species whose children go through a number of years when they are physically able to reproduce, yet are not ready to be entirely independent from their parents. The conflicts about premarital sex arise directly from this fact as well as from cultural and religious prohibitions that produce guilt.

One fifteen-year-old girl asked her mother, "What do you think about premarital sex?" This parent was fortunate because her daughter voluntarily opened the door to meaningful communication. We may often wish to start a discussion with our adolescent children, but at the time we want to, they may not be interested. They react with resentment or boredom and make it very difficult if not impossible to carry on a productive interchange. So take those golden opportunities when they arise and make the best use of them you can!

One might impulsively answer the vital question about premarital sex with a dogmatic reply that blocks further communication. Remember to answer instead in such a way that encourages further comments from your child. How many parents have regretted blurting out answers like "I don't approve of it one bit. It just leads to trouble and unhappiness. A girl can get pregnant and her whole life is ruined, and that's all there is to it." How can the child respond to such a statement except with discouraged silence or arguing, both of which lead nowhere?

A better answer would be: "Well, it's a complicated thing. I have some thoughts about it, and I'd like to know what you think, too." This lets the child know that you are willing to carry on a reasonable discussion, that the topic is open to being considered and talked about with you, that you are interested in what she (or he) has to say.

What are you confronted with in this situation? A young, not yet mature or experienced person, wanting to differ from your rules and develop her (or his) own, and filled with urgent feelings requiring some kind of expression as well as control. And what are you? A parent who loves this child and wants her (or him) to have a happy, productive life free from tragedy—an adult who through trial and error and sometimes bitter experience has learned about life and fashioned values and standards you believe are realistic and wise. And you want your child to adopt the same standards.

A mental-health clinic in a Boston suburb offered parents of high-school students a series of five discussion sessions with another child psychiatrist and me to talk about any problems or questions about understanding and living with their adolescent children. The parents were asked to give us some questions in advance that could be used as a starting point. I was struck by the number of questions beginning with "How can I make . . ." "*How can I make* my daughter come in at a reasonable hour?" "*How can I make* my son cut his hair?" "*How can I make* my daughter stop seeing a boy my husband and I don't approve of?" And so on. *The point is obvious: you cannot* make *teenagers do or not do anything*.

If you try to force them, they rebel all the harder because they resent being treated like little children. It is very easy when you feel panicky to try to coerce and resort to threats and ultimatums. But that only makes things worse. Try to keep cool and keep in mind that paving the way for a rational discussion with an honest exchange of ideas is by far the most helpful way to deal with differences of opinion between parents and teenagers. They can be belligerent and provocative and it takes much self-control not to blow up at them. We are all human, after all, and sometimes we do explode, but it's important not to explode as a regular pattern, but to aim for calm and reasonable communication. And it's extremely important to avoid lecturing and interrupting. Everyone hates being lectured. The kids will be turned off, and you will only get more upset. Give them a chance to express their views and don't interrupt. They are neither as knowledgeable nor articulate as you are. They are groping with strong, vaguely defined feelings and conflicts and it isn't easy for them to express what they are thinking and feeling. If the child feels s/he is really being listened to, s/he will feel much more positively toward parents and be much more responsive.

Here are two kinds of discussions between a teenager and her parents about the same issue, premarital sex. A fifteen-year-old girl, in blue jeans and shirt, with long hair covering her shoulders, sits at the kitchen table with her parents. She has read a magazine article about a popular, unmarried, young actress who has recently had a baby.

Girl: In the paper tonight it said _____ _____ had a baby and she's not even married. *(The girl leaves it at that purposely, being very interested in her parents' reactions.)*

Mother: Well, I think that's terrible. She should be so ashamed, I don't know how she shows her face. It's awful what's going on these days.

Girl: What's so awful about it?

Mother: Why, no *nice* woman would ever do a thing like that. The poor baby, with no father to give it a name. It will be teased and hurt about being illegitimate. The word, by the way, in common language is bastard——

Girl: (exasperated by her mother's condescending manner, interrupts) I *know* Mom. I'm not stupid. *(She needs to remind her mother that she is not a young child anymore, to let them know she is intelligent and has some ideas of her own. But this gets lost on her upset mother, whose anxiety pushes her to go on. She fears her daughter may end up the same way, thinking to herself that these things go on all the time.)*

Mother: Yes, but you don't know much about life yet. Let me tell you, no decent man wants to marry a woman who has had a child by another man. Men marry girls who keep themselves pure for marriage. They only fool around and have sex with the other kind——

Girl: (*more exasperated than ever with her mother's dogmatic response and resentful that no one seems interested in what she herself thinks, interrupts again*) Oh, Mom, you're back in the dark ages. Nobody thinks that way anymore. (*Her anger pushes her to upset her parents. Now Father becomes anxious; he worries that his daughter is indirectly letting them know that she has decided to be sexually free and active.*)

Father: Oh, no, young lady, your mother isn't back in the dark ages. These girls may think they're very smart and sophisticated, but you can bet on it that they're miserable inside. They're sorry for what they've done, but there's no going back. Once something like sleeping with someone or having a baby is done, it's done. Everyone looks down on a woman like that.

Girl: (*furious now and feeling rejected because of her parents' lack of interest in her thinking, stands up to put an end to the conversation and so rejects them*) Well, I don't look down on them. And the picture of her in the paper didn't look miserable at all.

The discussion comes to an abrupt, premature, and unfortunate halt as she leaves the room. Nothing good has been accomplished. The girl is angry and humiliated; the parents are upset, frustrated, and worried about their daughter. But their vehement, biased, preachy approach has not taught their daughter anything useful, and it will be a long time before she initiates another discussion about such matters with them. She will turn to others to exchange ideas and get information, to people who will not lecture but listen to her ideas as well as state their own. In all probability these people will be members of her own peer group, for they sympathize with her conflicted, uncertain feelings, since they feel the same way themselves. But they may not give her accurate information, being as inexperienced as she is. Perhaps she will talk with the parent of a close friend she admires. This can be very helpful, but her parents will have no control over what the friend's parent tells the child, and probably will have no knowledge of it, either.

These parents allowed their fears to make them autocratic, unreasonable, and thoughtless. What they actually said had some merit; it is still largely true that many men prefer a wife who has not been promiscuous before marriage, and it is very hard to be a fatherless child. But these valid statements were lost in the aggressive, anxious context.

Here is another discussion about the same issue. Again we have a long-haired, blue-jeaned fifteen-year-old girl and her parents sitting at the kitchen table. The girl has read the same article and it aroused much interest and feeling. At this point in her life she is preoccupied with sexual behavior and trying to figure out a code of ethics for herself. She wonders what her parents think about the actress's behavior and decision to keep the child. She feels safe bringing it up with them because the person who got pregnant was not her, but someone else. It's easier for her to talk about someone else's behavior. Her own is her private business.

Girl: In a magazine I read that _____ _____ had a baby. She's not married, either, you know. (*Pause. She waits to see what they will say. The parents wisely realize that here is an opportunity for real communication but that they must not preach or argue.*)

Mother: Well, it's not what a woman usually does, is it? (*She leaves the door open by ending her comment as a question.*)

Girl: (*responding to the invitation to state her thoughts*) No, but maybe it was what she wanted to do, what she decided to do.

Father: (*also keeping the door open by not being dogmatic and yet at the same time expressing his views*) Most women feel more secure having a baby when they're married. I wonder why she felt differently?

Girl: Nowadays a lot of people think marriage is old-fashioned. Today in psych class three or four of the guys said they don't want to get married, ever. They can't see staying married their whole lives to just one person. One boy said it would be like being in prison. A lot of kids think you shouldn't marry, but be with different people at different stages of your life.

Mother: I think that's because kids worry that no one person could ever be all they need. Maybe they think it would take several people to do that.

Girl: (*This is a new idea she hadn't considered before*) M-m-m. You know, I look at the boys in my classes and I think how could any one of them be the kind of husband I'd like someday? They all seem to have so many hangups. They're all so immature.

(The girl's statement shows she agrees with her mother without saying so directly; that would be too childish and she couldn't do that. If you see that your child is agreeing, let is pass and be glad; don't embarrass them by pointing it out. Also the girl is indirectly letting her parents know that she really wants marriage for herself someday, that she is rejecting the idea of living with a series of men by saying "the kind of husband I'd like someday." Again, don't point it out, but let it be.)

Mother: Everyone has faults; no one is perfect. At your age all the kids are working hard at finding out about themselves and life. They're not sure of themselves yet. It will be many years before they will be, if ever. (*Mother wisely directs her remarks to the anonymous group, and not to her daughter. If they were directed at her, the girl would want to defend herself.*) I remember the day your father and I were married. I was so nervous. I walked down that aisle and looked at him and thought to myself, "I'm making a terrible mistake. That's a boy standing there, and he's as scared as I am." He seemed so vulnerable at that moment. I wanted a strong, mature, all-knowing man to lean on. What human young man could be that to me? But my love for him got me through it. He smiled at me with such love in his eyes that I knew it would be all right. But I still felt unsure at times after that, for quite a long time.

Father: I felt love and fear at the same time. What a moment! Being young is exciting, but hard, too. (*This gives the daughter another opening to contribute to the discussion. At her age, she is the authority on how hard it is to be young these days.*)

Girl: Well, it is hard sometimes, I guess. A lot of girls wonder if they should go all the way with their boyfriends or not. The guys say to them, "It's old-fashioned to be a virgin. Get rid of it. It's nothing but a burden. You'll feel free without it, no more worry." Some of the guys say you're not grown up if you're a virgin, you're still nothing but a child. But I don't know . . .

(The parents' wise, calm, and open way of dealing with the discussion has encouraged the daughter to bring up this crucial issue. The parents refrain from jumping in with their opinions, and it isn't easy.)

Mother: What do you think about it?

Girl: I don't know . . . It's a big thing to a girl. I don't think boys really understand that. They think it's nothing, but it isn't nothing. I know a few girls who've had sex, and they act like they're perfectly fine and happy. But I don't know, I get the feeling they're putting on an act. The kids say they try to get their girlfriends to do it, too.

Mother: (giving the daughter a chance to express herself, and sensing the girl's confusion, expresses her own thoughts without being dogmatic. And she doesn't hesitate to use the terms the daughter has been reluctant to use, thereby opening up communication) I think the girls you speak of try hard to be casual about intercourse, but I wonder too what they really think about themselves, how they honestly feel? And I wonder if they try to get their friends to do it too so they won't feel guilt and regret? If they could get all the girls to be like them, they'd like it, I think.

Girl: *(appreciating her mother's keeping the conversation focused on other girls and not directly on her)* What's that saying? There's safety in numbers.

(All three laugh at the remark, and the laughter releases their tension. Now father feels he should mention how boys feel.)

Father: You know, teen-aged boys have a very great drive toward intercourse. They get excited at the least little thing—a sexy picture, the sight of a girl in a tight sweater. They are preoccupied with sexual fantasies and feelings a lot of the time. And when they're out on a date, any boy would be very tempted to go all the way if the girl let him, because he feels such a strong urge for it. Boys feel more strongly sexually than girls at that age. They get more excited.

Mother: And another thing is, they don't know about how

girls feel. Most of them are really ignorant about girl's bodies and sexual feelings. They're probably lousy lovers at that age!

Girl: (*intrigued enough now to ask a direct question*) Why are they lousy lovers? (*She isn't quite able to ask what a good lover is, so she asks this way, hoping to find the answer that none of her girlfriends have been able to supply.*)

Mother: They are so concerned about their own bodies and feelings that they don't really consider how the girl feels. They experience an intense need for intercourse as a release from almost unbearable sexual excitement and tension. That's what's occupying their minds. They don't always know what excites a girl or what is pleasurable for her. Most of them don't even know there's such a thing as a female orgasm, a climax in a woman. And the few teen-aged boys who do know don't have the faintest idea how to bring it about. So the girl ends up feeling upset and not satisfied or happy. This great ecstasy she hears and reads about doesn't happen at all. Intercourse is momentarily painful the first time it happens for a girl. And she has other things to worry about, too. (*She has provided a way of keeping the discussion going; the girl continues to be curious. What could those other things be?*) Well, you know about pregnancy—if a sperm meets a ripe egg then a baby begins to grow. Some women think they're safe at certain times of the month, but no one can be one-hundred per cent sure of that. Women have ovulated at any time during the monthly cycle. Some women think they can flush out the sperms by taking a douche right after intercourse. But that doesn't do any good because the sperms very quickly get up into the uterus where no douche water can reach them.

And so the discussion goes. It could lead to further talk about pregnancy before marriage, abortion, adoption, venereal disease, and forced, premature marriages. Don't worry if the discussion ends before vital issues are aired; because you have been open, accepting, helpful, and interested in your child's own opinions, more discussions will take place. No one covers everything in one session, and it is unrealistic to expect that to happen. Sometimes tough questions will be brought up again and again. Don't act bored or weary, and avoid commenting that you've talked about that before. Where there is anxiety and conflict, there are no easy answers. Be patient. Always respond to the cue, and take advantage of the opportunity to listen to and help your children.

From mid-adolescence on their questions will be triggered by events around them. They will read about something, see it on TV or in a movie, or something will happen to a neighbor, relative, or friend. They rarely ask parents questions directly, seeking a specific answer, as they did when younger. So keep your ears open for the hidden question in a seemingly casual remark. In school, especially in psychology and sex-education classes, teenagers are more apt to ask direct question. School is not home with its old ties and conflicts with parents. Adolescents are so eager to grow up, they intensely resent feeling like young children, yet they have many questions and want information. Often they hesitate to ask us parents because they don't want to feel dependent. It is hard for parents to see children grow up and away from us and we sometimes pretend they are still little. Teenagers won't tolerate a patronizing manner in a parent, and are very upset and hurt by derogatory teasing and joking. Even though some of their remarks and questions may seem absurd, be careful never to ridicule, for they will not turn to you again.

Even though teenagers don't want you to be autocratic and dogmatic in response to their questioning, they are looking for boundaries and guidelines. Too many sophisticated parents, eager to be accepted and liked, set no limits and are too permissive. In their need to feel youthful because our culture pays admiring attention to youth and beauty and not to age, some middle-aged parents dress and talk as though they were teenagers themselves, making it hard for their sons and daughters to rebel in quite ordinary and harmless ways. Give the child plenty of opportunity to talk, but when it is your turn, don't be afraid to state what you think is important and right. Don't worry if your teenager adamantly disagrees with you. A teenager must set up his or her own priorities and make his or her own judgments. If you are too vague, you are not really helpful. Let them disagree and argue if they need to, but if you believe in what you are saying, tell them so. I often advise parents to tell their adolescent children, "You and I probably have different ideas about things, so we won't always agree. But let's agree to talk, to communicate, and listen to each other. We both have more to learn about life."

Teenagers really want limits set on their behavior, even though they may protest loudly. Girls especially welcome limits about how late they can stay out if those limits are reasonable. It's easier if they can tell a boy who is pressing them to stay out very late that their parents have said they must be in at midnight and that's all there is to it: "Listen, I can't stay out any later. I have to be in by twelve. You know how *mothers* are! (accompanied by a grimace of distaste, but a distinct inner feeling of relief.) Or she could say, "I'm sorry, but I'll be grounded for *weeks* if I don't get home."

Limits give the child some external control over inner urges and impulses which may get out of hand. The girl mentioned above may be very anxious about mounting sexual feelings if she goes parking with a boy; her mother's time limit helps her deal with her own sexual feelings. Most girls formulate their own codes of behavior in sexual situations quite soon after they have begun dating. They talk among themselves, and sometimes with adults who are unusually understanding and helpful. Some girls will permit petting above the waist, some petting only with clothes on, and some will go further, but almost all will make a decision about how far to go and will try hard to stick to it.

If parents are a little old-fashioned in their views about petting, it doesn't do any harm. Remember the teenager's need to rebel against your standards and evolve his or her own. If you are too permissive in your eagerness to be "with it," you make it harder for them because they have to go even further to rebel against you. Don't be afraid to be a little square. Your teenagers need help from you, not competition, and they must see themselves as different from and more up to date than you. I remember teasing my mother about her prematurely white hair when I was a teenager, and urging her to have it dyed (as we said in those days), but I would have been horrified if she had.

It is crucial for us parents to be available to our children. Many times when I have asked adolescent girls if they ever talk to their mothers about sex, they look resentful and say "Talk to *her*? *Never*! She's always on the phone [*or* always out], anyway." And boys complain: "Ask *him*? Ah, he's always working, he's never home. And if he is, he's asleep on the couch, or watching TV and doesn't want to be disturbed."

How important it is for parents to be alert to signs that their children want to talk about something with them. It is rare for an adolescent to tell a parent that there is something they'd like to talk about or learn more about. They are so afraid of seeming childish or stupid. So they initiate the discussion in roundabout ways that can be easily missed if you are not aware of their meaning.

"This kid in school today said . . ."

"Bob has a new girl, and she's . . ."

"Have you ever heard of a book called . . ."

"This new girl in school, well, ah . . . I don't know if she wears a bra or not . . ."

"Joe was tellin' me about this jock strap he got . . ."

"One of the senior girls is pregnant and they say she's going to keep the baby . . ."

Not only are your words, manner and attitude extremely important, but also the way you conduct your life and the way you behave toward other people. If there is one kind of person an adolescent has no respect for at all, and cannot abide, it is a hypocrite. If a father takes all kinds of medication and drinks a lot and then tells his adolescent son never to try marijuana, the son will either inwardly or outwardly scoff at his father. If a mother secretly carries on an affair, unconsciously letting her teen-aged daughter know about it in a subtle way, and then tells the girl not to have intercourse with her boyfriend, the daughter will have no respect for her mother's views. The old adage, actions speak louder than words, is all too true here.

Children identify with their parents despite their rebellion. They fortunately don't turn out to be carbon copies of us, but they are like us in many ways as they grow into adulthood. If we treat other people with respect and consideration, if we are dependable, generous, and helpful, if we are honest and responsible, our children will most likely develop these qualities.

The Early Adolescent and Premarital Sex

Children in early or mid-adolescence are not usually ready for genital sexual activity with another person despite their feelings that they are. Girls in their early teens are more profoundly affected emotionally if they have intercourse than are boys. We child psychiatrists find that girls of this age are usually not mature enough to handle the psychological effects of intercourse adequately. They can easily become overwhelmed by anxiety and guilt which only push them to more sexual acting-out in the vain hope that if it becomes commonplace, it won't be so upsetting. They are so preoccupied with their conflict that other areas of emotional growth and learning are neglected and in the end we sometimes see limited persons with poor self-esteem. For this reason, I am against encouraging them to be sexually active at least until they are of college age, and even then they should be aware of the pitfalls and be fully prepared for love making. (See the section on contraception, pages 131-138.)

Boys are subject to frequent sexual fantasies and feelings during adolescence, at the same time that they are deeply concerned about their adequacy as males. They compete with peers and want to impress male friends with reports of sexual conquests. Their strong desires and anxieties make them more insecure and self-centered than they will be as adults. They need to be reminded about other people's feelings and needs because they get so caught up in their own, and this is where parents can be especially helpful.

Here is a discussion between a sixteen-year-old boy and his father:

Boy (going out to join his father, who is reading the newspaper on the porch): Hi, Dad, what's new?

Father puts down his paper and responds with a similar inquiry.

Boy: I heard in school today that a couple of the seniors are getting married right after graduation.

Father: Really? What do you think about that?

Boy: It's kinda soon . . . I'd rather have more time to have fun and get to know more girls before getting married. It seems awfully final.

Father: Do you think they might begin to feel tied down after a while?

Boy, pleased at his father's interest in what he thinks, is reminded that the girl as well as the boy might have negative feelings: Yeah. Some of the guys talk about just wanting to live with some girl when they get a little older. Then they don't have to have all the responsibility of supporting someone else, and if they get tired of each other, they split. No sweat.

Father: Sounds easy, but what if one of them wanted to leave when the other wasn't ready, didn't want it, and got all upset and sad?

Boy, thinking it over: Well, I'm not sure . . . It wouldn't be good to stick around if you didn't want to anymore.

Father: The one who did stay might feel angry, hemmed in——

Boy, eager to show that he understands: Like a prisoner.

Father: Yes, I agree, and that anger would undermine the love that had been there before. I think it's important to think pretty carefully about the other person's feelings, too.

Boy: I guess so, right. Like some of the guys, they brag about scoring with someone and they joke about it, and I wonder if they think at all about how the girl feels.

Pause. Father gives his son a chance to reflect.

Boy: You know, you listen to people talk about making out, and about all the divorces and stuff, and you wonder why they ever get married? I mean, how can you be sure you'll really be happy if you get married anyway?

Father, realizing that he has an opportunity to impart some important thoughts to his son, answers carefully: Well, if you choose someone who's easy to get along with, who's thoughtful and loyal and loving, it has a good chance of working out. And there's one thing that I feel is really important . . .

Boy: What?

Father: It's that both people be willing to talk over upsets and problems with each other, to communicate and understand and act on the understanding. Criticism is hard for all of us to take, and tact helps, but I think the only way to make something better is to be clear about what's the matter and how it got that way, and then you can do something about it.

Boy: Sounds better than yelling and fighting.

Father: If both husband and wife can see their part in what went wrong, and both try to do something about it, it's so much better than if one acts like they're blameless and it's all the other's fault.

Boy: That would only cause a lot of anger like we were saying before... but why couldn't all those things happen between two people who just decide to live together? I mean, why get married at all?

Father: You mean because sex is pretty easy to come by now, so what's the point of getting married?

Boy, relieved that his father verbalized this idea for him: Right. Isn't that why a lot of people got married in the old days?

Father: That was an important reason. But you know, when you live with a woman you've loved for a long time, and she's a good person and you've gone through many experiences and phases of life together and shared so much, a love is there between you that is deep and means so much to both of you, and it's kind of like a strong foundation, a bond that becomes the center of your life. And to be really cared about and loved by someone else through easy times and hard times is more important than anything else, I think. I'm glad I didn't miss out on that. But I guess it's hard for you to imagine yourself getting to that age, isn't it?

Boy: Right, but I can see what you mean about marriage. A lot of kids my age like the security of going with one person . . .

The boy would like to say that he, too, yearns to be loved as a man now, but holds back out of embarrassment and changes the subject. His father realizes the discussion has been useful and lets it drop, knowing that others will take place.

It seems to me that the old, conventional reasons mitigating against premarital sex are no longer as important as they used to be. A girl's life is not ruined by unwanted pregnancy; abortions are obtained quite easily and carried out correctly in an accepting atmosphere so that old fears about infection and pain and humiliation can be laid to rest. VD is treatable and curable, too, if detected early. Various kinds of contraceptives can be obtained easily. Men no longer feel as strongly about virginity in their brides. Why, then, shouldn't adolescents go ahead and freely express their sexual impulses through intercourse when and with whom they please? Frankly, I think the current trend toward this kind of behavior is harmful *emotionally* to both teen-aged boys and girls, for this degree of intimacy fosters dependence on the other person, a real wish to be cared about in a genuine way. It is very traumatic to lose the other person over and over again, to be left feeling bereft, hurt, and sad. One becomes more cynical and distrustful as these experiences are repeated. The end result is a young person who defends against deep feelings of loving and wanting to give and be committed to another, who keeps relationships too superficial to be really gratifying and meaningful. This pattern does not prepare a boy or a girl for the important kinds of devotion and caring necessary for marriage and parenthood.

Venereal Disease

"If a Girl [or Boy] Has Venereal Disease, Can You Tell?"

Adolescents have heard about VD and slang words like "clap" and "syph," and they know they are infections transmitted through sexual intercourse, but when you listen to their questions, it quickly becomes apparent that they have vague, hazy and erroneous ideas about VD.

"If a boy [*or* girl] has a venereal disease, can you tell?"
"How are gonorrhea and syphilis different?"
"Is it true you can get VD from toilet seats?"
"Can you get a disease from just kissing?"
"How can you prevent getting VD?"
"If a kid got VD and went to a doctor, would he tell the kid's parents?"

It is crucial that teenagers be informed about venereal disease for it is widespread now and increasing to epidemic proportions.

If it goes untreated, the results can be truly devastating emotionally and physically.

Gonorrhea

Gonorrhea is an infection of the reproductive tract caused by the gonococcus bacterium (germ) which looks like a tiny lima bean under the microscope. The first symptom for boys is a burning pain especially when urinating, for the bacteria multiply and grow rapidly within the warm, moist, and dark urethra. This occurs between eight and fifteen days after exposure through intercourse with an infected partner. It is soon followed by pus with an unpleasant odor dripping out of the urethra. If it is not treated, it can infect the eyes (gonococcal conjunctivitis) and/or the joints of the body, resulting in a painful, incapacitating acute arthritis accompanied by fever and requiring hospitalization (gonococcal arthritis). Inflamation of the epididymis (small tube within the testis) and abscesses of the prostate gland can occur as complications, the latter sometimes requiring surgical drainage. The lining and valves of the heart may be involved (gonococcal endocarditis). The most common complication is stricture or narrowing of the urethra necessitating dilation mechanically, often throughout the life of the patient, which is a painful process. Newborn babies have been blinded by having passed through the gonococci-laden vagina of their mothers and not having been promptly treated with silver-nitrate and penicillin eye drops.

Gonorrhea in all its forms is treated by a physician, with penicillin, either by intermuscular injection or by pills taken by mouth. The infection of the eyes is treated by penicillin eye drops.

Girls also experience burning pain on urination and vaginal discharge. They can also suffer complications. The infection spreads upward into the uterus and tubes and can pass out of the open ends of the tubes into the abdominal cavity causing a generalized infection and abscesses. By now there is fever and abdominal pain and the patient is acutely ill. She may have to undergo an emergency hysterectomy (removal of the uterus); but even if she doesn't, she may end up sterile because the disease scars as it heals, sealing off the small ovarian tubes, preventing the passage of sperms to the egg in the outer portion or stopping a fertilized ovum from passing through the tube into the uterus.

A rare and very serious complication is gonococcal meningitis which necessitates hospitalization and massive doses of penicillin.

Syphilis

Syphilis is an age-old disease which causes serious and lasting damage to inner organs, including the brain, if it is not treated. It is caused by a spirochete, a bacterium which looks like a corkscrew under the microscope, and is spread from one person to another through sexual contact. The spirochetes thrive on mucosal surfaces such as genitalia, lips, inner surface of the mouth, throat, and anus. With an increase in oral-genital and homosexual sex, syphilitic lesions of the anus and throat are being seen by physicians much more often than in the past.

The first symptom is the appearance, within a month after exposure, of a small, hard, painless ulcer, which is highly infectious. This lesion heals without any treatment and in two or three weeks the person may believe him- or herself cured, but actually the millions of spirochetes have migrated from the initial site to many places within the body, localizing mainly in the liver, spleen, walls of the arteries, heart, and brain.

After two to four months a rash over the body appears, which again is painless; but each spot of the rash teems with invisible spirochetes, so again the person is highly infectious. After weeks or months with no treatment the rash heals and the unsuspecting victim again believes himself well. Destructive lesions can occur in the bones and internal organs; fatal complications result from a weakening of the wall of the aorta, the main blood vessel leaving the heart, from which all the great arteries supplying blood to the body derive. This weak spot balloons outward from the pressure of the pulsating blood within and can rupture without any warning, killing the patient in minutes. The liver can become so involved that its normally functioning tissue is destroyed and the patient dies from liver failure.

The nervous system can become involved with dire consequences. These complications can take many, even thirty or thirty-five years to cause difficulty. All those years the person has thought s/he was essentially well, while within the body the relentless spirochetes have continued to multiply and destroy vital tissues. Both physical and mental deterioration can result. The brain tissue can be actually destroyed by the spirochetes, with resulting progressive mental deterioration. Strange behavior occurs which is not in harmony with the person's character; s/he may become surly, thoughtless, and careless, and show increasingly poor judgment and a failing memory. S/he may easily fly into rages or become afraid.

At the same time, paralysis takes place. Motor incoordination appears in his speech, writing, and gait; s/he stumbles and falls, becomes weak, and his or her speech after a time is no longer understandable.

Finally, perception, memory, and judgment all disappear. Memory fails so severely that s/he cannot perform the simplest calculation and cannot find his or her way around a house s/he once knew perfectly. Contacts with the outside world are lost and s/he connot recognize even his or her closest relatives. S/he finally meets with an early death, a vegetating, pitiful wreck of the person s/he once was.

Both gonorrhea and syphilis, the two most common venereal diseases, respond to adequate doses of penicillin, and the tragic complications can be prevented by prompt treatment.

Three other venereal diseases occur also: chancroid, caused by the bacterium Hemophilus ducreyi, manifested by genital lesions and responsive to sulfonamides and certain other antibiotics; granuloma inguinale, also manifested by genital lesions, and treated by streptomycin; and lymphogranuloma venereum, characterized by swollen, tender lymph nodes which sometimes drain in the groin, and responsive to treatment with sulfonamides.

Infants in utero are affected only by gonorrhea in the form of eye infection, and, more seriously, by syphilis. The newborn infant with congenital syphilis may have skin lesions of the mouth, face, and diaper area; the long bones may be infected; and the liver and spleen enlarged. If the disease goes untreated after the age of two, the teeth will be affected, the eyes inflamed (keratitis), the child may become deaf from infection of the auditory nerves, and the bones, joints, nose, and palate can be affected by destructive lesions. Congenital syphilis is treated with adequate amounts of penicillin.

With these technical details in mind we might look back at the questions high-school students asked me about VD. Usually a person can tell if s/he has a venereal disease from the symptoms of burning pain on urination and pus-like discharge from the urethra in gonorrhea and the appearance of the ulcerous lesion (chancre) in syphilis. But sometimes a chancre can occur inside the mouth, vagina, anus, or throat and not be detected by the victim. The only venereal disease that can be contracted from something like a toilet seat would be lymphogranuloma venereum, which can be transmitted via infected clothing or douche or enema nozzles or simply from being in the same bed with an infected person without any sexual contact. But gonorrhea and syphilis, which are far more common, cannot be transferred in this way because the bacteria which cause them can live only a few minutes away from a warm, moist mucosal surface. Syphilis can be contracted by kissing a person who has a chancre on the lips, tongue, or inside of the cheek.

VD does not result in blindness except in very rare instances of infants born infected with syphilis or gonorrhea who develop eye infections and go untreated. I have not heard of such a case for many years.

Venereal diseases are not hard to cure if they are treated promptly and adequately. It is terribly important for any teenager who thinks s/he might possibly have VD or notices any of the symptoms I have described to get to a doctor very quickly.

Many physicians now agree to treat an adolescent's VD without notifying parents if s/he requests. However, the teenager should remember that medical bills get sent to the house, and if s/he wants to be dealt with like an adult, s/he will have to make immediate payment.

VD is prevented to some degree by very careful choice of sexual partners. Boys and girls who become sexually active with people they don't know well are asking for trouble. The use of condoms helps protect the penis from disease in an infected vagina and also prevents gonococci or spirochetes present on the penis from entering the vagina of the partner. Washing with soap and water after intercourse may make an adolescent feel cleaner and safe, but is no way to kill these virulent bacteria. Clearly the most effective way not to get VD is to avoid sexual intercourse, but this is something adolescents in increasing numbers are reluctant to do.

Homosexuality

As children enter adolescence and their interest in sexuality greatly increases, they also become curious about deviations from conventional sexual behavior. They wonder why some people choose a person of the same sex as a sexual partner. All boys secretly worry that they may have homosexual tendencies, but girls show less anxiety about it. It is very common for a teen-aged boy to experience at least one fleeting homosexual contact, but rarer in girls. Here are some question asked by high school students:

"How does a homosexual get that way?"
"Does a person become a homosexual through genes or is it psychological?"
"Can a homosexual ever get back to normal?"
"Why do some men like men better than women, and some women like women?"
"How can homosexuals have intercourse?"
"I've heard that there are homosexuals who are married and even parents. How can that be?"
"What is a Lesbian?"
"What is AC-DC?"

Teenagers want to know why people develop as they do, what psychological forces push them in certain directions, partly because of a genuine wish to understand the causes of behavior and partly for reassurance that they are normal, for adolescents feel conflicted and at the mercy of strong feelings.

There are several theories about what causes homosexuality.

Some contemporary observers—especially those associated with gay-activist groups—believe there is no psychological or genetic "cause," that it is simply an expression of sexual preference.

One theory deals with the importance of a child's identification with one parent or the other. The usual course in a child's development within a family is that a boy identifies with his father and learns about being a male from him, and a girl identifies with her mother and takes on her feminine traits. Strong identification is fostered by a stable, harmonious relationship in which the child respects and likes the parents—despite occasional upsets and considerable rebellion during adolescence. A boy without a father to rely on, admire, and learn from has a difficult time identifying as a male. Many boys, feeling the need of a father figure, search for one, and find a teacher, uncle, neighbor, or friend's father whom they like and can spend time with. Sometimes a grandfather plays a paternal role. I remember a nine-year-old boy I saw in psychiatric evaluation a number of years ago who was refusing to go to school. It turned out that this fatherless child was spending all day standing beside a trolley driver who was friendly, told him how the trolley worked, and patiently answered his many questions.

If a boy is unsuccessful in finding a father-substitute or unfortunately loses those he manages to establish a relationship with, he may have a serious problem learning how to be masculine. The problem is sometimes compounded when his lonely mother turns to him too much for affection and closeness. One widowed young mother frequently clutched her son to her, kissing him with much feeling and saying, "My little man!" Sometimes mothers will have a boy sleep in the same bed with them. The seductiveness is usually quite unconscious, though obvious to observers. Under these circumstances the boy is pushed toward making a feminine identification.

It is also common for a boy to fear and dislike a cold or tyrannical father and move too close to his mother for warmth and acceptance. This also fosters a feminine identification and leads him in a homosexual direction, relating to men like a woman. He may be seductive and passive in a feminine way or he may be aggressive in his search for closeness with another man with whom he unconsciously hopes to identify.

Some homosexual men suffer from intense castration anxiety. Their own unconscious preoccupation with the dreaded idea of being castrated causes them to think of women as castrated creatures because they have no penis. Any genital closeness with a woman results in feelings of revulsion or, at best, a complete absence of sexual excitment. For them to experience sexual pleasure the partner must possess a penis so that castration anxiety is lessened.

It has been thought for a long time that relationships between homosexual men are characteristically fleeting and unreliable. Many are, and it is sad to think of people driven by a need for closeness and caring, picking up a stranger on the street, in a gay bar, or in a men's room for a few hours of pleasure. But as homosexuals "come out of the closet" and feel more comfortable about revealing their sexual preference, it is becoming apparent that many (no figures are yet available) have established long-lasting and very meaningful relationships with another man, similar in many ways to successful heterosexual marriages. It was once thought that all homosexuals were immature, abnormal people incapable of genuinely close and gratifying interaction, but that notion is being shown to be wrong and unjust.

Female homosexuals, or Lesbians (named after the Greek poetess, Sappho, who loved women and is said to have lived on the island of Lesbos in 600 B.C.), have often made a masculine identification because of problems relating to their parents as children. Their fathers did not value and develop a warm relationship with them and they feel that to be a man is the only way to be worthy. Some perceive men as hurtful and frightening. Other female homosexuals yearn for closeness and love from a motherly woman and take a passive role in the relationship.

In the January 2, 1974, issue of the American Psychiatric Association's newspaper, *Psychiatric News*, it was announced on page one that homosexuality does not necessarily constitute a psychiatric disorder or mental illness, but is now classified as a disturbance of sexual orientation. Most psychiatrists still believe that homosexuality cannot be regarded as a normal adjustment, for clearly there is a serious emotional conflict about intimacy with women, or in the case of female homosexuals, with men. But there is a growing belief that homosexuals should be protected by law against discrimination in employment, housing, and public accommodations, that they should be free to choose the lifestyle they prefer and find most comfortable and meaningful.

When homosexuals seek help from psychiatrists about sexual preference, it is for one of two reasons. Either they want to become heterosexual because they have found gay life frustrating and ungratifying, or they are anxious and guilty about their homosexuality and want to feel more comfortable about it. The conflict is defined and a goal established for the therapy toward which the patient and therapist work. I have dealt with both situations and feel if a homosexual chooses to remain one, that s/he has every right to do so, and I will work toward helping him/her feel happier and more secure in that role. If s/he wants to become heterosexual, we work to gain understanding of the underlying conflicts and fears interfering with the wished for adjustment and try to solve them to free the person from old binds and mistrust.

My own feeling is that homosexuals should be free to live their personal lives as they wish as long as they live together by mutual consent, keep their activities private, and do no harm to anyone. I think the same rules should apply to heterosexuals.

What parents fear about homosexuals is the seduction of a child and this occasionally occurs. We cannot supervise our teenaged children's every move. They need freedom and independence much of the time, and we do have to take some risks in allowing them freedom. The important thing is for the child to feel from past experience that he can talk over any upsetting event with his parents without their being shocked or condemning. The child who has been through a frightening experience such as rape or a homosexual seduction needs comfort and reassurance, not outrage. If you can cope with such an event as calmly and reasonably as possible, it will be much less traumatic for your child.

Let us return for a moment to other questions the high school students asked about homosexuality. Most have been answered in the preceding discussion, but some have not. One girl wondered about homosexuals she had heard about who were married and parents, and this confused her. Some people can experience pleasure with men and women. (The slang expression "AC-DC" means bisexual.) In their youth they were probably heterosexual much of the time, but as they reached middle age, they may have become more and more homosexual in their relationships and less interested in partners of the opposite sex. The usual situation is a young man marrying and fathering two or three children, keeping his homosexual activities secret. As the years pass, he feels more and more attracted to men and spends considerable time searching for homosexual partners. If his wife discovers his homosexuality, divorce often ensues. In fact, the man may become impotent with his wife, and potent only with men, severely straining the marriage.

Some married women may turn to other women for love and affection if they feel severely neglected by busy husbands. Overt homosexual activity, however, usually will not occur unless there is an inner psychological conflict. Women who are not employed can keep a homosexual affair secret more easily than men for they can meet with a partner while children are at school and the husband is at work. It is so common and accepted for two women friends to visit each other in their homes that no one thinks anything about it, while it is much more difficult for a man to meet regularly with another man.

Fostering Your Child's Self-Esteem

Fostering your child's self-esteem is one of the most crucial responsibilities of being a parent. Children are unsure of themselves, repeatedly needing reassurance that they are basically valuable, worthwhile human beings. If we parents have a good measure of self-esteem ourselves, it is very helpful, because our children identify with us. It is easy in moments of annoyance, disappointment, and fatigue to say something demeaning and rejecting to a child: "Boy, are you stupid!" or "Can't you ever do anything right?" or "Dummy" or "Can't you get anything through that thick head of yours?"

Children often remember these hurtful taunts for many years and may develop feelings of inferiority and inadequacy which they keep secret. Parents forget the taunting, but children don't. Many adolescent and adult patients have tearfully told me of such childhood incidents with a parent or teacher which made them feel stupid, unloved, and worthless.

The parents' general attitude toward the child is extremely important. Many parents are too depressed or preoccupied with their own problems to pay really full attention to a child. It always saddens me to see a young child eagerly talking to a mother who obviously isn't listening. Eventually the child feels that what s/he thinks or says is of little importance. The child then begins to think that *s/he* isn't important.

Some parents dislike themselves so much and feel there are so many things wrong with them that they tend to find fault a great deal with their children as though anything related to themselves must also be inferior. Other parents in their eagerness to be accepting and uncritical of the child do not urge him or her enough to do better. This is often true about school performance. A bright child will bring home a report card full of C's. The parents, reluctant to upset him or her or make him or her feel unloved, tell the child the marks are acceptable. But this isn't helpful to a child who has greater ability, for it may make him or her feel that the parents really think s/he's not very smart. It's more supportive to the child's self-esteem to tell him or her that s/he is smart and can really do better. (But it is also important that parents investigate the causes for the child's lack of achievement. Many bright children fail to receive good marks because they are handicapped by perceptual problems which, if recognized, can be corrected by physical treatment or special tutoring.)

Here are the reactions of two different families to such an incident. A family of four is gathered at the dinner table. The eleven-year-old sister does well in school and is proud of it. Her eight-year-old brother, though bright, has more difficulty. That afternoon he had brought home a report card liberally sprinkled with C's and comments from his teacher that he was not doing his best.

Sister: Well, Danny, how was your report? I want to see it!

Brother: It was O.K.

Sister: Where is it?

Brother: None of your business!

Sister: Oh, so it wasn't so good, was it? I guess you're the dummy I always knew you were, anyway.

(Parents, preoccupied with their own thoughts, are not paying attention to what is going on, and do not interfere.)

Brother: I am not!

Sister: Yes, you are. Oh, look at the tears! Oh, what a baby!

(Brother, angrily striking out at his sister, accidentally knocks over his glass of milk. Now the parents take notice and are angry at the mess.)

Parents: Danny! Look what you've done, Stupid! Well, don't sit there like a dummy. Go get a sponge and clean it up!

(The humiliated, sad, and furious boy sullenly gets a sponge and tearfully attempts to mop up the milk. Because he is so upset, he doesn't do a good job.)

Sister: (Gleefully) Look at that, he's so dumb and babyish he can't even clean up the milk right!

(At this, the child, hurt and angry beyond bearing, throws down the sponge and runs to his room, where he slams the door as hard as he can.)

Mother: Well, what's wrong with him?

Father: I suppose he feels bad about his report card.

Mother: M-m-m, but he doesn't have to act like that.

The boy, saddened by a mediocre report card, needs reassurance that he is not stupid and inferior as he secretly fears, and support that he has the capacity to do better. He is met by an older sister who for years has been resentful and envious because he was born and took a lot of the mother's time and attention away from her. She tries to get even by being derisive and critical; then for a brief time she feels superior to him. The parents' unfortunate lack of attention prevented them from seeing what was going on and doing something helpful. When anger resulted in the spilled milk, the exasperated mother's reaction confirmed the boy's fears that he was stupid and no good.

Here is another way the situation might have been dealt with.

Sister: Did you get your report card today, Danny? What did you get?

Brother: That's my business.

Sister: Oh, so it wasn't so good, was it? You're ashamed to show it, aren't you? I guess you're the dummy I always knew you were, anyway.

Mother: (realizing that the boy is being attacked, interferes) Joan, Danny is not a dummy.

Sister: Well, he's not very smart if he can't get a good report card.

Father: No, that's not true. Smart people sometimes don't get as good marks as they could.

Sister: Why? I get good marks.

Father: Yes, and we're proud of you. But something is interfering with Danny's doing as well in school as he should. Mother and I are thinking about talking with his teacher. Danny, would you like to be at the meeting and give us your ideas?

Brother: (relieved and pleased at the understanding and support from his parents) Well, yeah, I guess I would . . .

Mother: Good, Danny. Would you pass the butter, please?

(Danny reaches for the plate eagerly and knocks over his milk.)

Sister: (still wanting to vent her hostility at her brother) Oh, Stupid! Look what he's done now!

Mother: Accidents happen to all of us sometimes. Danny, there's a sponge on the sink.

(Danny gets up and mops up the milk. The family resumes eating dinner peacefully.)

In this instance the child receives the backing he needs from his parents. The parents make it clear that he is not stupid as he fears, and shield him from his envious older sister's aggression. They let him know they are interested in his problems and willing to try to help him. At the same time they give him the opportunity to be helpful by calmly pointing out that he can clean up the milk, so that he doesn't feel like a clumsy little boy. Also they let the sister know that they are proud of her accomplishments. In this way the parents increased the self-esteem of both children.

Adequate self-esteem is absolutely essential for any person to function at his best and be happy. Poor self-esteem affects everything one does and can last throughout life. School performance, competence at work, and interpersonal relationships are all profoundly influenced by self-esteem. And self-esteem comes primarily from the relationship with parents during childhood. Children need reassurance and bolstering repeatedly throughout their developing years.

Poor self-esteem causes great unhappiness. The person believes s/he is not bright or competent, not as good as other people, will not be liked and accepted, is not attractive or interesting. These negative expectations often become a self-fulfilling prophecy. People with low opinions of themselves often choose marriage partners who also have poor self-images and don't function optimally. Girls with this problem become involved with boys who do not measure up their family's standards, boys who may have a problem with drugs or alcohol or are school dropouts or get fired from their jobs. Sometimes people with poor self-esteem identify with someone they view as an underdog and try vainly to rescue him or her. They are often depressed, difficult, and dreary to live with, having little energy or enthusiasm. Sometimes they attempt to bolster sagging self-esteem by bragging and exaggerating. Certain girls with a low self-image are promiscuous because they feel the only way they can hold a man's interest is to go to bed with him. They are so self-demeaning that they invite rejection.

If a child is to make a happy sexual and marital adjustment, s/he must have good self-esteem. It's up to us parents to foster that vital feeling in our children. It's a constant task, but it's one of the most important things we can do for our children. Love enters into it; children who receive warmth and affection grow to feel that they are lovable people.

"Does Marriage Have a Future?"

Until very recently adolescents took marriage for granted. Boys and girls planned to go to school, work, and eventually marry. This is still the plan of the majority of teenagers, but a growing minority—especially in university cities and towns

—reject this role as outmoded and confining. Many high-school and college students tell me they have serious questions about whether traditional marriage is really for them, but they are conflicted too about living with someone without being married.

A sixteen-year-old boy said, "Marriage is a drag. I want freedom to move from one person to another when I need to without any hassle." A seventeen-year-old boy commented, "Marriage is like a ball and chain. All your life is too long to spend with one person." A seventeen-year-old girl added, "Living together is the only way to really know the other person." A sixteen-year-old boy was cynical about marriage: "At the beginning the wife will put flowers and candles on the table for about a week. Then one day you'd come home from work and you'd find last night's dishes in the sink. That's the way it is with most marriages."

Several high-school girls expressed doubts about living with a man without being married, focusing on how the girl could be hurt by the experience: "Boys screw around. Sex doesn't mean as much to them. Girls are scared. They have more to lose—like getting pregnant or feeling bad when the guy wants out." And "A girl's feelings are deeper. She wants to be loved."

One boy felt he couldn't be honest and vent his true feelings if he were living with someone without being married: "It isn't being honest. I mean if I was married and I got mad I could yell at my wife if I wanted to, but if I wasn't, I wouldn't let myself 'cause she might just walk out."

Each year for several years I have talked about sex and marriage with the seventeen-, eighteen-, and nineteen-year-old girls enrolled in a junior college in Boston. Until about two years ago the sixty girls crowded together in the room would vie with each other to ask me questions, arms waving in the air to get my attention. They wanted to know about premarital sex, contraception, abortion, what makes a happy marriage. Now they know more and prefer to state their ideas rather than ask questions. As a matter of fact, this year they let me know through one of their instructors that they would be glad to have me come if I didn't give them a lecture, but would listen to their ideas! But behind the sophisticated facades I could detect many unspoken questions.

They, like the younger high-school youths, were very much in conflict about whether or not to live with someone before marriage, a practice that is more and more widespread:

"Living together without being married is a lie because you're pretending you're married and you aren't. The kids I know who are doing it are scared to tell their parents, so they lie to them about it. Their parents don't know their roommate is a guy!" There was uneasy laughter from the group.

"It's hard to do something your parents disapprove of so strongly. Mothers understand better than fathers, though. Fathers get so uptight about what awful things could happen to *their* daughter!"

"Just breaking away from your family is hard."

Heads nodded at that.

"Why has living with a guy become such a big thing? Is it because people feel nothing's permanent anymore? Kids are afraid to commit themselves, they've seen too many marriages break up. I know so many girls just out of college who are divorced already."

"Well, I don't think marriage is necessary unless you want children."

"I want marriage because then you've got someone to hold on to."

"What about living together on a trial basis? Maybe you love each other but you can't stand little habits that are annoying that you wouldn't have known about unless you'd lived together."

One of the married girls expressed her thoughts about that: "Living together doesn't ask for that extra commitment that makes you work harder at the relationship. There *are* many little things that irritate, but if you're not married, there isn't that incentive to work them out."

"I may be old-fashioned, but I want the security of marriage. If I decided to live with a guy for two or three years and I really loved him and then he got interested in someone else and we split up, well, there I'd be, miserable, and that much older, too. I don't think it's worth it . . ."

"Oh, if you *really* loved each other, you'd get married in the end. I know a lot of people who have."

"Yes, but I know some who haven't."

"So do I."

I commented that they were living in changing times. The idea of living with a man without being married caused great conflict, because they had been brought up by parents who believed in marriage and expected their children to go that traditional route. I said it is very hard to cause protracted disappointment and distress to parents who have cared and given a lot, and it is a severe strain to live under the cloud of family disapproval for a long period of time.

I further told them that their statements revealed they had given this much thought—there are pros and cons—and what suits one person does not mean happiness for another. I let them know I felt the new practice of a man and woman living together without a permanent commitment, with an agreement that either could end the relationship when he or she felt the need, was unrealistic and immature because it did not consider the other person's feelings and needs. It is rare indeed when both people agree simultaneously that it is time to end an affair and find new love partners. I agree with the married student who had said that if one is married, more effort is made to work out difficulties. I told them I am seeing more and more young women in psychiatric consultation who are depressed following the breakup of a long-lasting relationship with a man they had been living with. They listened very carefully, both because they wanted to know what I as a psychiatrist thought, and also because I had listened to them. I said what they decide about their lives is up to them, but they should be aware of all the ramifications.

Unwanted Pregnancy and Abortion

The discussion of living together led naturally into questions about abortion. These girls have some knowledge of contraception but many are anxious about the Pill, having heard of complications that sometimes occur. Some are too embarrassed to go to an obstetrician to be fitted with a diaphragm or IUD (intrauterine device). They are all very much aware that boys expect them to take care of contraception, and many resent that.

They know that abortion is available and that is a great relief to them, but they worry about the possibility of going through such an ordeal, and are vague about the details. Their anxiety was intense enough to move them to actually ask me some questions.

"Just how do they do an abortion?"

"I heard about a new kind where they use suction or something?"

"Someone said if you're pretty far along, they put salt in your uterus and you go through labor and everything? That sounds awful to me . . . ."

"Does an abortion hurt?"

"If a girl got pregnant, just how would she find out where she could get an abortion?"

"I think abortion is wrong. It's killing a human life."

"Well, you can think what you want, but *I* think no woman should have to have a baby she doesn't want. It's terrible to bring a child into the world that isn't wanted. Besides, it's my own body, and I should be able to decide what happens to it."

I told them that during the first three months of pregnancy abortion is done by either gently scraping out the uterus or sucking out the contents mechanically. This is called a D & C, meaning dilation of the cervix and curettage, or scraping out. It is done in a hospital under general anesthesia, so the patient is asleep, or in an office or clinic with local anesthesia, injected into the pelvic area.

The general anesthetic most often used in the hospital is Pentothal, a barbiturate given intravenously. The procedure takes about a half hour. A woman goes into the hospital either the night before or early in the morning on the day of the operation. She is given a sedative to calm her and wheeled into the operating room, where the anesthesia is administered. When she wakes up later, she will be wearing a sanitary pad and may have some cramps and bleeding, much like a period which may last two or three days. If the procedure is done in an office, and the girl is awake during it, an attendant will be with her throughout to reassure her. Her cycles will resume normally. If the abortion is done properly she should have no complications and her ability to conceive and bear children will not be affected. No one can tell that she has had an abortion, and she should use her own judgment about whether she wants to let anyone else know.

There have been rare instances of infection, which can be treated with antibiotics, and very rare cases of accidental perforation of the uterine wall. In this case, an emergency hysterectomy must be performed.

After three months of pregnancy a D & C cannot be performed because the fetus has grown too large. The woman is admitted to the hospital. Her pubic area is shaved by a nurse and she is given an enema so that during delivery no accidental emptying of the rectum will occur, with possible contamination of the vagina and resulting infection. A sterile salt solution called saline, which is slightly less than one per cent salt in water, is injected through the abdominal wall into the uterus. The uterus reacts to this irritating substance by contracting, and labor begins, which may last several hours and is painful as it progresses. Medications to lessen the discomfort are given. Finally the cervix widens enough due to the pushing down of the fetal head and the fetus is expelled. It is too physically immature to survive. It is followed by the placenta. The uterus contracts down quickly. The woman can go home in two days when it is ascertained that no bleeding or fever have ensued.

Again, no one can tell that she has gone through this except an obstetrician observing the cervix during a pelvic examination. And this kind of abortion has no effect on her ability to have future children.

Until recently, abortions were against the law except where the life or health of the mother was endangered, where pregnancy was a result of incest or rape, or when the pregnant woman had contracted German measles during the first several weeks with a definite possibility that the baby would be born defective. Abortion laws varied from one state to another, and often girls traveled out of the country or had criminal abortions done which sometimes caused serious infections and even death. Even if no physical harm was done, women suffered for many years with feelings of having done something "dirty" and "bad."

The Supreme Court ruling of January 22, 1973, changed all this radically. It stated that during the first three months of pregnancy a decision about abortion would be a matter between the woman and her physician. After the first three months the state may regulate abortion procedure in ways relating to maternal health, such as requiring hospitalization. After the fetus can survive (the beginning of the seventh month), the state can determine whether an abortion is appropriate. One example would be to save the life of the mother.

The legal age of maturity, when an adolescent is no longer considered a minor, varies from state to state; Oregon sets it at fifteen years, many states at eighteen, Montana at nineteen, and still many others at twenty-one. Adolescents should know what the age of maturity is in their state, for most physicians are reluctant to treat a minor without parental consent, especially if it entails a surgical procedure, unless it is an emergency.

More and more pregnancy-counseling services are being established—especially in the larger cities—and can be found listed in the telephone book. They also advertise in many underground newspapers. The changes in abortion laws have certainly made it much easier both physically and emotionally for a girl who becomes pregnant. No longer will she find herself in the agonizing trap of not knowing where to turn for help. Abortion is rapidly becoming acceptable, and girls no longer feel the guilt and shame they used to be burdened with.

But it is a mistake to think that abortion is easy to go through, or that one will not be upset by it, for it is emotionally trying and very stressful. It's important for a girl to try to face her real feelings and think about it carefully. Many girls deny the seriousness of what they are going through and then find themselves depressed or anxious later, or compelled to become pregnant again. There may be an unconscious reason why a girl allows herself to become pregnant in this age of easy accessibility of adequate contraception. The abortion, though an enormous relief on a conscious level, may be a real loss unconsciously—the girl may have a wish to make up for that loss by becoming pregnant again. So it is very important for girls to do a lot of thinking about their problem if they find themselves in this situation. Counseling or therapy—even of brief duration—can be most useful in helping them get insight into their feelings and behavior.

Because abortion is usually not done after twenty or twenty-one weeks of pregnancy, it is important for girls to be realistic about the possibility of pregnancy if they have missed a menstrual period. Often girls deny the possibility until it is too late to be aborted. One girl told me, "I didn't know I was pregnant; I didn't think it could happen to me!"

Of course, parents should tell their adolescent children what they believe is right for them concerning the issues of premarital sex and pregnancy. But times are rapidly changing—our growing sons and daughters are living in a very different world from the one we knew at their age. Increasing numbers of young people are deciding that marriage is too confining, and many young women have clamored for repeal of restrictive abortion laws. More and more girls are getting abortions and the days of a girl being sent away to another town or state to a relative or maternity home to wait out a pregnancy and give up the baby for adoption are largely passing. Maternity homes are closing their doors, and adoption agencies are offering older children, handicapped, or racially mixed children to couples who apply for a child. Girls who decide not to abort often either marry or keep their babies after delivery. Some social workers predict that shortly a crop of toddlers will become available for adoption as adolescent unmarried mothers weary of the hardships of caring for a child.

How does one advise a son or daughter in these confusing times? Adolescents are often skeptical about marriage, seeing divorce all around them. With the ever-present threat of nuclear war hanging over them, they aren't sure they will live to an old age, and they want to live every day to its fullest; they are reluctant to postpone fulfillment. They worry about the population explosion and decide not to have any babies at all, or to adopt.

As I talked with and listened to the questions of the group of college girls about abortions, I raised the question of the emotional aspects of abortion. How would a girl feel about herself after having an abortion? What would it be like to be pregnant, to know that a fetus which could become a baby was beginning to develop inside, and then suddenly to end the process? What about the feminine longings for a baby that were in the girl even when she was little and played with dolls?

Adolescents respond well to such an approach. They like the challenge to their thinking, the interest someone else takes in their ideas, and they appreciate not being *told* things. Their thoughts poured out.

"It would be hard. I'd feel really awful, I know, even if I knew I had done the right thing."

"Even if you don't like to think it, you *have* decided to kill a living creature that is human, after all. I guess if it was very early in the pregnancy and it was just a little shrimp-like thing, I wouldn't feel so bad about it."

"But if it was moving inside you and you knew it had turned into a real *baby* even if it only was very small still, I don't know if I could do it then."

"Well, I don't really know . . . . It would be awfully hard to have to quit school and go away someplace and actually have the baby. My parents would be so upset, I don't know if they'd ever get over it . . . . I'm kind of scared of childbirth, too. I'm sure it's painful and I think about maybe getting torn down there . . . and the hardest thing would be to give the baby away and never see it again. I'd wonder about it all my life . . . ."

"I would definitely have an abortion. I wouldn't go through what she's talking about. I think an abortion, especially these days when it's done right, is much easier emotionally than having a baby."

"And I think the girls who keep their babies must have a very tough time. Just at the age when they should be going to school and having a good time they're changing diapers all the time and can't get out. And what guy wants to marry a girl who has an illegitimate child? I don't know any who would."

"Well, maybe a few would . . ."

"I think a girl would feel bad about it after the abortion even though she would be glad she did it. I mean, she might worry that she's a bad person, you know, feel guilty and sad. I guess there's no easy answer."

I agreed that there was no easy answer and that their thoughts were important. Whether a girl gets an abortion, carries through the pregnancy and gives the baby up for adoption or whether she keeps it and gives up school and a career, it is a very stressful time in her life. Abortion early by a D & C in a hospital is the easiest solution physically and emotionally, but it is still a trauma and affects the girl profoundly. It takes a long time to get over it, and it helps to have someone to talk to. I told them that I felt group therapy with other girls who had gone through the same experience would be very helpful, but too often girls who have had abortions try to put it out of their minds; then they don't gain insight into why they became pregnant in the first place and may go through the same thing again. I told them about a recent study of girls and women applying for therapeutic abortion at a large Boston hospital which showed that these women were unconsciously trying to make up for the loss of someone by becoming pregnant. They "forgot" about contraception because unconsciously they wanted a baby. But consciously they did not, and so were asking for abortions.

One of the girls expressed her conviction that an unwanted baby should not be brought into the world. I said I could sympathize with that because in my work I had dealt with unwanted, neglected, and abused children who suffered enormous emotional problems as a result. But I raised another question with them: what about the many couples who cannot conceive who long for a baby to love and care for, but are being turned away by adoption agencies because there are practically no babies as a result of widespread abortions and unmarried girls keeping their babies?

They felt it was unfortunate, but they didn't want to be the ones to provide the babies. "Well, it is a shame. I know if I were married and for some reason I couldn't get pregnant, like my husband turned out to be sterile or something, I'd certainly want to be able to adopt a nice, healthy newborn baby. But if I got pregnant before I got married, I know I wouldn't care at all about all those couples just dying for a nice little baby. I'd get aborted as fast as I could, I wouldn't want to go through the hassle of a pregnancy and giving birth and all that—never!"

Adoption

They raised questions as they talked about adoption:
"I think it must be harder to be an adopted child. I mean, you

must wonder why your real mother didn't keep you and what she's like."

"Do adoption agencies tell the adopting couples about the real mother and father?"

"And do they tell the real mother who is adopting her baby?"

"I read in the paper about this mother who went to court to try to get her child back that she had let be adopted. The couple were fighting it because they loved the child and felt like it was really theirs. It was really sad. I think I'd be scared to adopt a baby if I thought the real mother could come along later and want to take it away from me."

I commented that this happens on rare occasions and it is heart-rending for everyone, most of all for the child, who may end up being taken from the only parents s/he has ever known and placed with people who to him or her are total strangers. I told them about a new law in Massachusetts which protects adopted children and prevents the natural parent from taking the child later, for we know that great emotional harm is done by abruptly uprooting a child from parents, who mean so much to the child. S/he may be prone to depressions later and have a problem trusting others.

The agencies give out very little information to the natural mother and the adopting couple about each other. The mother is told that the baby is being placed with a loving couple who will be good parents; the couple is told of the general physical health of the natural mother and any hereditary conditions in her family background and in the father's background, if known. Identifying facts are not given out.

It is true that adopted children wonder about why they were adopted. But it is very foolish to try to hide the fact from the child, for s/he will learn of it sooner or later, and it is much better that s/he learn at four or five years of age from the adoptive parents than from a playmate or cousin. Adopted children do wonder about their natural parents; what did they look like, where are they now? In general babies are given up for adoption by unmarried girls who feel they cannot provide an adequate home for the child. The young adopted child can be told that his or her first mother could not be a good mother to him or her, though she wanted to. She had no husband and had to work and could not have been home to take care of him or her. She felt sorry and thought about it a lot because she cared about him or her and wanted him or her to be happy. She decided to let him or her be adopted because then s/he could have a mother who could take care of him or her and a father who would love him or her, too. You don't know where she is now, but she hopes that her child is happy. This reasurrance helps the child feel that the real mother doesn't hate or not care about him/her and that the adoption wasn't caused by something being wrong with him/her.

As the adopted child gets older, s/he may fantasize more about his or her natural parents, although some are so secure in the adoptive home they think little about their origins. During adolescence when the search for identity is going on, the child may wonder about the natural parent of the same sex. Adolescents are normally in conflict with their parents and during a time when there is frustration and resentment, it is easy for an adopted child to fantasize about the natural parents and think that things might have been happier with them. People who exist only in fantasy can take on the attributes the dreamer wants them to have, and frequently an adopted child begins to believe that the natural parents are ideal, wonderful people who are always beyond his or her reach. Living day after day with his or her adoptive parents with their faults fosters the romantic image of the unattainable natural parents. This makes it hard on everyone, and it is more difficult to be a parent of an adopted child, but if the adoptive parents try their best, providing the child with love and guidance, it will work out.

Some adopted teenagers actually go on a search for the natural parent and will go to town or city officials, trying to learn the identity and address of their mothers. They have wondered all their lives what she is like, and may go to visit her if they can find her. Usually the meeting is a surprise for both, for the mother does not match the child's fantasy and, because adolescents tend to do things impulsively, she may be entirely unprepared for the encounter. I feel that if an adolescent of fifteen or sixteen wants very much to meet the natural mother, it should be arranged, because clearly the child has a real need to answer some question within which s/he feels is imperative. The agency which arranged the adoption should be consulted by the adoptive parents and child together; in this way the child does not have to be furtive and the natural mother can be prepared. Adoptive parents should keep in mind that they really are the meaningful parental figures for the child and not feel that because s/he wants to meet the natural parent that s/he prefers her or loves her more. It is mainly that s/he doesn't want to live with a question mark throughout life.

The teen-aged adopted girl is especially apt to want to meet her natural mother, for she is trying to identify as a woman and wants to know what kind of woman her biological mother was and is. She is forging her own standards and personal philosophy and somehow needs to meet and question her mother to understand why she was given up for adoption.

Many unwed women who have given up a child for adoption later marry and have a family and decide to keep the earlier birth and adoption secret. If a woman suddenly hears from a child she gave up many years before, she should meet with the child at a social agency. This allows everything to be aboveboard and truthful, and the natural mother does not have to deal with her husband's and children's conflicts as she would if the child unexpectedly came to the front door one day. My feeling is if a woman wants to keep a past birth secret, that should be her decision.

The natural mother should be honest with the girl or boy and answer the child's questions truthfully, emphasizing that she cared for the child and wanted to do the best thing for her or him at the time of the child's birth. What all human beings basically fear is feeling unwanted and unloved.

Sometimes an adopted child wants to meet his/her natural father, but this may be more difficult, since the mother may have chosen to keep his identity secret at the time of the child's birth. Boys are more apt to seek their biological father as part of the process of working out their own identity.

If a girl finds herself pregnant and doesn't want an abortion, what options are open to her? She has three choices. She can contact a social service agency and talk with a social worker about her situation. The agency will either continue to counsel her and arrange for obstetrical care or will refer her to an agency that offers those services. As she verbalizes her conflicts and feelings to a therapist, she will arrive at a decision about her baby—whether to give it up for adoption or keep it. The ramifications of both decisions will be thoroughly explored with her. If she decides to give the baby up, she knows that she will see the baby frequently and feed it while in the hospital for three or four days following delivery, but after signing the surrender papers she will not see her baby again.

Some girls who find it extremely difficult to decide have the baby placed by the agency in a foster or boarding home for temporary care until a decision is made. The mother may visit the baby occasionally in the company of her social worker. Of course the more she sees the infant, the more attached she may become, and the harder it will be for her to give it up. But she should not make a decision until she is quite sure about it or she will be in a severe conflict afterwards and become depressed. But no matter what she decides, she will have a certain amount of conflict. She will inevitably feel sad and bereft if she gives the baby up, and if she decides to keep it, she may have to face the unhappiness and probable disapproval of her family and the community, despite changing attitudes, as well as the burden of caring for an infant without a husband's help and support while giving up many of the pleasures and activities she would ordinarily enjoy at her age.

If a girl wants to keep her baby, she must consider how she will manage. Will her family give her emotional and financial support, or must she go on welfare to survive? Will that mean adjusting to a different style of living with attendant deprivations? Has she ever lived alone before? How will she feel about caring for a helpless, demanding baby by herself? Will she be able to afford an occasional baby sitter? Day care? How will it affect her relationships with her friends? How does she feel about the baby's father? Will he help or not? How will being a mother affect her future relationships with men?

If she decides to give the baby up, should she keep the whole business secret or not? When she becomes deeply involved in the future with a man she loves and plans to marry, should she tell him about the child?

All these questions must be raised and considered to avoid possible chronic depression, conflict, and anxiety. How a girl answers them are her decisions to make and will vary according to the individual girl's needs. My feeling is that it requires a great deal of maturity and considerable self-discipline for a teen-aged girl to live alone and care for a baby happily and well. Most adolescent girls are not able to deal successfully with the stresses and deprivations inherent in such a situation.

If she gives up the baby and later decides to marry, should she tell her future husband about it? Again it is an individual matter. I put the question to the group of college girls:

"I would tell him everything. I want complete openness and honesty between us. If he couldn't accept it, then he wouldn't be the kind of man I'd want anyway."

"Well, I don't know. That sounds very nice, but if you loved him a lot and then he broke up because of what you confessed, I'm sure you'd feel just awful and sad."

"I hate to sound like my mother, but she says what you don't know won't hurt you and I think it applies here. Men get awfully uptight still about things like that. I think I'd keep it to myself because it would have no connection with our relationship anyway."

"Yeah, why rock the boat?"

I said that I felt it should be an individual matter requiring a judgement about the other person's attitudes and ability to accept and tolerate conflict. A mature, tolerant man could hear about it and still love and want the girl as much as before; a less mature and secure man might get very upset, feel threatened and betrayed, and the relationship could be severely strained.

The third alternative for a girl who does not want an abortion and does not want to give her baby up for adoption is marriage. This time-honored solution to the predicament is still widespread; almost half the brides under twenty-one are said to be pregnant at the time of marriage, but most are very early in their pregnancies, so the fact is not widely known until months after the wedding. I asked the college girls what they thought about getting married because of being pregnant:

"It's not good. What if the guy doesn't feel sure that this is what he wants or doesn't feel ready yet for marriage? Then he's bound to feel resentment sooner or later and there'll be trouble and it will probably end in divorce."

"And there's no time for just doing what you feel like together for a while before you decide to have a child. Right away you're tied down by a baby and there's no more freedom."

"Some guys get jealous of all the time and attention you give the baby and they feel left out and they get mad about it. The woman can't do everything at once. No, I think it's crazy, just asking for problems, and there are enough problems just getting adjusted to marriage . . ."

I told them I felt their comments were very astute, and then reminded them that some young people are having babies and living together—either as a family unit or in a larger group—without getting married. What did they think about that solution?

"Well, for myself, like I said before, I'd want the security of marriage. It would be very hard for me to live with someone *and* have a baby and still not be married. I mean, what would happen if he decided he was getting tired of it all and left? What would I do with a baby or a little child to support? I could never go to *my* family, they just wouldn't accept it. And I couldn't live on welfare; I couldn't stand having so little to live on. . . . I guess I sound like an awful snob, and maybe I am, but I just couldn't do those things!"

"I think if that happened to me, my family would help me financially, but they'd probably want me to live pretty far away from their town so I wouldn't embarrass them . . . . I think I could stand it, but it would be hard for the child. He would miss his daddy so much . . . . If you get married, there's more reason for the guy to stay, and you and the child wouldn't run such a risk of ending up alone."

"I guess some of those people do get married in the end, but I think I'd be so worried about whether we were going to get married or not that it would make for problems."

"Well, I think you all are terribly old-fashioned. I think marriage is a bind. Why are you all so scared the guy will get tired of it and want out? Why couldn't *you* get tired of it and want to leave? I think it would be the worst drag to be married and feel stuck and obligated. People should be free to make new relationships when they need to and get the old ones off their back when they're not good anymore, when you've grown out of them. Like if you mature a lot and the guy stays pretty much the same . . ."

At that point I said that different people have different needs and different capacities for dealing with changes and losses. What is important is to think honestly and carefully about what kind of a person you are, what you need to make you happy, what stresses and strains you can tolerate pretty well, and which ones you can't. If you feel that getting an abortion or carrying through a pregnancy and either giving the baby up or caring for it alone would be something you couldn't handle, then you should make sure you don't get pregnant in the first place. I reminded them that all these seriously conflicted situations we had been talking about could be avoided by faithful, consistent use of adequate contraception, and that they shouldn't worry at all about seeming unromantic by discussing contraception and making sure some form is used. They should think of their own welfare and take care of themselves.

Contraception

"How Do You Get Contraceptives? Can You Get Them Without Parents' Permission?"

Because adolescents are perhaps more active sexually than in the past, they need to have a thorough knowledge of contraception to avoid unwanted pregnancies and protect against venereal disease. Here are some typical questions that teenagers ask:

How do you keep from getting pregnant?
What is a contraceptive?
What is a condom (rubber, skin)?
What does the Pill do? Does it harm you to take it?
I heard about some foam stuff. What is it?
How do you get contraceptives? Can you get them without your parents' permission?
What is an IUD? How does it get inside? Does it hurt inside a girl?

What is the system the Catholic Church uses? I think it has something to do with music.

My mother told me about a rubber thing called a diaphragm that keeps sperms out of the uterus. How do you get it inside you?

What is it when the man interrupts intercourse so the woman won't get pregnant?

I feel that adolescents should know about contraceptives, but when you tell your son or daughter about them, be careful that s/he doesn't assume that you are thereby giving an immediate go-ahead sign to their having sexual intercourse. Emphasize the importance of being prepared for an event which may take place in the future, that people cope much better when they have some knowledge and have had time to think.

The Pill

The hormone medication containing carefully balanced small quantities of estrogen and progesterone, the female sex hormones, commonly called the Pill, is the most reliable contraceptive there is. The tablet is swallowed once a day at any hour a woman chooses, but it should be the same time every day in order to maintain a consistent blood level of the hormones. The hormones act on the pituitary gland at the base of the brain, suppressing its production of hormones that would ordinarily cause the ovaries to ripen immature ova. Thus, no ripened egg is available to the searching sperm and pregnancy cannot occur.

Many millions of women today take the Pill, and although there have been occasional reports of blood clotting, most obstetricians feel it is a safe and highly reliable form of contraception. The greatest asset is its convenience; a woman in the throes of an amorous embrace does not have to stop and think about protecting herself against pregnancy, or interrupt pleasurable activity to insert some kind of contraceptive device into the vagina.

The IUD

The intrauterine device, or IUD, is the next most reliable form of contraception. It is a plastic structure of varying shapes placed within the uterus by a physician. It prevents implantation of a fertilized ovum into the uterine wall, it is thought, or somehow causes the fertilized egg to travel so rapidly through the tube and uterus that implantation either does not take place or is insufficient. Usually it is entirely painless and a woman is unaware of its presence, but some women have complained of cramping and very heavy menstrual bleeding with it. Again, the advantage is convenience and the lack of having to do anything about contraception at a time when sexual feelings are running high and rational thought is not at its best.

The Diaphragm

The next most commonly used contraceptive is the diaphragm—a thin round rubber cap with a pliable metal rim which snugly covers the cervix, the opening into the uterus from the vagina. It is necessary to visit a gynecologist or obstetrician to be measured for this device, which comes in various sizes. Spermicidal creams or jellies must be smeared on the diaphragm to kill any sperm that might get around its edges. A woman lies on her back with knees bent and bends the diaphragm with her fingers and inserts it into her vagina as deeply as she can. She should be sure to tuck it up under the pubic bone (symphysis) in front, which she quickly learns to do. It should be put in not more than three hours before intercourse takes place, and should remain undisturbed for at least eight hours after. If intercourse is desired again before eight hours have passed, the diaphragm should be left undisturbed and an applicator full of cream or jelly inserted into the vagina. Many women like to douche when they remove the diaphragm, but it is not necessary. The normal cervical secretions gradually wash away the cream and semen.

The diaphragm, if used properly, is a reliable contraceptive; its major drawback is the necessity for its use at the time of intercourse. It does not interfere at all with the sexual pleasure of either the man or woman.

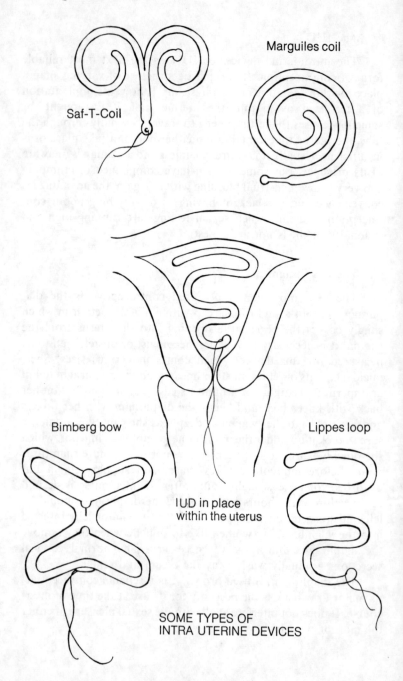

Marguiles coil

Saf-T-Coil

Bimberg bow

Lippes loop

IUD in place
within the uterus

SOME TYPES OF
INTRA UTERINE DEVICES

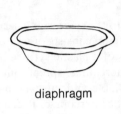

diaphragm

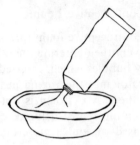

addition of spermicidal
jelly or cream

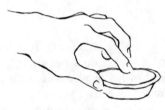

spreading of jelly or
cream over diaphragm

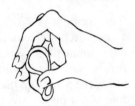

bending diaphragm
prior to insertion

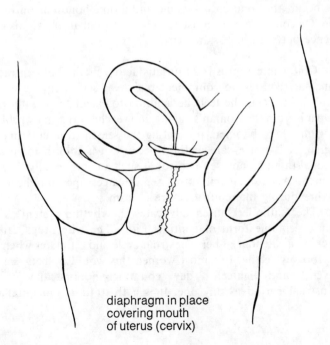

diaphragm in place
covering mouth
of uterus (cervix)

Contraceptive Foam

Contraceptive foam forms a barrier to the sperms and serves to prevent their entering the uterus. The foam consists of millions of tiny bubbles which, inserted by means of a plastic syringe-like applicator into the vagina just before intercourse, spread out to cover the cervix. Foam is not highly reliable and must be used conscientiously just before each episode of intercourse. It can be purchased without a prescription.

Condoms

The condom is a thin sheath of rubber which fits over the penis and catches ejaculated semen so that it does not enter the vagina. A man places it over the end of his penis and unrolls it toward the base. He should take care to leave extra space between the end of the penis and the condom to give the semen room. If the condom is put on too snugly it can rupture under the force of the ejaculating fluid. It is possible for the condom to slip off in the vagina during vigorous intercourse. If these unfortunate events do not occur, the condom is reliable and a time-honored contraceptive. Of course, a man must remember to put it on, so his conscience plays an important part.

Coitus interruptus is an unsatisfactory method of contraception that requires no equipment but great self-discipline on the man's part. When he feels he is about to ejaculate he withdraws his penis from the woman's vagina and reaches orgasm by rubbing it against her abdomen, preventing the semen from entering her vagina. It is not a safe method because it is foolish to rely on rational thinking and self-control at such an emotionally charged moment. Also, small amounts of semen can escape from the man's urethra during intercourse before orgasm.

The Catholic Church advocates the rhythm system as the only acceptable form of contraception. The wife keeps careful track on a calendar of her menstrual cycle and estimates when she is probably fertile. For most women this would be between the eleventh and eighteenth day, counting the first day of the menstrual period as day one. It is a frustrating and unreliable method of contraception because when the couple may feel like making love they cannot, and they begin to feel resentful that their sexual life together is ruled by the calendar. Also, many women are irregular in ovulating, and numerous Catholic wives, carefully following the calendar and its rules, have become pregnant.

While discussing contraception with a group of sixteen- and seventeen-year-old boys and girls in a psychology class recently in a large suburban school, I was told by several of the boys that they thought contraception should be the girl's responsibility. They really didn't want to be bothered with it. One said, "I'd be embarrassed to ask the guy at the drugstore for condoms." Another commented, "Rubbers take away a lot of the enjoyment for the guy."

Boys now expect the girl to take care of contraception, and daughters should be aware of this and, if they decide to have intercourse, they should not worry about speaking up about contraception. Girls must make sure that some reliable method is used to prevent pregnancy. Many unmarried young pregnant girls have told me, during psychiatric consultation in connection with their request for a therapeutic abortion, that they never thought about the possibility of becoming pregnant when they agreed to go ahead with intercourse. Others have told me that the possibility crossed their minds, but they were too embarrassed to say anything about contraception!

One of the boys in the high school class had heard about vasectomy and with considerable nervousness asked, "What is it when they cut the man? Like in India?"

I told him he was referring to vasectomy, a simple procedure performed under local anesthesia in the doctor's office. It consists of a small incision through the skin of the scrotum on each side and a painless cutting of the long, white, spaghetti-like tube inside, the vas, that transports sperms into the penis. This is a highly reliable method of contraception, but quite irreversible. Attempts have been made to undo the ligation in men who for some reason have wanted to father another child, but the results have been discouraging. Therefore, the man and his wife must think very carefully about the meaning of this procedure before going ahead with it. Also, the man should be reassured beforehand that the procedure will not affect his potency and sexual capacity for erection and intercourse, for some men have had problems later, due entirely to psychological and not physical causes. Many people confuse impotency with sterility, but the two have no connection. A sterile man, not producing viable sperm and therefore incapable of making his wife pregnant, can be a very competent lover, entirely capable of giving and receiving sexual satisfaction.

"Why Are So Many People Getting Divorced?"

Adolescents these days are very worried about divorce. They see it all around them, with their parents, their parents' friends, and among young people. They want to know why it occurs, and how they can prevent it from happening to them someday.

My feeling is that divorce happens for two basic reasons: people choose unwisely, and once married, get far too wrapped up in their own self-centered concerns. When problems arise, there is not enough real effort by both partners to understand and work on them in a sustained way.

Why do so many people choose unwisely? There is still a great deal of pressure on girls to marry, despite attempts of the women's liberation movement to free women from early bonds of marriage. Families and peers pressure girls from age eighteen or nineteen to find a man and get married. Many girls get panicky about becoming old maids. There is enormous status in becoming engaged and marrying. Many women feel that unless they are married they don't count.

Life in society is a lonely prospect indeed for the unmarried. Seventy per cent of the population lives in large, impersonal cities in apartment houses where neighbors are usually strangers to each other. We travel on subways and in buses where people avoid each other's eyes and remain silent, each wrapped up in his own thoughts. And yet Americans in their pioneer days were a gregarious people, banding together in small communities and forming meaningful relationships that lasted a lifetime. Now we move every five years on the average, leaving friendships behind, trying to adjust to a strange, new environment.

Young people, once they are out of school, have a difficult time meeting each other. Men and women in their twenties despair of meeting anyone despite the fact that they live in crowded cities. Small-town dances and socials used to perform this function. Young women go to singles bars only to be approached by men who often turn out to be married or interested in only a brief sexual encounter. They shy away from computer-dating systems, feeling the only people who would turn to them must be undesirable. Their loneliness and desperation increase, and each birthday becomes a day of panic and depression. All these pressures may push them into unwise marriages, for often they feel if they turn a person down, there will never be anyone else.

Some men fear the responsibility of having a wife and children and resist marrying until the depression from chronic loneliness overcomes their anxiety.

And there is another important factor of which most people are unaware. People often choose someone to marry for unconscious neurotic reasons. Some unconsciously hope for a mother figure to take care of them; people with unresolved Oedipal ties search for the longed-for yet unattainable parental figure; men and women with conflicts involving anger and dependency seek someone with whom they can continue to struggle in the old neurotic way they fought with their parents. People are unaware of these urges, but they play a very important part in any relationship a neurotic person establishes and often lead to serious difficulties.

Parents can best prevent their children from having unconscious conflicts which push them into neurotic, problem-filled relationships by providing a stable, warm (but not seductive), and helpful environment in the home which fosters self-esteem and maturity. Children indentify with their parents. If you can cope with and solve problems successfully, they will learn from you and at the same time feel capable themselves. If you make efforts to understand, to think of others' feelings, and to be helpful, they will learn to do this too.

One sign of maturity is the ability to admit making a mistake, to be able to say one was wrong. Immature people find it very hard to take criticism, to admit that they might not have been right about something, to apologize. The now-famous saying in a recent very popular novel and movie, "Love means never having to say you're sorry," is absurd.

"What Makes a Happy Marriage?"

How can this question be answered? Perhaps the following family discussion between two middle-aged parents and their adolescent son and daughter will give you some ideas.

Daughter: I read in the paper that＿＿＿＿＿＿＿＿ is getting divorced again! Don't movie stars ever stay married?

Mother: Yes, some do, but the divorces get in the papers because they're news.

Son: Talking about divorce, Don's parents are splitting up. And they've been married since the year one, for Pete's sake!

Daughter: How can people stay together all those years and then decide to get divorced? I don't understand that. You'd think if they were that unhappy they'd have been that way long before.

Son: Some people stay together even if they hate each other for the sake of the children, I hear. What a lousy idea! The kids know it and feel awful. I hope you two never do that.

Father: Don't worry. You mother and I love each other and we're not going to get divorced.

Daughter: Well, I didn't think you were. But sometimes when I hear about so many people getting separated and divorced, I get a little worried. I think what if Mom and Dad did that? It'd be pretty sad and lonely around here.

Son: Why do so many people get divorced anyway?

Father: I suppose there are different reasons, according to the individuals involved. What might get one person all upset another person might be able to overlook. What do you think?

Daughter: Well, I think——

Father: Wait a second, give your brother a chance.

Son: Yeah, like I notice at school some guys are so quick to get mad at some little thing that really isn't that important. They're always on the defensive.

Mother: Does that mean they feel attacked, criticized too easily and take offense too quickly? What do you think, Ann?

Daughter: I know some kids like that. They get into a lot of fights that way and other kids get fed up. I can see how that kind of person would be very hard to live with. I wouldn't want a person like that to be my husband.

Father: What kind of person would you like to marry?

Daughter: Well, I guess someone who would be easy to get along with, someone who wouldn't get all upset and mad real easily like we were saying. Someone I could talk to if there was a problem, who would really listen and try to understand.

Mother: What do you think of this idea, to maybe say to him that you've both been at fault and you will try to do things differently from now on, and you hope he will, too. So all the blame doesn't get onto one person. I don't think it's ever good when one person feels like the good, perfect one and the other feels like the bad one all the time. The one who feels like the bad one over and over would resent it after a while.

Son: Yeah, that makes sense.

Father: What do you think feeling angry at the other person a lot would do to a marriage?

Daughter: It'd be pretty unhappy. Angry feelings lead to quarrels and fights.

Father: Yes, and misunderstandings. When a person is really mad, he's not able to be rational and accurate in what he says. He exaggerates and accuses and causes all kinds of hurt and angry feelings in the other person.

Mother: It takes a pretty mature person to say, "Look, I'm getting angry and I'm not happy about it, let's talk and see if we can solve it."

Daughter: We've been talking a lot about unhappy marriages. What makes a happy marriage?

Mother: What are your ideas about it? It's a very important question.

Daughter: Well, first of all, it would help if you married someone you like and who likes you basically. I'd hate to live in a country where my parents chose a husband for me and I had to marry him whether I liked him or not—ugh!

Mother: What kind of person would you be apt to feel attracted to?

Daughter: I guess like what we were talking about before—someone who would be good to me and understanding and not get teed off easily, someone I could count on . . . and someone I could be proud of. I don't care if he makes a lot of money or not, but if he likes what he's doing and he feels proud of it, then I would, too. Oh, yes, and someone who would be a good father to my kids!

Father: I'd agree with those ideas, Ann. John, what do you think?

Son: Yeah, makes sense, I guess. Those things are important in a person if you're going to be happy with them. Sounds kinda mushy, but I'd want a wife who would be loving, too, and who wouldn't fool with other guys if she got mad at me. I'd want her to be able to talk about problems. Over at some of the guys' houses there's screaming and yelling all the time. It's really awful. What a way to live! I'd want to be sure it wouldn't be that way in my house.

Mother: I agree, but you'd be part of that; if you can keep yourself from blowing your top, then your wife won't be so likely to do it. When one person gets really furious it's awfully easy for the other person to get all upset too.

Son: Yeah. So we'd both have to try to keep our tempers and discuss things.

Daughter: What else makes a marriage happy? I suppose if you feel loved by your husband and he's thoughtful and cares about you, then you would feel the same way back. That would be a pretty happy thing, I think.

Father: I think you've hit the nail on the head, Ann. I think a happy marriage is where two people really care for each other and think about each other's needs and feelings and do thoughtful things for each other. What would be some examples?

Son: Let's say a guy comes home real tired from his work and his wife has the house looking nice and a good meal that he likes ready. That would make him feel good and yet he'd let her know he appreciated it to make her feel good. No flowery speech or anything, just a little remark that it was good and he liked it.

Daughter: All right, you male chauvinist, how about a wife who works *and* takes care of the house and she's really dead from working hard, so he helps her with the housework and he doesn't feel stupid about it either. He sees that she's tired and he wants to help and he feels good about it.

Mother: What if she's really tired and he doesn't notice, so he doesn't think to help. Should she make some sarcastic remark to him or what?

Daughter: Well, it would be a temptation if she was feeling mad about it. I guess the mature thing to do would be to tell him that she's really pooped and would he help her.

Father: Do you think it would help if she asked him to do something specific rather than being vague about it?

Daughter: Yes, I can see it would be a good idea. Then he could do that and it really would be a help. Otherwise he might do something that he thinks is a help but it wouldn't be what she wanted at all.

Mother: You know, this is important, I think, because a lot of people act as though their husband or wife should be able to read their minds, and that's just ridiculous. I've heard wives say to their husbands, "You should have known how I felt," and be really mad that they didn't know what was wrong without anything being put into words and made clear.

Of course, there is much more to be said about marriage, but this is the kind of discussion that can take place when parents throw out thought-provoking ideas and give teenagers a chance to express their thoughts without interrupting or joking.

If a discussion ends because the phone rings or someone has to do something or the participants get weary, think over what has been said and determine what important areas still need to be talked about. The conversation above centered mainly on how a man and woman living together can relate to each other in a mature and giving way that promotes happiness. It did not get into the sexual life of the couple, coping with misfortune, dealing with other family members, adjusting to getting older, handling money, settling any religious or cultural conflicts, and interacting with others socially. It did not touch on the deepening devotion and meaning of a relationship between two people who have lived together for many years through both fulfilling and difficult times, and how very special and desirable that experience is. It did not include the area of childbearing, the decision to have or not have children and when, adjusting to pregnancy and the new baby, and bringing up children.

Some things adolescents will have to deal with are so far in the future that they may not be very interested in discussing them. Planning when to have children, getting along with in-laws, managing money, and getting middle-aged seem very distant to a sixteen- or seventeen-year-old. But the problems of choosing someone to marry and wanting a happy relationahip are of great interest to the teenager. Their own sexual drives focus much of their attention on how to establish a sexual relationship. They wonder what married people do about sex; do they have intercourse just about all the time or how often and who decides when it will happen? They can be told that this is an individual matter, that each couple decides what is best for them and the frequency and styles they choose may be quite different from what another couple enjoys. Healthy, loving couples carry on an active, satisfying sexual life throughout their lives.

What people do in the privacy of their own bedrooms is, in my opinion, up to them. If both partners agree that a certain sexual act is enjoyable and desirable, then I think they should feel free to indulge in it. Oral-genital sex, for example, is increasing and now occurs regularly among fifty per cent of married couples. Teenagers hear terms pertaining to this and may ask what they mean:

"What is fellatio?" (Usually mispronounced—don't laugh!)
"What is a blow job?"
"What does eating a girl mean?"
"What is sixty-nine?"
"What is fornication?"
"What does adultery mean?"
"What is cunnilingus?" (Also invariably mispronounced.)

Most parents feel embarrassed and anxious when asked these questions. The best way to answer is to be factual and brief.

Fellatio is when a woman takes a man's penis into her mouth; the man moves his penis back and forth, causing pleasurable feelings. It is sometimes a preliminary to or substitute for intercourse. "A blow job" is a slang term for fellatio.

"Eating" is a slang word for oral-genital lovemaking in which a man's mouth comes in contact with the woman's genital area. His tongue moving over the clitoris or entrance to the vagina causes exciting sensations for the woman. Care should be taken NEVER to blow air into the vagina, for it can travel into the uterus and into her bloodstream and deaths from air emboli to the heart and brain have occurred. The correct term for this kind of oral-genital lovemaking is cunnilingus.

Sixty-nine refers to the sexual act in which both the man and the woman make mouth contact with each other's genitals at the same time.

Fornication is the legal term for sexual intercourse between a man and woman who are not married to each other.

Adultery refers to sexual intercourse between a married man and a woman other than his wife, or between a married woman and a man who is not her husband.

Teenagers hear all kinds of terms, often accompanied by leers and smirks, that tend to give an unfortunately negative feeling about sex. For many years sex has been widely regarded by many people as dirty, wrong, or bad. It is so important that we parents try to counteract that attitude and talk with our children about sex as a pleasurable, gratifying aspect of love between two people, a positive, good force in life. They should learn that a satisfying sexual relationship cements a marriage, creates a bond of mutual trust and gratitude, and promotes a wish to remain devoted and loving to each other. Adolescents who grow up in a stable and loving home, who observe their parents behaving in a thoughtful and devoted way to each other and to their children, and who hear about sex and marriage from their parents as positive forces in life are well on their way to establishing happy, fulfilling relationships in their adult lives.

When Children Don't Ask About Sex

Not infrequently parents ask me what they should do about a child who just doesn't ask questions about sex. How should they get important information and attitudes across to such a child? They don't want to give an unsolicited lecture, nor do they want to plunk the child in the pediatrician's office for a talk.

First, it is essential that children clearly know that it is perfectly all right to ask questions about anything that concerns them or that they want to know something about. It is very common for children to feel that it really isn't permissible, to think that parents would be upset or embarrassed, or that it is wrong to bring up sexual topics.

It is helpful to make a comment like "You know, Dad and I will be glad to answer any questions or talk about anything you'd like to know more about." Or "So many things are going on in the world today, it must be hard growing up to decide what to do sometimes, how to live when people are living all kinds of different ways." This kind of statement is open-ended, leaving plenty of opportunity for a response from the child. Try to avoid flat statements which do not encourage response.

You might leave one or two books on sex education aimed at chidren casually lying around the house. No comment is necessary; the title of the book is a clear message to the child that you would like him or her to read it. But it is helpful to remind the child that you would be interested to know what s/he thinks about the book, and then use any remark from the child as a starting point for a discussion.

A very useful way to do some sex education with your teenagers is to bring up in conversation something that was in the newspaper or on TV or in a movie that bears on sexual mores. Again, the important aspect of this approach is to make an open-ended comment that expresses a thought of yours and invites your child to express his ideas. Be sure to listen carefully without interrupting, and your child will be encouraged by your interest and willingness to put other things aside and really hear him or her.

In the end, the way you live your life is the most effective way to teach sex education to your child. Your attitudes and behavior have a very great influence indeed. If you want your child to conduct his sexual life along lines that you believe are satisfying and fulfilling, your hopes will have a much better chance of being realized if your demonstrate in your own life what a loving relationship is. Relationships with other people are the most vital ingredient in our lives and teach our children more than any words we can say.

Bibliography

This is not meant to be a complete bibliography of books about sex and reproduction, but suggested titles which I like and have found useful.

J.G.S.

Books for Pre-Teen Children

A Baby is Born: The Story of How Life Begins by Milton I. Levine, M.D., and Jean H. Seligmann, Golden Press, revised edition, paperback, 1962, $1.00.
How Babies Are Made by Andrew C. Andry and Steven Schepp, Time-Life Books, 1968, $3.95.
Growing Up: How We Become Alive, Are Born, and Grow, by Karl de Schweinitz, MacMillan, revised edition, 1965.
The Wonderful Story of How You Were Born by Sidonie M. Gruenberg, Doubleday, revised edition, 1970, $3.95.
The Wonder of Life: How We Are Born and How We Grow Up by Milton I. Levine, M.D., and Jean H. Seligmann, Golden Press, revised edition, 1964.

Books for Adolescents

Girls and Sex by Wardell B. Pomeroy, Ph.D., Delacorte Press, 1969.
Boys and Sex by Wardell B. Pomeroy, Ph.D., Delacorte Press, 1968.
A Teenager's Guide to Life and Love by Benjamin Spock, M.D., Simon and Schuster, 1970.
Love and Sex in Plain Language by Eric W. Johnson, Bantam Books, paperback, 1970.
Sex and Birth Control: A Guide for the Young by E. James Lieberman, M.D., and Ellen Peck, Crowell, 1973.

Index

Literature and the American Tradition

Literature and the American Tradition

LEON HOWARD

Doubleday & Company, Inc.
Garden City, New York
1960

Library of Congress Catalog Card Number 60–5933

For
Michiko and Toshio, Guido, Pat, Tauno, Bernard Kao,
Monique and Isabelle, Mustafa, Broder,
and the many others
with whom I have sought the ethos of America
beneath the surface of its literature

Preface

THIS book had its origin in an experiment in the writing of literary history, and it was completed under pressure. The experiment was made in response to a challenge, issued by an eastern university a good many years ago, to discover and define in a public lecture the distinctively American qualities of a seemingly incongruous group of nineteenth-century writers who were strongly affected by the European literary tradition yet maintained an independent existence within it. The pressure developed in later years when I lectured in various universities in Japan, England, France, and the Scandinavian countries and realized how eagerly many foreigners looked to imaginative literature for an understanding of the United States and how confused or misguided they often were by the raw facts with which the imaginative writer deals and the raw ideas he sometimes expresses. Would it be possible, I wondered, to write a short history of American literature which would be comprehensive and at the same time analytic enough to seek out those attitudes of mind which controlled the creative imagination and helped shape the country's literature toward a recognizable national character?

Imaginative literature is one of the richest and most

revealing expressions of the human mind; but an attempt to survey its whole national history, for this particular purpose, created its own problems. The first involved the concept of history itself. Should it be simply a philosophical interpretation of known facts and such new ones as I could discover? The older writers on national characteristics in literature had assumed so, reasoning in terms of analogy and causation or from some arbitrary critical approach. Yet it seemed to me that such a concept placed artificial boundaries on our knowledge of the past, diverting part of its richness into a predesigned channel to serve some useful purpose, perhaps, but without attempting to estimate its natural force. As I continued to experiment with the problem, most directly in a series of lectures at a midwestern university, I began to see the past less as a stream of water which the historian could observe or control and more in terms of a shifting flow of lava, consisting of a hardening surface and of undercurrents of energies and unformed beliefs which were the true basis of what I sought to describe. The history of America was to be found as much in these undercurrents of impulse and belief as in their recorded expression, their solid surface and visible symbols; and the peculiar value of literature, as the material for historical research, lay in its impulsive energy, which kept it alive and distinguished it from the less imaginative records of its time.

Such a concept of history, however, was not easy to handle. Its special difficulty was that the lava stream behaved too naturally: near its source it was all impulse and no solid surface, near its end it was still roiling with lumps whose solidity was not yet determined. In short, the first two centuries of America, when the national character was in the process of formation, produced little pure literature in the conventional sense of the word; whereas the canon of literature for the last half century, at least, is so unsettled that it is impossible to determine which authors reflect the values which posterity will call "permanent." Only in the middle period was there a solid body of writing beneath which one could perceive a dominant and reasonably consistent moving impulse. Accordingly I was forced to divide my investigation into three major sections. The first followed the pattern of what is often called intellectual history. The second consisted of somewhat conventional literary interpretation. The third is an exploration of the mass of recent writing in an effort to see whether my interpretation of the earlier period revealed a force of sufficiently enduring character to continue into the present the recognizable power of the past.

The story I have finally tried to tell was inevitably affected by the pattern of investigation upon which it was based. It differs from the research pattern, though, because of the conflicting currents of impulse and belief which became evident in America after the Civil War, when an earlier attitude of mind had come to the surface and become hardened into a symbol, the visible evidence of an established tradition. Consequently I felt compelled to devote the third part of my narrative to the evidences of conflict between the older tradition and a new one which threatened to emerge and dominate it. I reserved for an Epilogue such evidence as I could find among recent writers which bore firmly upon the question I originally set out to answer: Does the literary history of America reveal the existence of an attitude of mind consistent and durable enough to be called an aspect of the national character?

I would not have spent so much time upon so short and in some respects so ordinary a book (filled, as it is, with dates and titles) had it not been for my experience in teaching abroad. My dedication of this volume to a representative group of foreign students and personal friends expresses something of the gain one feels in seeing his own country through other eyes. But my indebtedness to the many students in this country whose researches and reactions have improved my knowledge and judgment is great, and I want to acknowledge a special debt to those friends who read the manuscript—Ralph Cohen in part, and Robert Falk, Robert Kirsch, Norman Holmes Pearson, and Walter Rideout *in toto*—whose suggestions and corrections have improved its quality and would have improved it more had I been capable of following all of them.

L. H.

Los Angeles, May 12, 1959

Contents

PART ONE

Background and Beginning
1608–1828

CHAPTER ONE

The Law and the Land

I

THE story of American literature begins deviously, for to be told it must begin with a developing attitude of mind of which the earliest writings were evidence rather than products—an attitude which developed over a period as long as that of the memorable literature itself. Yet without this attitude the literature would never have acquired the distinctive national character that makes a coherent story possible, and so we must begin with a people whose minds were more involved in religious, economic, and political problems than in matters of esthetics, in order to see what they acquired and left to posterity as an intellectual and cultural heritage upon which a literature could be based.

The first writers were explorers, one of whom (George Sandys of Jamestown) was engaged in what was to become a famous translation of Ovid, although most of them were like Captain John Smith, who reported on his Jamestown experiences in *A True Relation* (1608), encouraged new settlers in *A Description*

of New England (1616), and defended and romanticized his activities in *A General History of Virginia*
(1624). After them came the Pilgrims from the English
colony in Holland under the leadership of William
Bradford, whose *History of Plymouth Plantation* was
written for posterity rather than for a contemporary
public and perhaps for that reason proved to be one of
the most moving of early American narratives when
the manuscript was eventually published in 1856. Finally came the Puritans of the Massachusetts Bay
Colony, a thousand strong in the summer of 1630,
bringing with them their own charter and therefore a
greater independence than the other colonies possessed as well as a firm determination to establish a
new way of life in the exile they chose in preference
to oppression at home.

These were people with a peculiar heritage which
had given them the name they had just begun to accept as a term of distinction rather than of contempt.
They were devoted to the great reformation which
would prepare the way for the second coming of Christ
on earth, and they represented its second phase. As
self-designated "Doctrinal" Puritans, they had inherited the fruits of the first reformation in the form of the
Calvinistic doctrines which had recently been systematized by the Synod of Dort: they believed that mankind was totally depraved in its heritage of Adam's
original sin but that a limited portion of the race had
been mercifully and unconditionally elected to salvation by the vicarious atonement of Christ, and they believed that for these chosen Saints God's merciful grace
was a gift which could be neither refused nor aban-

doned. As English followers of such "Old" Puritans as
Thomas Cartwright, William Perkins, and William
Ames, they carried their doctrinal reform further by
insisting that they were New Testament Christians
who lived under a "Covenant of Grace" (made with
Abraham and confirmed in Christ) rather than under
the "Covenant of Works" (made with Adam and violated by him), which they identified with the Roman
Catholics, Lutherans, and Arminian heretics. Yet, use-
less though they considered good works to be as a
means of salvation, as "Moral" Puritans they were obedient to Biblical law as the revealed will of God, convinced that it was binding upon the unsanctified mass
of mankind and disposed to make it the only law of
the new colony.

But as representatives of the second stage of reformation they were mostly preoccupied with their role
as "Ecclesiastical" or "Church" Puritans, whose great
calling was to remake the church in the image of the
primitive New Testament congregations, which were
gatherings of confirmed believers rather than catholic
assemblages like the Old Testament Jewish church to
which all members of the nation were initiated in in-
fancy. Their acceptance of this aim—into which they
were hastened by the mere fact of their voluntary
emigration and by the necessity for taking with them
the unsanctified servants and artisans needed in the
wilderness—was actually somewhat premature, for the
English Puritans as a whole had not yet decided
whether the Bible dictated a "gathered" church of
Saints or a reformed "national" church like that of
Scotland. Some, who were called "Political" or "State"

Puritans by their contemporaries, believed that the state itself would have to be purified before the character of the church could be established, and the only firm area of agreement at the time of the migration was opposition to such relics of Romanism in the church as the episcopal hierarchy and clerical vestments, although there was widespread opposition to a set liturgy and kneeling for communion.

The earliest literature of the emigrants reflected their dominant interests. Quite properly, their responsibilities as Moral Puritans were set forth before their departure by the Reverend John Cotton, who was to join them later and become the most prolific writer in the early settlement. In a sermon on "The Christian Calling," later printed in *The Way of Life* (1641), he summarized the Puritan ethical system inherited from the previous generation. Its primary virtue was industry. A good man would not rest until he had found some warrantable calling—a particular employment which would enable him to serve the public good as well as his own, which would be agreeable to his talents, and into which he could enter readily without deceit and without undermining others. Their second virtue was dependence upon their Divine Creator: "Faith saith not," explained Cotton, "give me such a calling and turn me loose to it; but faith looks up to heaven for skill and ability." Having found his calling and sincerely committed himself to God, the Puritan had other formal virtues to practice—the virtue, which Shakespeare had allowed Sir John Falstaff to mock, of laboring faithfully in his profession; the virtue of humility, which he practiced by embracing "any

7 virtues

homely service" he was called to give, "although a carnal heart would blush to be seen in" it; the virtues of cheerfulness, modesty, and, when he came to lay down his work, resignation.

These seven Puritan virtues were the guiding principles which the colonists were expected to accept in the same way that John Milton was to accept them in his sonnet "On His Blindness." They constituted a stabilizing system of ethics, designed for a conservative society in which God's immutable law was supreme. For those who lived under the dispensation of God's mercy as well as his law, the Reverend Thomas Shepard set forth a higher ideal in *The Sincere Convert* (1641), which was to prove the most popular of all collections of early colonial sermons. In one of the most memorable of these discourses he preached against sloth, carelessness, and formality in religion and taught that "the way of self-love"—in which a man, out of fear, "useth diligently all means whereby he shall be saved" —was an "easy" way to hell. There were easier ways, of course, for the irreligious strangers who had joined the colony for material reasons and were more interested in economic than in religious freedom. But the leaders believed that all men should be kept acutely aware of their insignificance before God.

Such sermons as these (and there were many of them on ethical and spiritual subjects) were printed for the edification of all readers, English and American alike. But there was one subject, often labored in extensive manuscripts circulated for years before being printed, which became of primary importance because of English curiosity concerning the New England way of doing things. This was the new reformation in church government. Richard Mather's *Church Government and Church Covenant Discussed* (1643), John Cotton's *The Keyes of the Kingdom of Heaven* (1644) and *The Way of the Churches of Christ in New-England* (1645), John Norton's Latin *Responsio ad Guliel. Apollonii* (1648), Thomas Hooker's *A Survey of the Summe of Church Discipline* (1648)—these were the books from the new world which caused excitement in England, for the Americans expounded and defended a new way of church government, which freed each congregation from all external state or ecclesiastical control and guaranteed that freedom by allowing each to call and ordain its own ministers and officers and by giving each the absolute power to admit, release, admonish, or excommunicate its own members. Such freedom was unimaginable to most Englishmen, who were accustomed to a church regulated by the state and who found it difficult to distinguish between the "New England Way" and the Independency of the Brownists, or Separatists (represented in America by the Plymouth Colony), who refused communion with the Church of England because of its "impurity," and the independence of the various sects who refused communion with each other because of differences in doctrine.

The New Englanders, however, maintained that theirs was a middle way between Independency and a national establishment, and they were convinced that they were following the Lord's way of maintaining a uniform discipline without institutionalized control. Their confidence was based upon an absolute acceptance of the will of God as revealed in the Scriptures as the supreme law and upon a belief in the law-abiding sincerity of those Saints who formed the churches and whose exclusive right to the franchise made them the only full-fledged citizens of the new commonwealth. Their problem, as it quickly developed, was the purely human fact that a sincere Saint might also be a zealot who placed his own interpretation of the law above that of his fellows. Their first unfortunate experience was with the Reverend Roger Williams who became "teacher" (or minister of doctrine) of the church at Salem in 1631 but soon removed to Plymouth, only to return and engage in so many attacks upon the legality of the colonial charter, the rights and responsibilities of the magistrates, and the propriety of communing or even praying with unregenerate persons that he was banished from Massachusetts Bay in 1635 and became the founder of the Rhode Island Colony. Their second was with Mrs. Anne Hutchinson, a cousin of the English poet John Dryden and a woman of ready wit and great energy. She followed John Cotton to New England in 1634 and became the private interpreter of his sermons to a large group of followers whom she convinced that Cotton was the only minister preaching the true Covenant of Grace in a colony of legalistic heretics. She, in turn, was accused of antinomianism (or of denying the binding force of Biblical moral law) and after much turmoil—which included the public disarming of her followers—was exiled to Connecticut.

Both affairs stirred the colony deeply, for each involved numerous meetings of ministers in an effort to convince the troublemakers of their errors and each provided a test of the Puritan confidence in the efficacy of revealed law. In one affair, Williams at first admitted error and then returned more stubbornly than ever to his own interpretation of the law. In the other, neither Mrs. Anne Hutchinson nor the Reverend John Wheelwright was convinced; but John Cotton was, and he participated in Mrs. Hutchinson's excommunication and became the official spokesman for orthodox New England in the later controversy which followed the publication in 1644 of Williams' *The Bloody Tenent of Persecution, for Cause of Conscience.* The crux of this basic Puritan problem, originally so involved in personalities and now so surrounded by historical implications that it can hardly be seen clearly, was the meaning of "conscience." Williams and Mrs. Hutchinson evidently thought of conscience as a somewhat intuitive quality, which in Mrs. Hutchinson's mind came very close to private revelation. Cotton accepted the more widespread Puritan view that it was a rational faculty, subject to information from without, and that a "rightly informed conscience" was informed primarily by the Word of God. Furthermore, he tacitly accepted, as Williams emphatically did not, the principle of a judicious review of his own individual interpretation of the Word.

The civil action of banishment which concluded each affair also had its effect in helping convince the leaders of the Bay Colony that the power of the churches, even over their own members, was not sufficient to keep the peace. For eight years they tried to get along without a body of civil laws, handling all problems by means of a General Court of citizens who met to elect a governor and other magistrates and deal with such civil problems as were important enough to come before it. But the growing extent and population of the colony and the increasing amount of business made a democratic assembly inconvenient and unwieldy and compelled a decision that the General Court was "like a parliament" to which representatives should be elected. By the end of a decade, in short, State Puritanism had been forced upon the refugees from English politics, and it was becoming easier to have recourse to a secular arm in any effort to put down troublemakers.

II

It was against this background that the Americans responded to the Puritan Revolution, which began in England in 1640 when the ill success of King Charles I in his Scottish war forced him to assemble a Parliament for the first time in eleven years. The New Englanders had worked hard to establish themselves as a Christian commonwealth. They had founded Harvard College in 1636 for the education of future ministers, brought over a printing press, and published their first book—a new metrical translation of the Psalms from the original Hebrew, called *The Bay Psalm Book*—in 1640. They had been obliged to fight the Indians in the Pequot War of 1637 and had suffered internal troubles, but, in general, they had managed to keep peace and were prepared to look with sympathy upon their English brethren when active civil war broke out between Parliament and King in 1642.

But their sympathy was not wanted, they discovered, as they found themselves in a completely unexpected psychological relationship to their mother country. Instead of being pioneers in the second stage of the reformation, the Puritans in exile discovered that they were considered escapists by the Puritans of the resistance. State Puritanism became the dominant movement in the England of the Long Parliament, and, when the Westminster Assembly of Divines was called in 1643 to make recommendations for a reformed church, the Scots moved in with their Presbyterian discipline, and the idea of a national church came to dominate both the assembly and Parliament. Only five "dissenting brethren" at Westminster were willing to advocate the New England way of Congregationalism, and they never brought in a formal report, because, as they protested, the assembly violated its instructions by seeking guidance from human experience rather than exclusively from the Word of God. But political expediency was the order of the English day, and when the battle of Marston Moor, in July 1644, effectively demonstrated the superiority of Oliver Cromwell's sectarian Ironsides not only to other English troops but to the Presbyterian Scots, the military leader of the Revolution was under practical compulsion to tolerate a variety of sects which made Anne Hutchinson and Roger Williams seem comparatively orthodox. The New England middle way of church government thus found itself in the middle of a violent political controversy, damned by the Presbyterians for its independence and by the Independents for its intolerance; and it is not surprising that the New Englanders should have gone on the defensive in their writings and actions.

Their defensiveness was both particular and general. Cotton replied to Williams' attack in *The Bloody Tenent* with *The Controversie Concerning Liberty of Conscience in Matters of Religion Truly Stated and Distinctly and Plainly Handled* (1646) and *The Bloody Tenent Washed and Made White in the Blood of the Lambe* (1647), and he and others supplemented and defended the expositions of the New England way of church government which had been circulating in manuscript and were beginning to appear in print at this time. The latter also sometimes contained a more general defense of New England, most explicitly in a little pamphlet called *A Defense of the Answer* prepared by Thomas Shepard and John Allin and published in London in 1648. The Preface protested against the settlers being "judged as deserters of our Brethren, and the Cause of Christ in Hand: with whom (excuse us if we now speak plainly) it had been far more easy unto many of us to have suffered, than to have adventured hither upon the wilderness sorrows we expected to have met withal." The American settlers "surely all were not rash, weak-spirited, inconsiderate of what they left behind, or of what it was to go into a Wilderness," they assured the critical stay-at-homes. What was needed was a proper history of the settlement: "If we were able to express and recount the singular workings of divine Providence for bringing on this work to what it has come unto, it would stop the mouths of all that have not an heart to accuse and blaspheme the goodness of God in his glorious works."

Certainly no writer at that time had produced or was in the process of producing the sort of history Shepard required. Francis Higginson, for example, who had come over in 1629 and written his *New-Englands Plantation* (1630) in order to encourage others to follow him, bore no witness to the hardships and sorrows of wilderness adventure when he boasted of his improved health and digestion in America—even though he died before his book was published. Nor did William Bradford or John Winthrop in their histories do more than barely list the undeniable sufferings they had witnessed. Shepard's call was answered two years later, however, when Edward Johnson began his *Wonder-Working Providence of Sions Saviour in New England*, which was completed and published in 1654. His account of the building of Concord made the soldiers of Christ in America appear as heroic as those in England who had captured the town of Bristol. Lying in the open air or in smoky dugouts, wet and cold in day and night, the men and their wives and children—"every one that can lift a hoe to strike it into the Earth"—struggled with the land while they "cut their bread very thin for a long season." Johnson's settlers had not escaped to the land of peace of which Shepard had boasted only ten years before. The English had no grounds for criticizing the sort of people he portrayed.

A certain amount of self-righteousness was implicit in this defensive portrayal of the settlements, but it was more apparent in the official New England attitude to-

ward the religious toleration which was spreading in
the mother country. During the middle forties, when
John Cotton and others were regularly advertising the
New England way or middle way of church government as a way of compromise between the English
Presbyterians and Independents, the colonists made no
secret of their feeling of superiority to their contentious
brethren at home. In a letter to a friend in England on
December 10, 1644 (printed in 1645 as *New England's
Lamentations for Old England's present Errours and
Divisions*), Thomas Shepard had expressed a widespread American sentiment: "To contend, and divide,
and grow drunk, and stagger with novelties, and every
new device of unstable minded men, while the common Enemy is in the field and the Sword of the Lord
stands at every man's door almost, this argues deep distempers, close hypocrisies, and such unreasonable
wantonness and abuse of liberty that the Lord Christ
will not pass by without darkening the Sun and turning
the Moon into blood, which will and shall continue
until the Lord hath made the remnant which shall escape a poor, weak, humble, pliable-spirited people
unto the good ways of grace." In comparison with conditions in England he boasted: "We wonder at God for
our peace that the Lord gives us in these parts, we
know not how to improve it. The reports of the divisions in *New-England* are fables; the Churches are
here in peace; the common-wealth in peace; the Ministry in most sweet peace; the Magistrates (I should
have named first) in peace; All our families in peace;
We sleep in the woods in peace, without fear of the
Indians, our fear is fallen upon them. When we travel

abroad, we rise up, and lie down in peace; yet this peace giveth us no rest, while our dear *England* is in trouble, for which we would weep, and we wish our heads fountains in this wilderness, for our sins there as well as others."

But such peace was not easily maintained. Governor John Winthrop (whose Journals provide the best contemporary record of life in the Bay Colony) tried to keep it by judicious flexibility in the enforcement of strict laws and found himself charged with exceeding his powers as a magistrate. After his acquittal by the General Court, on July 3, 1645, he made a "little speech" on the causes of "such distempers as have arisen amongst us." They were basically questions "about the authority of the magistrates and the liberty of the people," he declared; and he made it clear that in his own opinion the magistrates, though elected by the people, derived their "authority from God, in way of an ordinance, such as hath the image of God eminently stamped upon it." They might err from lack of skill for their offices, but if they were faithful in their calling and erred in good faith the people "must bear it." Liberty, he added, was of two sorts—the natural liberty to do as one pleased and the civil or federal liberty to do "that only which is good, just, and honest"—and of the two the latter was "the proper end and object of authority," for which the people should hazard their goods and their lives.

Such was the attitude of a people who had as one of their literary spokesmen the Reverend Nathaniel Ward who called himself *The Simple Cobler of Aggawam in America* (1647) when he set out "to help 'mend' his Native Country," which he considered "lamentably tattered, both in upper-leather and sole." His "honest stitches" got him an invitation to preach before the Presbyterian Parliament, and they included an outright attack on the principle of religious toleration. Four things, he wrote, his heart naturally detested: the standing of the Apocrypha in the Bible, foreigners dwelling in his own country, alchemized or counterfeit coins, and "Tolerations of divers Religions, or of one religion in segregant shapes." As the "Herald of New England" he proclaimed in the name of the Bay Colony "that all Familists, Antinomians, Anabaptists, and other Enthusiasts, shall have free liberty to keep away from us, and such as will come to be gone as fast as they can, the sooner the better." He expressed his contempt for any colony—such as Roger Williams' Rhode Island—which would provide "free stable-room and litter for all kind of consciences, be they never so dirty or jadish," and added that if England should "either willingly tolerate or weakly connive at such course," the church would soon become "the Devil's Dancing-School" and the civil state a "Beargarden."

Ward of course was like the English Thomas Coryate and Robert Burton in being one of the eccentric literary wits of the seventeenth century, but the resemblance between his attitude and that of the colony as a whole was revealed when the New Englanders undertook to set Old England an example of unity. They called a synod of churches in Cambridge in June 1648, to draw up A *Platform of Church-Discipline* for their own use and for the guidance of their brethren in England.

They signified their desire for unity by a unanimous acceptance of the English Westminster Confession "in matters of doctrine" and confined themselves to an exposition of the New England way of church government on which they hoped the warring factions of Presbyterian and Independent might compromise. The result was accepted by the Massachusetts General Court in August and published for "public edification" with a Preface which made clear its intent. "The more we discern (that which we do, and have cause to do with incessant mourning and trembling) the unkind, and unbrotherly, and unchristian contention of our godly brethren and country-men in matters of church government"; the Preface stated, "the more earnestly do we desire to see them join together in one common faith; and ourselves with them."

The authors of the Cambridge Platform displayed a considerable amount of self-righteous humility when they addressed to the English Puritans such words as these: "And if the example of such poor outcasts as ourselves might prevail, if not with all (for that were too great a blessing to hope for) yet with some or other of our brethren in *England* . . . we hope in Christ it would not only moderate our harsh judging and condemning of one another in such differences of judgment as may be found in the choicest saints; but prevent (by the mercy of Christ) the peril of distraction and destruction of all churches in both kingdoms. Otherwise, if our brethren shall go on to bite and devour one another . . . it will be to the consuming of them, and us all; which the Lord prevent."

The example of the "poor outcasts" had no effect.

Before the Cambridge Platform could be printed, Cromwell had declared for "union and right understanding" among all "godly people, Scots, English, Jews, Gentiles, Presbyterians, Anabaptists, and all." And by the end of the year Colonel Thomas Pride had purged Parliament of its Presbyterian members, whose understanding of union, like that of the Americans, was not "right," and a court was being constituted to try the King and order his execution on January 30. Only such temporary followers of the New England way as William Hook and Sir Harry Vane and such dissenters from it as Hugh Peter and Roger Williams were friends of Cromwell and the new order in England. The solid builders of the Bay Colony became not only conservative but reactionary.

The reaction took a form that Roger Williams had expected—the use of civil authority and sometimes bloody punishment to enforce unity of religious belief. Taking Nathaniel Ward's position "that God doth no where in his word tolerate Christian States, to give Toleration to such adversaries of his Truth, if they have power to suppress them," the secular authorities of the Bay Colony had Obadiah Holmes publicly whipped in 1651 for being a Baptist, and two of his fellow visitors from the colony of Rhode Island were fined. Three years later, the Reverend Henry Dunster, the learned and faithful president of Harvard College, was indicted by the Grand Jury for "disturbing the ordinance of infant baptism in the Cambridge Church" and was forced to resign his office and remove to the Plymouth Colony. When the Quakers began to make their appearance in 1656, the Boston authorities were prepared to move quickly against them under laws forbidding heresy; and the first arrivals were placed under arrest before they left shipboard and had an opportunity to create a civil disturbance. When whipping, branding, and ear-cropping failed to keep others out, the united colonies of the orthodox New England Confederation threatened economic sanctions against Rhode Island for standing on liberty of conscience and thus providing a "back door" for the admission of religious enthusiasts into Zion. Massachusetts passed a law in 1658 providing for the death penalty against Quakers who returned from banishment, and two male Quakers were hanged in 1659 and a woman (a former follower of Anne Hutchinson) in 1660. No one in the orthodox colonies of New England could any longer disclaim the bloody tenet of persecution for cause of conscience or attempt to wash it white. The signs of the times had been so clear as early as 1652 that John Clarke could say that while Old England was becoming new, "New England is become Old."

III

The primary reaction of the New Englanders to the events in Old England during its Puritan period was a determination to make the law prevail even though they had been forced to go beyond God's law in their effort to free their society from those persons who refused to accept the sort of judicious interpretation of the Word to which John Cotton had yielded in the early years of the settlement. But always opposed to the law was the land—a land which had compelled the original Puritan immigrants to bring with them settlers whose qualifications lay not in saintliness but in their skills. It had thus impelled the Saints toward a system of church government which was in itself disposed to place more reliance upon individual character than upon institutionalized authority, and it continued to attract great numbers of settlers whose interests were material rather than religious. Most of them were welcomed, for the early Saints of New England, like the later landowners of the South, knew that neither divine grace nor material wealth gave a man the ability to grind corn, thatch a roof, construct a plow, or build a boat; and they had to recognize the value of a man who could do these things, else their own grand designs would fail because the social fabric was too weak to sustain them. The recognition was practical rather than theoretical, but it was conscious on the part of colonial leaders who regularly protested the inflexibility of regulations sent over from England or who displayed, with John Winthrop, an apologetic feeling for not having codified their own laws for "want of sufficient experience of the nature and disposition of the people." Their ideology was rigid enough, but they knew that man did not live by ideas alone, and they were prepared to make tacit compromises with the practical demands of a new country.

In literature a quiet movement toward individuality may be seen in the differences between the early and later poetry of Mrs. Anne Bradstreet. The poems in the first edition of *The Tenth Muse Lately Sprung Up in America*, most of them written some seventeen years before their publication in 1650, were conventional and perhaps nostalgic reflections of her reading in the Elizabethan poets before she left England. The new poems that appeared in the posthumous second edition of 1678 were, with the exception of "The Four Ages of Man," reflections of her individual emotional experiences—"Contemplations" of external nature and the pleasures of the imagination, expressions of affection for her husband and children, or the display of emotions aroused by a burning home. The human experiences of daily life had come to mean more than books to her when she sat down to express herself in verse.

But other writers who occasionally produced verse during this early period were inclined to remain conventional, and it is impossible to generalize from a single case. Yet Mrs. Bradstreet's way of poetic development was the real New England way of ordinary living. The plan of settlement in self-sufficient communities required a mutual recognition of the dependence of individuals upon one another. In towns so small that a dozen individuals might undertake to form a church, every person was well known. His opinions and character were familiar to his neighbors, and his strong points and shortcomings were generally discussed and carefully estimated. The result was that no matter how he might stand in the eyes of the Lord, he had an independent standing in society. And no Puritan was so impractically pious as to deny that a good reprobate might be a useful citizen.

Such good but unsanctified citizens, in contrast to the English custom, were forbidden the privileges of the church. They were permitted and eventually re-

quired to attend divine worship, but it was the worship
of a God who had turned his face away from them for
all eternity; and the temporal signs of reprobation were
always with them in their inability to select the minister whose word they heard, to choose the elders who
supervised their conduct, or to vote for the men who
represented their material interest in civil affairs. New
immigrants who had been church members in England, baptized children who had grown to maturity
without the experience of grace, and persons who had
once been of "the poorer sort" but had found a ready
means of advancement to prosperity and respectability—all were in the same outcast position. The spirit of
piety was too prevalent in New England for them to
demand admission to the church for selfish reasons; but
hypocrites had crept into the church with unsanctified
designs, and honest men on the outside were a disturbance to the conscience of honest men within.

The Puritan Saints who accepted the obligation to
be their brothers' keepers, in fact, knew their brothers.
Such ministers as John Cotton and Thomas Shepard,
especially, were acutely aware of the hypocrisy within
the church and were candid in admitting its existence.
Their clear-sightedness, at times, tempted them to
abandon the teachings of William Ames and other
Puritan fathers by preaching that the "gathered"
church of visible Saints was not a reality but an appearance, that formal and superficial evidences of
grace were all that should be required for admittance.
Another impulse was to compromise rather than abandon their principles, and in that spirit the Cambridge
Platform of 1648 recommended the admission into

church fellowship of "those with weak measures of faith" and advised against "severe examinations."

But such measures could not solve the problem. The individuals whose plight was so bothersome were not of the sort who could be induced into the church by easy examinations of half-hearted professions of faith. As their numbers increased and their pressure became genuinely insistent, the modesty of their demands became evident: those who were baptized wanted nothing for themselves, but they did want the privilege of baptism for their children in order that they might enjoy the protection of the church while awaiting the experience of grace. An association of ministers, in 1657, met and offered a solution to the problem, and, after five years of discussion and debate, it was formally adopted by a synod in 1662: the doors of the church were opened halfway in order that baptized but unsanctified persons might claim the sacrament of baptism for their children but not the sacrament of the Lord's Supper for themselves. Such halfway members thereby gained the right to vote in civil elections but not in matters of church government. The Puritan church in America never adopted the semicatholic principles of the Anglican and Scottish churches, nor did it accept the principles of sectarian toleration which flourished in Cromwell's England. It did, however, adapt its ideology to the requirements of individuals whose importance in the land was great enough to compel a reinterpretation of divine law.

This "Half-Way Covenant," as it was sardonically called in a later period, destroyed the unity of the Congregational churches and kept some of them apart for

more than a century. It had temporary political implications inasmuch as it gave the civil franchise to a
considerable number of respectable citizens who might
otherwise have formed an influential opposition to the
theocracy. But there is no evidence that it was adopted
for political reasons and very little indication that it was
passed under the illusion that it would strengthen
rather than weaken the church by an increase in its
membership. The synod of 1662 did not gather to dwell
upon statistics. Its members gathered to consider the
spiritual situation of the children of their friends and
neighbors and of their own grandchildren, whose
names they knew and whose rights as individuals to
the protection of the church they felt a strong compulsion to recognize. The fact that the claims of the individual were strong enough to modify a rigid and reactionary ideology without raising a rival system to
oppose it shows that the seventeenth-century Puritans,
through the force of their environment, were being impelled to follow what was later to become a characteristic pattern of American intellectual behavior.

IV

The pattern of individualism did not appear, however, in the literature of the late seventeenth century.
On the contrary, the prevailing tone of Puritan writing
in America from the Restoration of 1660 to the Glorious Revolution of 1688 was one of uneasiness and
strain. This tone may be perceived in the tendency of
the later Puritans generally to substitute dogmatism
for assurance in their expression of religious beliefs, in

their emphasis upon fear rather than faith in their attitude toward the Divine Being, and in their obsessed search for evidences of God's providence, which they seemed no longer able to take for granted. For three decades and more their literature became a literature of fear, motivated by a suspicion that God had turned his face from them and directed by an effort to find symbols of evil abroad in the land.

The restoration of the ungodly Stuart dynasty was a blow which they did not formally admit but which they could not avoid feeling, especially as it soon strengthened the position of tolerant Rhode Island and brought an investigation of religious persecution in Massachusetts. Michael Wigglesworth may have been responding to it when he redirected the attention of New England from the contemporary successes of the unrighteous to the future triumph of the Saints on Judgment Day. At that dreadful time the illusions of "carnal reason" would be confounded, and those who "put away the evil day and drowned their care and fears" would be "swept away by vengeance unawares." *The Day of Doom* (1662) became one of the most popular books printed in seventeenth-century America, for its tone was peculiarly fitted to the uneasy spirit of the times. The year 1662 was also the time of the great drought, which was visited only upon New England; and Wigglesworth celebrated it too in a poem entitled *God's Controversy with New-England*, which represented God's contempt for the falling away from grace of his chosen people yet was not published—perhaps lest it inspire similar expressions of contempt from worldly men unfit to echo the divine sentiments.

At the end of the decade Wigglesworth allowed himself to become slightly more hopeful about the present
state of the world in his *Meat out of the Eater or Meditations Concerning the Necessity, End, and Usefulness
of Afflictions unto Gods Children* (1670); but in 1675
the Indian King Philip's war broke out, and the New
Englanders had new evidence that the devil was walking abroad. Observations to that effect poured from
their printing presses in the form of personal narratives,
sermons, and even an epic poem by Benjamin Tomp-
son called *New England Crisis, Or a Brief Narrative,
Of New-Englands Lamentable Estate at present, com-
par'd with the former (but few) years of Prosperity*
(1676). It is no wonder that the Reverend Urian Oakes
should have felt called upon to preach vigorously on
"The Sovereign Efficacy of Divine Providence" or that
Increase Mather became eager to push to completion
An Essay for the Recording of Illustrious Providences,
the ambitious effort to demonstrate God's guiding
hand in human affairs which was supposedly begun in
England before the Restoration and was finally published in Boston in 1684. But even in their search for
evidence of God's goodness they kept their eyes open
for the devil's work, and the section on witchcraft
which the book contained helped prepare the way for
the witchcraft hysteria of 1692 and the outburst of excited literature that accompanied it. By this time, England had permanently disposed of the Stuarts with
Roman inclinations, and acquired a king of unquestion-
able Protestantism; the prospects of Massachusetts,
after an unhappy succession of royal governors, were
improving; and the colony should have been psycho-

logically ready to return to the progressive world from which it had exiled itself. But the Puritan disease had profoundly affected the New England spirit, and the malady could not be thrown off without the experience of catharsis.

The catharsis of witchcraft hysteria was, on the whole, effective. It led to the attack on the Mathers by the Boston merchant Robert Calef, whose *More Wonders of the Invisible World* (1700) bore witness to an awareness of human values, which were more important to him than were the evidences of supernatural activity. It led to a reappraisal of his attitudes by Judge Samuel Sewall, whose *Diary* records his public confession of error and whose pamphlet, *The Selling of Joseph* (1700), and a later essay against slavery were signs of a new humanitarian spirit among the Puritans. Cotton Mather, like his father Increase, tried to preserve the old attitudes; and his "providential" history of New England, the *Magnalia Christi Americana* (1702), was a monument to the Puritan belief that God took an active part in the affairs of men. Yet Cotton Mather himself was a sort of Puritan Janus, looking before and after. His primary interest was in the relationship of God to man, but his *Bonifacius* or *Essays to Do Good* (1710) and his later volume of advice to young ministers revealed the concern for human relations which was to be characteristic of the new century. Furthermore, his essays in *The Christian Philosopher* (1721), although designed to show the unity of science and religion, offered natural science as a support to religion in a way that would have profoundly shocked his grandfather Richard, who probably never thought that religion needed a support from any source. The old specialized interest in religion was dying out as the dominant and almost exclusive interest of literary minds.

Even when it survived, as it did in the private manuscripts of America's finest colonial poet, Edward Taylor, it began to take on the emotional color of a new humanism. For Taylor was one of the few poets at the turn of the century to "preach Christ" in the old-fashioned way, and in the manuscript sermons of his *Christographia* (1701–3) he was as passionately orthodox as Thomas Shepard. Yet he rejoiced in the union of human nature with God's through Christ and found in that union justification for asserting man's superiority to the angels, and he found in Christ a pattern for human imitation despite man's inability to achieve spiritual regeneration by his own efforts. His own desire to realize God had a formative effect upon his poetry—especially upon the *Sacramental Meditations,* which provided an emotional climax to the intellectual processes of his prose discourses—for he suggested in some of them the possibility of rising through thoughts and words, reason and rhetoric to the verge of comprehending the incomprehensible. And it was perhaps this effort to find in poetry a means of knowing which went beyond reason that made his poetry so suggestive of the earlier English metaphysical poets in its unexpected juxtaposition of ideas and images which strains and shocks the ordinary and familiar processes of the mind.

But Puritanism as a solid and coherent force was rapidly disappearing. The land had won over the law, and as the descendants of the Puritans spread out over the expanding country their heritage of moral Puritanism was to become dissipated in a mist of propriety which was occasionally precipitated in revivals of State Puritanism through spasmodic attempts to regulate personal morality by law. Doctrinal Puritanism was to survive more in the catechisms of the institutionalized Puritan churches than in the active beliefs of their members whose independence in many instances under the Congregational system enabled them to abandon all traditional doctrine and become Unitarian. Perhaps in the final analysis the most profound effect of the movement was to create in the American consciousness a greater trust in written law than in legislative assemblies and a willingness to accept a judicial interpretation of the fundamental law as a final recourse for stability and the supreme authority in government. But before Puritanism was completely broken down into its residual elements, American society had to go through a major shift of interest, involving a more active preoccupation with human affairs, during which its literature was to reflect an entirely different quality of mind.

CHAPTER TWO

Ways of Reason

I

THE new quality of mind reflected in the literature of the eighteenth century was the distinguishing characteristic of the period some historians call "the Enlightenment" and others call "the Age of Reason." In its essence, it represented a profound cultural change, which occurred later in America than in other parts of the Western world—a shift in the focus of men's attention from the divine mind to the human mind, a new confidence in the ability of man to solve the mysteries of nature by his own efforts, an exciting disposition to follow the dictates of reason rather than those of revelation, and a belief in self-determination rather than in providence and predestination. Its immediate cause, perhaps, may be found in the great intellectual achievements of the seventeenth century, particularly those of René Descartes, Isaac Newton, and John Locke. But, because it reflected an attitude of mind rather than a generally accepted system of ideas, the Enlightenment is one of the most complex periods in intellectual history and one of the most difficult to explore.

43

In America, however, the Enlightenment was clearly heralded by certain changing concepts of logic. The Puritans had been followers of the impetuous French rebel against Scholasticism, Petrus Ramus. They followed a system of logic which modern philosophers are reluctant to consider logic at all. It assumed that truth had some sort of absolute existence and that the function of the human mind was merely to perceive it. The Ramean system of logic was no more than an attempt to present a systematic way of searching out the truth and making it evident to others, and the way of seeking was one of considering alternative possibilities, or "dichotomies," between which the mind could choose. Reason, therefore, was equated with choice, and formal logicians became more subtle only as they multiplied the possibilities of choice.

The most important subtlety that developed in the Ramean system, during the century of its use in England, was that which explored a multiplicity of causes, any number of which might be independently adequate or "efficient" causes of a particular effect. It was especially useful to the Puritan followers of John Calvin because it enabled them to avoid the practical difficulty of reconciling such apparently contradictory doctrines as those of predestination and moral responsibility; for, although they believed that God operated both as a first cause and through various immediate or proximate causes, they shared with John Milton the opinion that the chain of causation was a mystery with which the human mind could not profitably concern itself. Neither Puritan theology nor Ramean logic was greatly concerned with the temporal relationship of cause and effect.

The Reverend Urian Oakes had made an exhibition of characteristic Puritan logic in a sermon on "The Sovereign Efficacy of Divine Providence," which he delivered in 1677. In it he insisted that human will and seemingly blind chance were parallel causes, either of which might operate according to God's determination. But the determining agent was always God's mysterious will and not an unbreakable sequence of causes and effects. The manuscript verses of Edward Taylor consistently illustrated the same way of thinking. His metaphysical poem "Huswifery," for example, found as many different things contributing to man's salvation as were needed for the spinning of thread and the weaving of cloth; and his most ambitious work, "God's Determinations Touching His Elect," described so many means to the realization of grace that some readers have been willing to believe that it preached universal salvation. But Taylor's logic was clear to him if not to his later readers: whatever devices He may have chosen to use, God personally wove the cloth of salvation and elected those sinners who were to be saved by such various means.

By the early part of the eighteenth century, however, a new formal logic, better adapted to the world of Newton, was becoming known to the English-speaking countries. Basically Cartesian, it was disseminated in the American colonies by the French *Port-Royal Logic*, which had been translated into English as *The Art of Thinking*. Benjamin Franklin remembered it in his old age as one of the particular books he had read in his

45

youth, and its influence had been strong on his first ambitious literary work. For Franklin, as a young typesetter in London, was given to reflecting upon the books he set up in print, and he was offended by the old-fashioned reasoning of a book he was putting into a second edition. The book was William Wollaston's *The Religion of Nature Delineated*, which attempted to place an ethical obligation upon human beings to discover truth by the observation of "things as they are" and to act freely in accord with their discoveries. Franklin undertook to answer it according to the more modern art of thinking.

His answer took the form of a published dissertation on *Liberty and Necessity, Pleasure and Pain* (1725), in which the nineteen-year-old philosopher denied the distinction between good and evil, on the ground that both were the results of the same first cause, and denied the moral responsibility of the individual human being, on the ground that he was the predetermined product of a chain of causation. It was a strange work for a young man who had already shown in his own life so much independence and self-reliance, and he later looked back upon it as one of the serious mistakes of his youth. So it was, in fact, because it represented an intellectual denial of all the principles by which he guided his mature life, but his ability to make such an error is an indication of the grip the new mode of thinking could get on eighteenth-century minds.

The mind which fell permanently into this sort of rationalism was that of Franklin's precocious contemporary Jonathan Edwards. At the age of sixteen, when he was beginning his senior year at Yale College, Edwards wrote his father to send him *The Art of Thinking*, which he was persuaded would be as profitable as his textbooks would be necessary to his education. He had been "mightily pleased," he wrote in one of his college notes, with the study of the "Old Logicke" because it had enabled him to order his thoughts and distribute them into classes and subdivisions after what seems to have been the fashion of the Ramean system. But the sort of reasoning to which he became devoted was the new system he described in another note: "All our reasoning, with respect to Real Existence, depends upon that natural, unavoidable and invariable disposition of the mind, when it sees a thing begin to be, to conclude certainly that there is a *Cause* of it; or if it sees a thing to be in a very orderly, regular and exact manner, to conclude that some *Design* regulated and disposed it." "*Knowledge* is not the perception of the *agreement*, or *disagreement*, of ideas" (as the Ramists suggested by their system of dichotomies), he concluded, "but rather the perception of the *union*, or *disunion*, of ideas" (as in a chain of reasoning).

Edwards was to give up his early scientific and miscellaneous speculative interests and devote himself to theology for thirty-five years before he published his *magnum opus*, in 1754, as *A Careful and Strict Enquiry into the Modern Prevailing Notions of that Freedom of the Will which is supposed to be Essential to Moral Agency*. But he did not give up the method of reasoning from which he had anticipated so much profit. "The first dictate of the common and natural sense which God hath implanted in the minds of all mankind, and the main foundation of all our reasonings

47

about the existence of things, past, present, or to come," he said, in laying the foundation of his argument, seems to be "that whatsoever begins to be, which before was not, must have a Cause why it then begins to exist." And "if this sound principle of common sense be taken away," he added, "all arguing from Effects to Causes ceaseth, and so all knowledge of any existence, besides what we have by the most direct and immediate intuition, particularly all proof of the being of God, ceases."

Edwards had asserted his own direct and immediate intuition of God in his autobiographical *Personal Narrative* and elsewhere, but he had also learned, through his connection with the evangelical movement known as the Great Awakening, how difficult it was to distinguish between a personal revelation and an emotional illusion. In his most mature work he placed his dependence upon reason. We may suppose an intuitive knowledge of God possible, "but," he wrote, "we have not that strength and extent of mind to know this certainty in this intuitive, independent manner." The true method of knowing, as he described it in a passage which was an unconscious echo of *The Art of Thinking*, was by the movement of reason backward and forward along the chain of causation: "We *first ascend* and prove . . . from effects, that there must be an eternal Cause; and then *secondly* prove by argumentation, not intuition, that this Being must be necessarily existent; and then *thirdly*, from the proved necessity of his existence, we may *descend*, and prove many of his perfections *a priori*."

How completely Cartesian Edwards was in his

point of view and how utterly dependent he was upon the rational chain of causation may be illustrated by another passage in which the author became almost as eloquent over his logical system as he had been in his Northampton sermons: "Yea, if once it should be allowed that things may come to pass without a Cause, we should not only have no proof of the Being of God but we should be without evidence of the existence of any thing whatsoever but our own immediately present ideas and consciousness. For we have no way to prove anything else but by arguing from effects to Causes; from the ideas immediately in view, we argue other things not immediately in view; from sensations now excited in us, we infer the existence of things without us as the Causes of these sensations; and from the existence of these things we argue other things on which they depend as effects on Causes. We infer the past existence of ourselves, or any thing else, by memory only as we argue that the ideas which are now in our minds are the consequences of past ideas and sensations. We immediately perceive nothing else but the ideas which are this moment extant in our minds. We perceive or know other things only *by means* of these, as necessarily connected with others, and dependent on them. But if things may be without Causes, all this necessary connection and dependence is dissolved, and so all means of our knowledge is gone."

It has often been said that Edwards' logic is so good that if we grant him his premises his conclusions become inevitable. Actually, though, if we grant the logic and its applicability to theological matters, either his or Franklin's premises and conclusions would both be inevitable. But few Americans would consistently grant him his logic. He acquired a limited number of followers for his "new light" theology, but many orthodox Calvinists would have agreed with the Reverend Chauncer Whittelsey who feared that the teaching of Edwards' system at Yale would lead students into deism or atheism by substituting "necessity" for an "intelligent Moral Governor." They preferred the relics of dogma to the fine structure of the new logic. The new light of Edwards' severe rationalism struck most of his contemporaries blind.

Much of the distrust of Edwards was founded upon the natural frailties of the human mind—its resistance to systematic discipline and its limited span of attention. Yet his critics did not consider themselves antirational, for they thought within a logical framework which was older than his and considerably more respectable in New England if not in the other colonies. It had been provided by Francis Bacon, whose name had high authority in colonial America.

Bacon's logic, in a sense, was negative rather than positive. He was severely antagonistic toward the system of classical logic (into which Descartes' method was fitted by the Messrs. de Port-Royal) because he distrusted words as vehicles of thought, and he was contemptuous of the basic Ramean assumptions. Yet he agreed with the Ramists in his belief that "a faculty of wise interrogating is half a knowledge" and in his approach to truth by their method of "invention" or exploration guided by a systematic arrangement of classifications or "topics."

The real quarrel of Bacon with the Ramists was that

of a scientist with Platonic abstractions. He observed that "topics are of two sorts, general and special," and he was thoroughly impatient with people who concerned themselves with the abstract "originals of things" and rejected all thought of specific things because they were considered secondary and variable. The Ramean method was one of induction, but Bacon had thoroughly damned it in *The Advancement of Learning:* "The induction which logicians speak of, and which seemeth familiar with Plato . . . their form of induction, I say, is utterly vicious and incompetent." His own method of induction was different in that it was based upon specific observations rather than perceptions of general principles, and he emphasized his attack upon the Ramean schoolmen with the caustic opinion that "men are rather beholden to a wild goat for surgery, or to a nightingale for music, or to the ibis for some part of physic, or to the pot-lid that flew open for artillery, or generally to chance or anything else than to logic for the invention of arts and sciences." Bacon's method of thinking was not foreign to his age. His attitude of mind was simply critical, practical, and realistic.

This attitude had made a strong appeal to the tough-minded Puritans, who might be obliged to consider general principles in their theological meditations but were concerned with specific things in their daily lives. There was no inconsistency of pattern between the Ramean approach to intellectual generalities and the Baconian approach to specific material problems, and they could admire the wisdom of the Viscount St. Albans while deploring his moral and spiritual limitations. And so, when the formal Ramean logic died out, its substantial pattern of thought lingered on as a sort of practical inductiveness which was traditionally satisfying to the mind. It was also, as a sort of everyday logic, useful in the ordinary affairs of life.

Among these ordinary affairs in America, however, religion continued to be one of the most important—not only among the sons of the Puritans but in the Dutch, Quaker, Roman Catholic, and Anglican colonies to the south. Religious belief was by no means uniform, but belief of some sort was almost universal. Often it assumed a human capacity for the direct apprehension of abstract or supernatural ideas, and although this assumption was far older than any formal system of logic, the actual transformation from an implication of logic into an explicit theory of knowledge can be traced through the writings of Samuel Johnson, who graduated from Yale four years before Jonathan Edwards and discovered the new learning of Locke and Newton before he discovered the new logic of the Port-Royal *Art of Thinking*.

Like Edwards, Johnson undertook to compose an undergraduate compendium of human knowledge in an "Encyclopedia of Philosophy," which, in its earlier version, dealt with the art of reasoning entirely in Ramean terms. After he had read Locke, shortly before graduation in 1716, he revised his consideration of the intellectual powers in order to stress the importance of "ideas" and recognize the faculties of perception and reflection, or, as he called them, "apprehension" and "reason." But he retained "judgment," or choice, as the basic intellectual process because it was a "perception of the agreement or disagreement of any two or more ideas" and consequently the only secure foundation for any knowledge other than the simplest sort, and he continued after graduation to recommend the study of Ramus as the best introduction to logic for college students. For the next three decades, while he made his way from New England to New York and from the Puritan into the Anglican church, he strove to absorb the new learning without changing the pattern of thought fixed in his undergraduate mind. By the time he published his *Elementa Philosophica* (1752), the first textbook in philosophy to be printed in America, he was sufficiently under the influence of Bacon to stress accuracy of observation and perception more than he had in his youth but still determined that this accuracy should be achieved by the use of Ramean dichotomies. He had also become acquainted with Cartesian logic and rejected it in favor of the simpler intellectual process of judgment.

But judgment upon those philosophical matters which were of more interest to him than science, he now realized, required some absolute basis which Bacon did not provide. Sensory experience was not enough. Something more was needed. To fill this need, Johnson reaffirmed the general topics that Bacon had denounced, explicitly developed the Platonic notion which was implicit in Ramean logic, and asserted the existence of "a kind of intellectual light within us" which affects our minds so strongly that "they can no more withstand the evidence of it, than they can withstand the evidence of sense." Thus the basis of judgment might be intuitive as well as sensuous. And, having given his allegiance to an intuitive "intellectual light," Johnson had less use than ever for the elaborate reasoning process he now called "demonstration" and had once called "reason." In a rhapsody entitled "Raphael," composed a decade or so later, he could epitomize his mature thought by having "the Genius of the English America" represent man as a rational being whose knowledge of truth was an apprehension of "things as they really are." He would have to apprehend them in "their beings and relations, connections, and dependencies as they stand variously situated one to another," but it was a direct apprehension rather than the acceptance of a demonstration. For a mind was not absorbed in its own true interest, he suggested, if it "must needs be continually worried in endless mazes of anxiety" and was "ever fluctuating in doubt, skepticism and uncertainty, or under a perpetual delusion,—mistaking sounds for things and grasping at shadows instead of substance." This antispeculative character of his logic was strongly opposed to both the old Scholastic and the new Cartesian method, but it brought Bacon into accord with Ramus by explicitly affirming a new means of perception which balanced the light of sense with the light of intuition and thus anticipated the nineteenth-century notions of a sensory understanding and a Transcendental reason.

There had developed, in short, two patterns of logic which provided quite separate ways for the human mind to follow into the Age of Reason. The new method which Descartes systematized had proved invaluable in the development of a new cosmology and a new mathematics—and Jonathan Edwards tried to use it as an instrument for the creation of a new theology. It was primarily deductive and concerned with general principles. The other method, as Bacon had presented it, provided a sound basis for the solution of practical problems relating to the architecture of fortune and the relief of man's estate. It was primarily inductive and concerned with specifics. But it permitted the inclusion and development of an intuitional heritage from the older Ramean system which enabled men's minds to accept simply and readily certain general ideas—especially those relating to religion and morals—which were actually beyond Cartesian demonstration. All of the major ideas and attitudes of the later Enlightenment and the self-conscious Age of Reason were to appear within these two logical frameworks, and the American inclination toward one or the other—an inclination which gave lasting character to the national way of thinking—was to be determined by certain qualities that developed under the influence of the American environment.

II

If there was any single predominant impulse which led men to seek out the American environment it was a concern for the architecture of fortune. The leaders of the Puritan colonies had come to New England for religious reasons, and there were many other religious refugees among the thousands who followed them across the Atlantic—especially to such tolerant settlements as Rhode Island, Pennsylvania, and Maryland. But the vast majority of the immigrants, as the tenor of the promotion literature (designed to encourage their settlement) has shown, were seeking a land of opportunity where they could get a new start in life and enjoy a new sort of existence. They were a self-selected lot of people who were willing to take a chance for their own betterment; and even their idealistic leaders and encouragers, from John Winthrop of Massachusetts Bay to James Edward Oglethorpe of Georgia, would have been willing to admit that their leadership and encouragement was directed toward the relief of man's estate. The Baconian impulse was overwhelming, and neither the static system of Puritan morality nor the inherent laziness of the gentlemen adventurers in Jamestown could resist it for long.

The desire to improve one's place in the world achieved its most spectacular success in the southern colonies, especially among those settlers who had enough capital to invest in substantial areas of wilderness and to import bound servants to develop their estates. They were the sons of goldsmiths and woolen drapers and the offshoots of gentry who were forbidden English land by the laws of primogeniture but who had a consuming ambition to be landed gentlemen in the tobacco country. Many of them achieved their desires, and the great plantations of the Fitzhughs, the Carters, and the Byrds developed a pattern of civilization which was also realized in the rice and indigo plantations of South Carolina and the manorial estates of New York. The entire seaboard south of New England and the river country which adjoined it became dotted with the holdings of a gentry who were mostly self-made.

These new gentlemen of the new world differed from their English brethren. The American tended to be expansive rather than conservative. However large his possessions were, he wanted to increase them; and he was, by necessity, the steward of his own estate with an active interest in trade. He could not despise commerce and live upon rents derived from well-established tenants. Instead, he marketed his own produce through his English agent and was constantly engaged in purchasing laborers—bound servants, who had to be replaced every five years, and Negro slaves. If he speculated in lands distant from his home plantation, as most of the gentry did, he had to recruit settlers to make them profitable. Money was always necessary for his many expenses, and to obtain it he was not above playing the part of the tradesman himself, importing rum and manufactured goods for the yeoman farmers in his neighborhood and sometimes sending out deputies to trade with the Indians. He watched the expenditures of his trans-Atlantic agent, collected fees for his services to the colony, and kept a close eye on the rulings of the English Board of Trade, which controlled the tobacco monopoly and tried to control all colonial commerce. Every successful planter had to be a merchant of sorts, and his sons, who were generally sent to England for a gentlemanly education, normally spent some time in an English commercial house before coming home to look after their many affairs.

The literature which reflects their lives provides a revealing record of gentlemanly leisure and business-like activity. The *Secret Diary* of the second William

Byrd of Westover, kept in his own private shorthand, is a copious and intimate account of everyday activity which reveals the dual nature of the eighteenth-century Virginia gentleman. The son of a large land-holder, Byrd was educated in England, where he acquired a proficiency in learning and a taste for literature which he carefully cultivated after his return to America. Each morning before breakfast he devoted an hour or more to reading Latin, Greek, or Hebrew—or, on rare occasions when a ship arrived from England, to reading the latest books in English or French. Afterward he entered into a busy round of plantation activities, as a supervisor of agriculture and handi-crafts and as doctor and judge to his bond servants and slaves. He was a rollicking host to his many friends and a colonial politician of considerable eminence. He said his prayers, kept a record of his diet, and devised schemes for exploring and settling the western regions. But above all things he was the architect of the family fortune, scheming for advantages over enterprising rivals and increasing his large inheritance fivefold. His one major ambition was to die in a position greater than that to which he had been born.

There were variations, of course, from the gentle-manly pattern revealed by William Byrd. His brother-in-law, Robert Beverly, author of the *History and Present State of Virginia* (1705), was more aggres-sively American, furnishing his house with articles of home manufacture and showing as much interest in the Indians as Byrd had shown in the white back-woodsmen in his *History of the Dividing Line* between Virginia and North Carolina. In Puritan New England, properly enough, the pattern was more Spartan, if it can be judged by the Reverend John Adams' poetic representation of "The Contented Man" or Benjamin Church's "The Choice." New Jersey's William Livingston professed a desire for a life of "philosophic solitude" in a retreat full of good books rather than costly furniture, and he was content to grow his own grapes rather than import Madeira; but the dream of a private estate with a well-filled cellar was widespread, and the surviving colonial homes of New York, Pennsylvania, and Maryland bear witness to the fulfillment of the dream by many persons who did not give it expression in writing. The common quality of these dreams, however, was that they were of a position to be achieved rather than of one in which the dreamer could settle.

The dream of individual progress toward some higher estate, of course, was far more widespread than the gentlemanly ideal. The majority of colonial Americans either were or aspired to be yeoman farmers, and the small estate, held through a nominal quitrent or in fee simple, represented the most common aim of colonial ambitions. George Alsop had been its spokesman in the seventeenth century. *A Character of the Province of Maryland* (1666) described a poor man's paradise, in which the equity of the laws made even bondage agreeable and every bound servant could look forward to the early achievement of fifty private acres and the possibility of their increase. These could be improved and passed on to children who, by virtue of their property, would proudly call themselves free men and enjoy all the rights and opportunities of freedom. The aspirations of the small farmers rarely found such direct expression in literature, but they lay back of such social ferment as that represented by the manuscript accounts of Bacon's Rebellion in seventeenth-century Virginia and the published protests against Oglethorpe's excessive paternalism in eighteenth-century Georgia; and they paralleled, in a modest but more pervasive way, the ambitions of the landed gentry.

The mechanics and artisans of the small but flourishing towns did not find a literary spokesman until the eighteenth century, but when they did, theirs was the clearest voice in colonial America. It came from Benjamin Franklin, who, while a mere boy, wrote a series of "Dogood Papers" for the Boston *Courant* which satirized the pretensions of the gentry and attacked the obstacles that the Puritan conception of a static society placed in the way of a mechanic's aspiration to higher education. After his settlement in Philadelphia and his brief period of logical intellectuality—a period which extended from his London *Dissertation on Liberty and Necessity* through his *Articles of Belief and Acts of Religion* in 1728—Franklin became the persistent and articulate opponent of all forms of deterministic philosophy and especially of that precept of the Puritan ethic which taught that a man's duty was to labor contentedly in a humble calling unless he found a ready and easy entrance to another. When he ran away from his apprenticeship and deserted the colony of Massachusetts, Franklin abandoned the static implications of the Puritan ethical system; and his action was not an uncommon one, if we can believe the observations of Ebenezer Cook, author of *The Sot-*

Weed Factor, in Maryland, at the beginning of the century. His distinction lies in the fact that he made a career of discreet opportunism, achieved fame by the exercise of a practical inductiveness, and expressed on a high literary level the devotion of a humbly born individual to material ambition.

Franklin quickly learned "the Way to Wealth" as a printer and publisher and expounded its simpler aspects in Poor Richard's widely read *Almanack.* The practical results of his observations concerning ordinary life and the possibility of improving it were soon evident in his own city: a street lighting and sewage system, warmer homes with fewer smoking chimneys, the first circulating library in America, a philosophical society for the advancement of learning, and an academy for its dissemination which was to become a college and eventually a great university. His broader observations and inferences from them led to the publication of his *Experiments and Observations on Electricity* in 1751 and to European fame as America's first scientist. When he became involved in international politics, in England on the eve of the American Revolution and in France during the actual war, he acquired a notable reputation for ironic good sense and developed the pose of sophisticated simplicity which made him a successful negotiator in the French court; and his last service to his country was that of the wise and witty compromiser of differences in the Constitutional Convention. More than any other single person he became the new world's representative of the Enlightenment.

It was enlightenment, however, in the Baconian

rather than the Cartesian sense. Franklin's interest was in immediate causes and immediate effects, not in the chain of causation. There is little speculative reasoning in Franklin's writings, and, after the philosophical *errata* of his youth, almost nothing that could be equated with logical demonstration. His method of reasoning was that of observation, classification, and judgment. Perhaps this is nowhere more evident than in his *Autobiography,* a book dedicated to that belief in "the truth of things as they are" which had so offended him in his youth but to which he had become as devoted in practice as Samuel Johnson was in theory. For the private benefit of his son, he showed how closely the architecture of his fortune was related to the ways of the world and how practical and immediate was his concern for the relief of man's estate. It is a narrative of shrewd perception and generally shrewd choice.

And one of the most interesting sections in the *Autobiography,* from the point of view of American intellectual history, is that in which he explains his scheme for attaining moral perfection. His was no speculative plan directed toward the perfectibility of mankind. Instead, it was a down-to-earth system of individual improvement. To achieve it, Franklin drew up a list of accepted virtues—a systematic group of "topics"—scrutinized, one by one, his week-long efforts to practice them, and passed judgment upon his success. The virtues themselves were either identical with or subdivisions of those found in the Puritan system of ethics. The only thing lacking was the Puritan dependence upon God and the sense of piety which pervaded the whole Puritan system. In its empirical concern for improvement by the light of "sense" it was the sort of scheme that Bacon might logically have drawn up had he been interested in moral advancement, but in its failure to admit any other light it went only partially along the intellectual way which Americans were to follow during the latter part of the eighteenth century.

For Franklin's mind was a secular mind, public-spirited and progressive but lacking in that peculiar quality sometimes called "American idealism" and often associated with such of his younger contemporaries as Thomas Jefferson. It was a quality which might be described as a sort of religious perception brought to bear on human affairs, but the weight of evidence seems to be against any theory that it represents a transfer of religious training into secular thought. Instead, it represents a pattern of thought which could be used alike by the Puritans of the seventeenth century and the skeptics of the eighteenth— equally adaptable to a belief in the depravity or in the perfectibility of man.

III

An independent United States of America, in fact, might never have come into existence during the eighteenth century had the colonists not shown a widespread willingness to follow, along political as well as religious lines, what Samuel Johnson called "a kind of intellectual light within us"—an intuitive light which began to dawn long before Johnson formally defined it in his *Elementa Philosophica*. Identified as the light of nature, it may be recognized as a reflection of many aspects of seventeenth-century thought in Europe; and in America it seems to have made its first literary appearance in *A Vindication of the Government of New England Churches* by the Reverend John Wise in 1717.

In such a religious context the light of nature might easily be confused with the supernatural light Jonathan Edwards saw when he became aware of his regeneracy, for Wise was indeed writing about a church made up of God's elected Saints. But he actually professed to have discovered it in the works of the German jurist, Samuel von Pufendorf, and he specifically disregarded the question of man's moral turpitude while assuming a close relationship between man's "natural" and "civil" being and asserting his subjection to the "law of nature" in both civil and church government. This law he described as "the Dictate of Right Reason founded in the Soul of Man"—a dictate apparently revealed by the same "light of nature" which made self-evident man's inherent liberty and equality and which did "highly value" democracy as a form of government. It was not a law hypothesized by the sort of speculations which led Locke to assume a state of nature preceding the social compact but a law which was intuitively perceived.

The mystery surrounding this concept of natural law in eighteenth-century American thought is that it was so rarely used. The colonial architects of fortune were aggressively concerned with their "rights," but they obviously preferred to defend their rights as "freeborn Englishmen," whose immunities and privileges were solidly founded on precedents identifiable by the light of sense rather than that of intuition. Such is the attitude, at any rate, found in such early landmarks of American political thought as the Maryland resolution of 1722, the Connecticut election sermon by Jared Eliot in 1738, and the 1747 sermon by Charles Chauncy which the Massachusetts General Court tried in vain to suppress. It was also the attitude taken by the great colonial lawyer, Andrew Hamilton, in his famous defense of the freedom of the press during the trial of John Peter Zenger who was being prosecuted with all the power of the New York colonial government. The English constitution, unwritten but firmly incorporated in legal precedent, provided a more solid basis for judgment than anything to be found in an intuitively perceived law of nature.

Yet when constitutional law failed to achieve some practical end, the law of nature found its advocates. As a last resort in the Maryland controversy, for example, Daniel Dulaney used it as the basis of a pamphlet insisting upon *The Right of the Inhabitants of Maryland to the Benefits of English Law* in 1728, and an anonymous New England clergyman who called himself Philalethes asserted it in behalf of the Church of England in a pamphlet on *The Essential Rights and Liberties of Protestants* in 1744. But both founded their arguments upon John Locke, and it is doubtful whether they considered this law spontaneously perceptible to all men. The person who left no room for doubt was the Reverend Jonathan Mayhew whose *Discourse on Unlimited Submission,* on the centennial anniversary of the beheading of Charles I, called it "treason" manifold "to say that subjects in general are not proper judges when their governors oppress them and play the tyrant." To Mayhew the powers or rulers were not so much limited by English law as by "the eternal laws of truth, wisdom, and equity, and the ever-lasting tables of right reason—tables that cannot be repealed, or thrown down and broken like those of Moses." In placing the dictates of natural reason not only above legislative acts but above the Ten Commandments, Mayhew elevated the law of nature to the highest position it had yet achieved in the American colonies.

Nevertheless, English common law held its superior place in the minds of most Americans until the very eve of the Revolution. It dominated John Dickinson's *Letters from a Farmer in Pennsylvania to the Inhabitants of the British Colonies* (1768), which vigorously defended the constitutional right to representative government and proved to be the most popular expression of American political thought during the decade. Yet the concept of intuitively perceived natural law was lurking in the background, and Dickinson himself had alluded to it in a pamphlet of 1766. Accordingly, when the First Continental Congress met in Philadelphia in September 1774, its members were in practical agreement concerning their attitude toward the regulatory powers of the British Parliament—but were not in agreement concerning the ideological grounds for their attitude. John Adams later recalled that he wanted to insert into the declaration of principles "an appeal to those general ideas of natural right so clearly and broadly laid down not long afterward in the Declaration of Independence" but that his desires had been opposed by the delegates from Pennsylvania,

Virginia, and Maryland. This restrictive attitude, however, was soon to change. At some time during that same year the Philadelphia lawyer James Wilson decided that the times required the publication of his earlier manuscript *Considerations on the Nature and Extent of the Legislative Authority of the British Parliament* and so publicly announced his conclusion from "the law of nature" that "all men are, by nature, equal and free." In the fall, when the "Westchester Farmer" began to address his *Free Thoughts on the Proceedings of the Continental Congress* successively to the farmers, the merchants, and the members of the legislature of New York, the young Alexander Hamilton took his quill in hand to refute him with "a more comprehensive view of the dispute." To the citizens as a whole he recommended an application without delay to the study of the law of nature as expounded by Hugo Grotius, Samuel von Pufendorf, John Locke, the Baron de Montesquieu, and Burlamaqui; and in a later pamphlet he insisted that "the sacred rights of mankind . . . are written, as with a sunbeam, in the whole volume of human nature, by the hand of divinity itself, and can never be erased or obscured by mortal power." There is a strange irony in the fact that Alexander Hamilton should have preceded Thomas Jefferson in a public expression of inviolable attachment "to the essential rights of mankind" and of a conviction that "the whole human race is entitled to" the blessings of liberty. But the political writers of the time were dipping their pens in the ink of human interests rather than of abstract philosophy, and Hamilton, as later events were to show, had a quicker eye for interests than Jefferson ever did.

For the fact seems to be that the light of nature had little inherent appeal to Americans, who were inclined to accept its guidance only toward some material end and only after the light of sense had failed. They preferred to be empirically progressive and chose to think their way forward by other means only when they became impatient with their rate of progress. Accordingly, when hostilities had broken out with England and the American cause was failing to progress, it was perhaps natural that they should leap toward independence under the guidance of an Englishman who had not arrived in America until the latter part of 1774 when the appeals to legal precedents had failed and the expediency of the law of nature was becoming widely recognized. Thomas Paine's argument for independence as a "natural right" was supported by a combination of realistic observations and false analogies, but in January 1776 it was an almost inevitable expression of the "common sense" of a people who were in a desperate state of transition from civil war to revolution. In any case, Paine's *Thoughts on the Present State of American Affairs* was a pamphlet which cleared the way for a document which was remarkably in part what its authors intended it to be—an expression of "the American mind."

The greater part of the Declaration of Independence is, of course, a piece of temporary political propaganda designed to divert American antagonism from the British parliamentary government to the king and so destroy the sentimental basis of colonial loyalty. But its whole argument provides the best illustration to be found in literature of an emergent American way of thinking. It opens with an appeal to Cartesian logic in a subordinate clause—a reference to that progressive "course of human events" in which a certain action "becomes necessary" in order to reach an end made legitimate by "the laws of Nature and of Nature's God." But the "causes" which were declared to "impel" that action bear no relation to the linked Cartesian pattern of ratiocination. The logic of the Declaration was of a quite different sort. One efficient cause of the action was that "all men are created equal," and operating with it as additional efficient causes were the "certain unalienable Rights" with which men "are endowed by their Creator." Of these Rights, the principal ones were "Life, Liberty, and the pursuit of Happiness"; and the cause helping men to secure these rights was the institution of "Government," which derived its inner impulse from "the consent of the governed," who possessed a further inherent "Right" to change the government if it did not perform its proper function. The occasion or pretext for change was a cause operating from without—here described in the elaborate bill of particulars drawn up against George III, listing the acts of tyranny which formed the greater part of the document—and the instrument of change was the solemn publication and declaration contained in the concluding paragraph.

The formal logical structure of the Declaration (which happens to correspond with John Milton's analysis of the "Efficient Cause" operating "singly and with others") was probably uncalculated and is relatively unimportant. What is important in American intellectual history is, first, that the Declaration avoids any attempt at elaborate reasoning or mathematical demonstration and follows a pattern of simple inferences from basic truths. Second, and equally important, these "truths" are held to be "self-evident"—immediately perceptible by some light which was obviously not the light of sense or experience but the intellectual light of intuition. The Declaration of Independence is not only a milestone in American political history; it is a milestone in American intellectual history as well. For it reflects a calculated judgment upon what was called "the American mind" by three temperamentally different but extraordinarily shrewd eighteenth-century observers: Thomas Jefferson, John Adams, and Benjamin Franklin. And their judgment is clear. If "the American mind" was compelled to abandon the solid ground of experience, it would take off on a leap of intuition rather than along a chain of ratiocination.

With the framing of the federal Constitution, twelve years later, the American mind returned to things as they were and to the perception of the light of sense. The Constitution was an ingenious compromise of material interests and working methods, designed to meet the need for a "more perfect union" which had been made self-evident by years of experience with instability and civil unrest. The *Federalist* essays (1787–88) which argued for its ratification followed a pattern of drawing simple inferences from observable conditions or from possibilities readily conceived on the basis of recent experience. The chain of argument occasionally found in the essays rarely contained many links, and their authors—Alexander Hamilton, James Madison, and John Jay—made few appeals to abstract principles intuitively perceived. The new form of federal republican government was experimental but not speculative in its conception, expedient rather than inspired.

During all the violent controversies that marked the concluding decade of the eighteenth century in America, the pattern of thought revealed both in the boldness of the Declaration and in the conservatism of the Constitution was never seriously challenged. The speculative rationalism of revolutionary France created panic among many Americans, especially after 1792, and such literary men as the Reverend Timothy Dwight thundered against philosophy and vain deceit. Dwight himself retreated—in the verse of *Greenfield Hill* (1794) and the prose of *The True Means of Establishing Public Happiness* (1795) or *The Duty of Americans at the Present Crisis* (1798)—into an almost hysterical defense of things as they are. But he was actually able to discover in America few speculative philosophers of the Continental sort.

Joel Barlow, poet, promoter, and pamphleteer, perhaps came nearer than any other American to being a thinker after the French fashion. In his *Advice to the Privileged Orders* (1792–93) he assumed that a "necessary" effect of the French Revolution would be the spread of the revolutionary movement throughout Europe, and he undertook, from France and England, to persuade the privileged classes to face this fact rationally. He had absorbed enough of the Continental rationalism to trace the evils of contemporary society through a chain of causation to their origin, but he was too American to project his chain of argument into the future. Of the three ways of knowing which he described in the introductory part of his *Advice*, one was by experience and another by intuition; the other method was by collateral experience or analogy. It was less absolute but more applicable to politics than the others, and in his various political pamphlets addressed to European readers Barlow tended to draw more upon the American experience than upon demonstrative logic for the reforms he advocated.

The most intellectually interesting of Barlow's writings was the long philosophical poem *The Columbiad*, which was a revision of his earlier *The Vision of Columbus* (1787) made mostly in France in 1802 and published in America in 1807. For in it the American who for thirteen years had been intensely exposed to French thought surveyed the intellectual progress of the human race and made his own choice between the Continental and the Anglo-American ways of reason: Nicolaus Copernicus and René Descartes represented two great milestones in the progress of thought, but it was Francis Bacon who had most effectively taught men "what to learn, and how to know." The "moral science" of the future—which included the science of government—would be an inductive science, and the state of nature which mankind would eventually achieve would be a world-wide utilitarian state politically organized after the pattern of the federated states of America.

By the close of the Revolutionary era, then, that intangible cultural quality which Jefferson and his colleagues had called "the American mind" had settled upon the way of reason by which it would move toward enlightenment. It had rejected Cartesian logic, and, with it, the probability of any profound intellectual achievement in such fields as mathematics, theoretical science, and philosophy. Instead, it had chosen the logic of Bacon with its practical emphasis upon observation, inference, and judgment and with its bias toward such material and humane concerns as the architecture of fortune and the relief of man's estate. But it persisted in holding on to some of the "general topics" that Bacon had rejected—in considering "good" some of the abstract ideas which the English philosopher had called intellectually "vicious"—and so turned away from his cold conception of the New Atlantis. In religion and morals some of these abstract ideas were widely accepted, fervently by the devout and the conventional but only tolerantly by men like Franklin who privately considered them "impractical" and hardly worth arguing about. In political thought they were frequently useful for the purpose of achieving ends which experience could not justify and dialectic might obscure. They freed the ordinary mind from complete bondage to materialism and introduced into it that quality of idealism which was to puzzle European intellectuals for generations to come.

The result was an intellectual disposition which was usually stubbornly practical, often erratic, and sometimes extraordinarily flexible. The ordinary man was habitually given to following his own judgment, and if he suffered from the illusion that one man's judgment was as good as another's, he was also able and willing to grapple experimentally with questions beyond the range of his formal intellectual training. Occasionally he found the answers. But in any case he was probably inclined to feel a certain pride rather than shame in his awareness that his notion of what was "reasonable" differed somewhat from that of his fellows, for by the end of the eighteenth century intellectual authority seems to have become as abhorrent to most Americans as institutionalized religious authority had become at the end of the seventeenth.

CHAPTER THREE

The Naturalization of Symbols

I

IN his two-volume *Brief Retrospect of the Eighteenth Century*, published in 1803, the Reverend Samuel Miller of New Jersey wrote of the United States—along with Russia and Germany—as one of "the nations lately become literary." He paid his respects to the religious literature of New England and to the political literature of the late colonies and the new nation, and he tried to explain why poetry and fiction languished in a country where popular education and newspapers flourished. The impoverishment and inadequacy of the American colleges was one reason he offered, and the scarcity of books throughout the country was another. But both of these conditions might be improved with an increase in wealth. The desire to increase wealth, however, offered obstacles of its own. The pressure of business allowed little leisure for the cultivation of literature, and the commercial spirit of the American people offered no encouragement to learning in the form of academic fellowships and other rewards. Booksellers in the small American cities were too poor to serve as patrons of native writers, especially when they could reprint freely the established authors of Great Britain. Yet he "confidently predicted" that in time to come the United States would achieve cultural conditions comparable to those of Europe and "letters will flourish as much in America as in any part of the world."

But in the meantime the new country would have to go through a literary revolution which Miller could neither imagine nor anticipate. It had already achieved its basic freedom from religious institutional authority by the very efforts of the Puritans to establish their own peculiar institution in a land which gave people more freedom than they consciously sought. It had acquired freedom from intellectual authority through the same environmental compulsion toward direct and simple thinking leading to individual judgments. And, finally, it used these slowly developed and yet undefined attitudes of mind in gaining a political freedom from Great Britain which enabled it to incorporate in a written Constitution assurances of permanent freedom from religious establishments and from governmental interference with fundamental human rights. But these underlying attitudes of mind had not yet been generally brought to bear upon the more subtle and tenuous problems of literary expression.

For the art of literature is the art of communication by symbols that are rarely defined explicitly in the minds of either writers or readers. In their larger and grosser forms these symbols are subjects, themes, or interests which have some special value at a particular time and therefore help inspire linguistic symbols with the living vitality that is the essence of literature. During the late eighteenth century and early nineteenth century the values found in the new subjects of popular interest tended to be emotional rather than intellectual, eccentric and personal rather than traditional and social—in short, Romantic—and the most popular themes were the attractions of external nature, the fascinations of the past, and the rebellion against tyranny. Like most people in the process of escaping narrow provincial interests and acquiring an international literary consciousness, the Americans of this period were acutely sensitive to what was grossly "new" on the literary horizon, and the country "became literary" in terms of the English Romantic movement.

Aside from a newborn nation's enthusiasm for politics, in fact, an interest in nature was one of the most widespread qualities exhibited in late eighteenth-century American verse. At the end of the Revolution, Colonel David Humphreys, in *A Poem Addressed to the Armies of America* (1780), had tried to cheer and quiet the continental soldiers by describing the beauty and productivity of the Ohio lands which had been promised them and in which they were assured that the "golden years" would "anew begin their reigns." But usually, as in his poem "On the Happiness of America," Humphreys was less practical: nature was simply a fashionable symbol for the poet to use, and, like most of his contemporaries, he followed the fashion. Philip Freneau had already dwelt proudly upon the subject of natural abundance in "The American Village" in 1772, had written enthusiastically about the

77

natural beauties of Santa Cruz in the West Indies, and was engaged in writing a variety of nature poems ranging from the grandeur of "The Hurricane" to the simplicity of "The Wild Honey Suckle." These poems grew out of the poet's own experience. But the attractions of a popular symbol led other writers far afield, and in 1788 Richard Alsop completed but did not publish a long poem *The Charms of Fancy* which "rang'd o'er nature's wide domain" from the Atlantic seaboard to the Ohio country and crossed the seas, through the medium of travel books, to dwell upon the charms of Tahiti, the peculiar animal life of Australia and Africa, the fireflies and upas trees of Siam, and the gardens of Shiraz.

Such poems as these dealt with nature in an appreciative way rather than in the meditative way which was to become a Romantic fashion. At most the external scene refreshed the American poet, as it had James Thomson in earlier eighteenth-century England, or gave the same pleasure to his imagination that it had given to Mark Akenside's. But a more philosophical consideration was already beginning to emerge. As early as 1772, Timothy Dwight, a young tutor at Yale College who had recently published a poem on America in the manner of Alexander Pope's *Windsor Forest*, began to think of nature as a means of escape from literary tradition. In "A Dissertation on the History, Eloquence, and Poetry of the Bible," delivered at a public commencement of the college, he attacked the neoclassical rules and praised the biblical writers for allowing "their imaginations an unlimited range," giving "life to the whole inanimate creation," and thereby

finding "the shortest passage to the human soul."
During the years that followed, Dwight studied and
taught the *Elements of Criticism* by Henry Home,
Lord Kames, and found in it a systematic esthetic,
which he used in his biblical epic *The Conquest of
Canäan* (1785). From Kames he learned to make his
images "distinct," "complete," and "lively" by having
the reader stand as "a real spectator" at "the very place"
from which the scene was to be described and to
achieve his effects by following the "course of nature"
in his descriptions. The results were pedantic, for
Dwight was more of a schoolteacher than a poet, but
he persisted in what was at least a theoretical revolt
against pedantry. "Nature ought to be consulted in
reference to Aristotle," he wrote in an anonymous series
of critical essays called *The Friend* (1786), for "on this
plan the wings of genius would be no longer clipped,
and . . . the writer who produced pleasing selections
of images and sentiments from the widely extended
and endlessly diversified paradise of nature, would be
assured of regaling the taste of his readers." Two years
later, in the locodescriptive poem afterward published
as *Greenfield Hill,* he put his critical theories to practice in what was perhaps his most varied and successful poetic work.

The most interesting of the meditative writers on
nature, however, was Thomas Odiorne, who attempted
to treat the subject philosophically in a blank verse
poem unhappily called *The Progress of Refinement*
(1792). Believing that the human mind was formed
to bear a delicate relationship to "external things,"
which were, in turn, admirably formed "the mind to

amuse and raise the bliss of thought," he anticipated his slightly younger contemporary William Wordsworth in an attempt to explain this mutual adjustment in terms of the associationist psychology of David Hartley. Accordingly, he carefully portrayed the development of the mind, under the influence of external nature, from its state of sensory perception through its acquisition of imaginative ideas into the increasingly complex region of ideas of ambition, self-interest, sympathy, God, and morality. Furthermore, in a true Hartleyan and Wordsworthian fashion, he dwelt upon the reciprocal influence of these complex ideas upon simple sensation, holding that a man not only grew intellectually under the influence of nature but learned by his growth to find a greater and more mature pleasure in the natural scenes that stimulated his development. Two years before this, in the Preface to the ninth edition of his poem on the happiness of America, David Humphreys had also made the Wordsworthian suggestion that the minds of American poets were "imperceptibly impressed with the novelty, beauty or sublimity of surrounding objects," which thus "gave energy to the language which expressed our sensations." But neither Humphreys nor Odiorne became a Wordsworth. In fact, the one quality they had in common with Freneau, Dwight, Alsop, and their other nature-loving contemporaries was that their language distinctly lacked the living energy of poetry.

Had they been right in their assumptions concerning the direct connection between objects and words —either by Platonic correspondence or Hartley's material vibrations—they might have shown, even within the range of their limited talents, a bit of the life they fondly hoped for. But they fooled themselves by over-estimating the specious values of a fashionable subject. However poetic or philosophical they may have felt in the contemplation of natural surroundings, they could not have been stirred—even had they possessed the capacity—to the depths of the great English poets who found in nature a purer font of inspiration. For nature meant escape, peace, and a restoration of nerv-ous energy to the troubled Wordsworth, the perse-cuted Shelley, and the world-weary Byron; and, no matter how they may have attempted to rationalize their relation to it, the experience of escaping from the haunts of men provided them with a release of creative energy which did vitalize their language with new qualities of sensitivity and suggestiveness. But to country-bred Americans, for whom the lowing kine were often reminders of their daily chores, nature of-fered no such psychological values. It was a popular symbol, large enough for them to grasp and use with no appreciation of the way it was beginning to revital-ize the verbal symbols of English Romanticism. While crossing the Atlantic into a new cultural environment it suffered a sea change and became something arti-ficial rather than alive.

Among the other gross symbols of Romanticism, the fascination of the past had little to offer Americans during the first flush of their incipient nationalism. They knew little of their own history at the time of the Revolution, for the period of historical investiga-tion was just beginning and that of popular myth-making was to come a generation later. Yet they strove to grasp and use the past as they were using nature. As an undergraduate at the College of New Jersey Philip Freneau contemplated "The Pyramids of Egypt" with poetic awe and made efforts at an epic and a descriptive poem on Christopher Columbus. But for his public commencement poem he turned toward the future and in collaboration with a classmate, Hugh Henry Brackenridge, wrote on "The Rising Glory of America." He set the precedent for other young poets who made commencement programs ring with prophecies of the achievements of the new country, and the idea of progress became far more prevalent than pictures of the past in late eighteenth-century American verse. Poets were acutely aware, however, of the popular symbol. They versified such events from the French and Indian Wars as the capture of Louisburg and Arthur St. Clair's defeat, and stories of the ancient mound builders of the Ohio country attracted the *Anarchiad* poets, who called themselves "the Wicked Wits" of Hartford and fascinated the anonymous author of *The Returned Captive* (1787). But only Timothy Dwight, in "The Destruction of the Pequods" in *Greenfield Hill*, succeeded in achieving anything like a Romantic tone in a treatment of the American past. Their difficulty was that progress was a part of their experience. The past was not. And in dealing with this Romantic symbol they were beginning to realize that something which made sense in terms of their own experience was a more valid source of poetic inspiration than something which did not.

The best representation of this conflict between the attractions of the past and the future, symbol and belief, is Joel Barlow's philosophical poem *The Vision of Columbus* (1787), which he was later to revise into *The Columbiad.* The actual experiences of Columbus did not interest him, and so he made his poem principally a "vision" of American colonial and Revolutionary history. But to it he added a survey of the pre-Columbian civilization of the Incas in Peru and a prophetic survey of the future when the nations of the world would be brought together by improvements in transportation and peoples would be united by the progress of thought toward the discovery of those "general laws in every breast, Where ethics, faith, and politics may rest." One survey was designed to display the highest achievements of human society under the direction of "the laws of Nature and Reason." The other foretold the future for a people who had the benefit of revelation and were following the divine plan. Each, at the time, had a genuine intellectual value for Barlow as a Romantic symbol; but each, in these insecure days of his ambitious youth, was relatively cold in its attractions. The significance of the conflict did not appear until he began to revise the poem fifteen years later. By then he was ready to leave the pre-Columbian past as he had originally described it and devote his greatest effort to a revision of his idea of progress and incorporation into it of his mature belief in the power of human effort and the self-determination of mankind.

If the symbolic value of the past was translated into a dream of the future when it crossed the Atlantic, the symbol of rebellion against tyranny suffered a more drastic change. For the tyrannical monarch—who, as exemplified by Percy Bysshe Shelley's Jove, was to become the climactic symbol of this sort in English Romanticism—had been placed in contempt before the American people by the authors of the Declaration of Independence and squeezed dry of its emotional force within a decade. By the time the federal government was being formed, the mob had a more powerful effect than the monarch as a moving symbol of tyranny. Yet the sensitiveness to new fashions was strong, and the antidemocratic young poet Richard Alsop, while reading Claude Étienne Savary's *Letters on Egypt* the year after its publication in English, was as impressed as the yet unborn Shelley was to be by the irony of the ruined statue of the tyrant Ozymandias. Alsop, too, in *The Charms of Fancy,* versified his impression. But instead of holding the monarch up for execration as Shelley did, he merely treated his "pompous claim" to unlimited power as a curious irony. The emotional value of the symbol had almost completely disappeared.

II

The decay in value which marked the passage of the grosser symbols of Romanticism did not cause them to disappear from American literature. On the contrary, they flourished on its surface as fashionable manifestations of interests which the writing of the new world reflected from that of the old. Even the least valuable among them—that of rebellion against tyranny—became commonplace in the political satire which was so characteristic of the era. In the first in-

stallment (1775) of his Revolutionary satire *M'Fingal*
John Trumbull had undertaken to mock the Tories,
but in the last, composed at the end of the war, he
became more indignant at the tyrant mob and eventually joined the Wicked Wits of Hartford in a concerted attack upon the rule of Anarch, which they saw
foreshadowed by the pre-Constitutional turmoil. Philip
Freneau moved in the opposite direction politically
and in the last decade of the century sacrificed most
of his early Romantic promise to satiric journalism in
which he versified his opposition to the aristocratic
tyranny implicit in the Federalist policies as he saw
them from a Jeffersonian point of view. Descriptions
of nature became increasingly evident in American
verse as the symbol acquired greater depth in the poetry of England, and the past was being brought into
everyday consciousness by a dozen state historians and
by such myth-making biographies as Parson Mason
Locke Weems's of George Washington, David Humphreys' of Israel Putnam, and John Filson's less pretentious biography of Daniel Boone.

But the basic problem of the American writer remained unsolved. Unable to resist the current of influences from abroad, he could not adapt his borrowed
symbols to the attitude of mind which had become his
native heritage. The deepest and most original values
of the symbols did not make sense in terms of his own
experience. Empirical and practical by adjustment to
the environment in which he lived, he was frustrated
by his inability to find a practical meaning in the material which so evidently had a profound significance
for authors abroad. The nature of his dilemma can per-

85

haps be best illustrated by Charles Brockden Brown, for three years the most prolific of early American novelists. In his effort to achieve popular success, Brown turned to the Gothic tradition, generally neglected or scoffed at in matter-of-fact America, and in *Wieland* (1798) produced a tale of terror which included death by spontaneous combustion, mysterious voices, and a multiplicity of senseless murders. He tried to adapt his sensationalism to a new environment by offering a rational explanation of his mysteries, but it was not a successful attempt, for there was evidently no union of sensationalism and reason in Brown's mind as he composed the novel. With more preparatory awareness, he attempted such a union in *Arthur Mervyn* (1799) and *Edgar Huntley* (1799) by drawing upon the terrors of the yellow-fever epidemic in Philadelphia in the one and upon the dangers of the American forest in the other, but his effects were those of absurdity. That he had too little talent and too much fluency is obvious, but *Ormond* (1799) reveals a deeper reason for his failure. Here he followed William Godwin in an attempt to present an unvillainous villain, but he could not, as Godwin did in *Caleb Williams*, hold society responsible for the evil he was unwilling to attribute to an individual. The society he saw around him was not the society of classes and pressures which Godwin observed in England, and, as a result, Brown's novel was a motiveless imitation which was like Godwin in everything except the strength of belief.

A more successful writer of prose fiction was Hugh Henry Brackenridge, the classmate and collaborator of Philip Freneau, who eventually found himself observing the rising glory of America from the vantage ground of the western Pennsylvania frontier. American democracy rose, he discovered, only to heights of demagoguery and pretentious ignorance, and he sought to boost it higher by satire in the manner of *Don Quixote* and Henry Fielding's *Tom Jones*. His long-continued *Modern Chivalry* (1792–1815) outrambled its earliest prototype and outdid *Tom Jones* in its essays in explanation. But it is more alive than the writings of Brown or of the many sentimental novelists of the period, partly because of its interest as social history and partly because Brackenridge almost succeeded in mastering his material by his point of view. He found an inspiring symbol in the national scene and in his dream of a national future. But he found the reality of the scene disillusioning and his dream apparently frustrated. So he laughed—somewhat in bitterness, somewhat for relief, and somewhat in the hope that his satiric laughter might help his dream come true.

The unconscious escape into laughter and the conscious desire to achieve an idealistic aim through satire may, in fact, be one of the reasons why the mocking spirit was so strong in American literature during the late eighteenth and early nineteenth centuries—in the later essays of Benjamin Franklin, in the verses of the Wicked Wits, the political poems of Philip Freneau, the essays and allegories of Francis Hopkinson, such novels as Royall Tyler's *The Algerine Captive* (1797), and such dramas as Tyler's *The Contrast* (1790). In any event the mockery of the early Knicker-

bocker group in New York—William and Peter Irving,
James K. Paulding, and others—prepared the way for
the first successful solution of the American writer's
problem of dealing with the native past in a way which
enabled him to adapt a conventional symbol to a new
sense of values and thereby in effect find a literary
advantage in his own apologetic self-consciousness.

Washington Irving, who was to become one of the
most conventionally Romantic of American writers, began as a somewhat old-fashioned satiric humorist with
contributions in the manner of Joseph Addison and of
Oliver Goldsmith to New York newspapers under the
signature of Jonathan Oldstyle (1802–3). A few years
later he was associated with his older brother William and James K. Paulding in the composition of
the *Salmagundi* papers, professedly designed to "in-
struct the young, reform the old, correct the town, and
castigate the age." In the same spirit, he and William
undertook to parody a contemporary guidebook to the
city. But when the older brother gave up the project,
Washington Irving, affected by a personal grief at the
death of his fiancée, allowed his mind to escape into
the past and produced a *History of New York* (1809)
which was primarily concerned with the Dutch rule
of the colony and was purportedly composed by a
queer Dutch character named Diedrich Knickerbocker. Through at least one book of it ran a strong
strain of contemporary satire, but on the whole it was
a humorous treatment of a Romantic subject which
Irving could not handle in a grave or earnest vein. He
undoubtedly found in the past a means of escape from
the weary weight of an unintelligible world, but the

associations formed in his mind were neither lofty nor sober. His native past was something that he could take seriously but not solemnly.

Much of the humor in the Knickerbocker *History*, of course, reflected the cultivated character of Irving's youthful mind. Yet his later writings were to show that his basic temper was not that of a humorist, that the primary charm of the past to him was Romantic, and that his humor was mostly evident in his treatment of contemporary subjects and American history and legend. In *The Sketch-Book* (1819–20) his humorous cast remained evident in his observations on the English scene but was most obvious in the two American stories, "Rip Van Winkle" and "The Legend of Sleepy Hollow," attributed to Diedrich Knickerbocker. In *Bracebridge Hall* (1822) he began to mellow, and in the *Tales of a Traveller* (1824) he tended toward the serious treatment of the Gothic and the grotesque except in the American setting of "The Devil and Tom Walker." After he had become seriously interested in Spanish history and turned to Spanish legendary material for fiction, in *The Alhambra* (1832), there was little in his writing to suggest that he had ever made his reputation as a humorist. Successive revisions of the Knickerbocker *History* gradually eliminated many of the passages which had provoked laughter in the first edition, and an examination of his later writings on the American West shows that he tended to cut the comedy out of his actual experiences as he recorded them in his Journal and remove it entirely from his published *Tour of the Prairies* (1835). It took him a quarter of a century to learn to contemplate his own country without concealing his mixed emotions behind the mask of laughter.

His friend and former collaborator, James K. Paulding, was also slow to learn, and back of them both lay not only the conflict between a borrowed Romantic symbolism and an inbred attitude of mind but a theory of esthetics which exaggerated the American literary dilemma. This was the belief that literary quality depended upon the natural associations which existed in the author's mind as he wrote and which he shared with his prospective readers. It was based upon John Locke's notion that all ideas were the products of sensation and reflection and upon David Hartley's exposition of the psychological processes by which these simple ideas were combined by association. Thomas Odiorne had used this psychology in his philosophical poem on *The Progress of Refinement*, but it did not have any great effect upon literary practice until it had been systematized into esthetic doctrine by Sir Archibald Alison in 1790 and spread abroad in the early nineteenth century. Its most unhappy effect upon the American writer was to make him feel self-consciously limited, in comparison with the European, by his own nationality. Since America had no familiar past, he could either stay at home and make shift with the humdrum associations of his natural surroundings, or he could go abroad and make a belated attempt to acquire associations with a past which American readers could not share and into which he himself could not fit as naturally as could a European. Such intimate friends as the minor poets Joseph Rodman Drake and Fitz-Greene Halleck parted company over this problem—Drake to write artificially about "The Culprit Fay" in Hudson River surroundings and Halleck to go abroad and become a second-rate Byron in "Marco Bozzaris."

Irving, of course, found his serious literary inspiration abroad. But William Cullen Bryant, who was America's first successful writer in verse as Washington Irving was in prose, kept his at home. Like Irving, Bryant's first endeavors were in the field of contemporary satire, and his poem *The Embargo*, published in 1808 when the author was only fourteen, was an attack upon the Jeffersonian administration comparable to the one Irving was preparing for the fourth book of his Knickerbocker *History*. But Bryant struck his most congenial note a few years later in "Thanatopsis," a poem which in its first version represented the melancholy outpourings of a young man brooding upon an early death, when he would lie down with the wise and good of ages past and all nature would be his sepulcher. Bryant was fascinated by both of the major and by now well-established Romantic symbols, but he could find little in the American past which moved him deeply. He was to search for Romantic associations in Indian legends, in the events of the American Revolution, and in the fancies he wove about the ancient mound builders in "The Prairies," after he had paid tribute to the abstraction of "The Past" in 1828. The identifiable wise and good of ages past, however, were not buried on American soil, and there were few spontaneous associations with this theme that he could share with his fellow countrymen.

Nature, perforce, was the subject best suited to the

solemn chords he had learned to strike so successfully in "Thanatopsis." He approached it in the manner of James Thomson in an "Inscription for the Entrance to a Wood" (1817), learned the art of suggestive description in "Green River" (1820), moralized it in numerous poems, and eventually pantheized it in "A Forest Hymn" (1825). He seems to have reached his greatest maturity about 1820 when he began to realize the constructive rather than the limiting implications of the associationist esthetic and, as in "A Winter Piece," allowed his descriptive verses to flow along trains of thought like those of Wordsworth with a coherence which appeared spontaneous rather than predetermined. Soon afterward he put "Thanatopsis" in its final form by giving it a framework of sixteen and a half new lines at the beginning and fifteen and a half at the end, making the sonorous lines of the original poem represent "the still voice" of Nature rather than the melancholy outpourings of youth and thereby giving them more dignified and philosophical associations. Four years later, in a lecture "On the Nature of Poetry" (1825), he distinguished between the imitative arts of painting and sculpture and the "suggestive art" of poetry, which dealt in words as arbitrary symbols and appealed to "the mind" rather than to "the senses." The success of a poem depended upon the capacity of its reader's imagination to pursue "a path which the poet only points out, and shape its visions from the scenes and allusions which he gives. It fills up his sketches of beauty with what suits its own highest conceptions of the beautiful, and completes his outline of grandeur with the noblest images its own stores can furnish." In practice and in theory, Bryant succeeded in naturalizing one of the great symbols of Romanticism by insisting that nature poetry make sense in terms of the American writer's and reader's mutual experience.

Through Irving and Bryant American literature began to move toward the solution of one of its greatest problems in achieving a character of its own. As a subordinate part of a much greater literature in English, it was inevitably subject to the dominance of the interests and fashions which developed across the Atlantic—those great and readily recognizable symbols which had the power to stir new depths in creative spirits and at the same time give some assurance of communication. Provincial Americans needed this assurance badly and grasped at the means of getting it without realizing that these symbols lost much of their power when transferred to a different cultural environment. But Irving discovered that the American past actually did possess vitality if he adapted his treatment of it to the temper of his own mind and reassured himself and his readers, during his early years, with the knowledge that he did not take it very seriously. Bryant discovered that he could make serious use of external nature if he adapted his treatment of it to the stream of associations he found in his own mind and could normally anticipate in the minds of his readers. Both conscientiously referred their borrowed symbolism to their own individualities instead of accepting it superficially at its face value, and neither stirred any considerable depths in their personal reference. But they gave the lesser symbols of their language a greater vitality than can be found in their predecessors and

93

marked the way for the eventual triumphs of their successors. It remains to be seen, however, what could be done seriously with the American past.

III

James Fenimore Cooper became a novelist almost by inadvertence. A landed gentleman by inheritance and a former naval officer whose energies could not be absorbed by farming and business, he wrote and published *Precaution* (1820) at the age of thirty-one in a burst of irritation over an English novel on manners on which he thought he could improve. Its Jane Austen-like portrayal of life in an English vicarage, however, was foreign to his experience and temperament, and he turned almost immediately to a story of the country he knew and in *The Spy* (1821) told a tale of border activity in the American Revolution in the manner of Sir Walter Scott which is memorable for its yeoman hero, Harvey Birch, who was much more alive than the major historical figures who stalked its pages. Neither book wholly satisfied him, however, and so with some qualms but considerable ambition he combined the method of one with the material of the other and undertook a novel of distinctively American manners representing a typical aspect of the American past. The result was *The Pioneers* (1823), a story of frontier settlement in the Otsego country of central New York state. Its substance was drawn from the periphery of Cooper's own childhood memories, for his father had founded such a community, represented it in the federal Congress, served as its judge, and reared his family there. Young James had known its geography and inhabitants intimately and its early history by vivid hearsay.

The book, then, was the closest that American fiction had yet come to the reality of personal experience. Through it ran a romantic plot, which created a background of mystery and ended with the reconciliation of two old friends through the marriage of a recognized and a missing heir, but most of its characters were realistic representatives of frontier types—the substantial but venturesome promoter and his dependents, the shrewd and opinionated Yankees who formed the great body of settlers, the emigré French storekeeper and the wandering German, the retired soldier whose wife kept the tavern, the minister and the schoolteacher, the former British sailor who had gone into service, the humble Negro, and the professional wood chopper. On the outskirts of the settlement Cooper placed two other representative types—the "Indian John" hanger-on, Chingachgook, last of the once-great tribe of Mohicans, who died in a forest fire bravely singing his death song; and the hunter in buckskin jacket and leather stockings, Natty Bumppo, scrawny and old and wise in Indian ways, whose unfailing rifle saved the heroine from a wild panther and accompanied him on his solitary flight into the western forest after he had fought his battle with civilization and resolved the plot. From the lives and mannerisms of these people and from the opportunities for construction and entertainment on the frontier Cooper drew the real substance of his tale.

But the life of the story was not entirely of his determination. For he wrote and published at a fortunate time, when the mythology of America was just coming into being. A score of historians had by now made the American past and the American scene more familiar to the general public, and many of them had followed the example of St. John de Crèvecoeur's *Letters from an American Farmer* (1782) and of Thomas Jefferson's *Notes on Virginia* (1784–85) by struggling consciously against the European myth of the "degenerative effects" of the American climate. The "man of America," settler and savage, was being ennobled in reaction to the theories of the Comte de Buffon, Abbé Guillaume Raynal, and others in France and England. Chauvinism was growing more widespread after the successful conclusion, in 1815, of a second war with England. The war itself had discovered a new type of hero, quite unlike the gentlemanly generals George Washington and Nathanael Greene of the Revolution, in "Old Hickory" Andrew Jackson and his hunters of Kentucky, who were credited with winning the dramatic Battle of New Orleans. The buckskin-clad hunter, in fact, had already begun to emerge in literature as the distinctive man of America. John Filson's *The Discovery, Settlement, and Present State of Kentucke* (1784) had attracted wide attention to its supposed author, Daniel Boone, as the prototype of the pioneer who opened up the wilderness west of the Appalachians, and Boone had been made the hero of an epic poem in Daniel Bryan's *The Mountain Muse* (1813). The poem had been too poor to catch the public fancy, but the public fancy was ready for a self-sufficient frontiersman who seemed at the same time both real and wonderful.

Cooper caught the wave of readiness. Natty Bumppo in his original appearance might have been too uncouth for the prepared pattern of a hero myth, but he was introduced to the public in the panther-killing episode, which was published in advance of the book and which helped sell the entire first edition in a single day and establish its author as America's first successful professional novelist. A primitivistic symbol, growing out of the national past, had finally developed in the new world.

Yet Cooper may not have been aware, at the moment, of what he had created. Natty Bumppo (or Leatherstocking, as he came more frequently to be called as the irony gradually disappeared from his characterization) certainly grew upon his creator in the course of the story and acquired dignity in *The Pioneers*. But Cooper's next book was another tale of the American Revolution, *The Pilot* (1823), built around one of the most daring ventures of John Paul Jones and centered upon the character of Long Tom Coffin as a sort of Leatherstocking of the ocean. The self-sufficient sailor, however, was not a part of the common consciousness of the American people, and it was in Natty Bumppo that Cooper found the symbol of communication as well as power. Before he left for Europe in 1826 he wrote and published *The Last of the Mohicans*—an exciting adventure story rather than a novel of manners, dealing with Natty and Chingach-gook's maturity—and in Europe he completed *The Prairie* (1827), which dealt with the beginning of the

97

westward migration and Natty's death on the Nebraska plains. Later he was to involve Natty in a self-sacrificing love affair in *The Pathfinder* (1840) and fill out the complete series of the Leatherstocking Tales with an account of Natty's youth in *The Deerslayer* (1841). With the noble young Hawkeye of that book his portrait of Natty Bumppo was complete.

As one follows the evolution of Natty's character through these books, in the order in which they were written, it becomes evident that he did not spring full-blown from Cooper's mind. His first appearance in *The Pioneers* is almost comic—a scrawny, snaggle-toothed fellow who is so absurdly dressed that his name is obviously ironic. He is more closely akin to Irving's Ichabod Crane than to Daniel Boone, as though Cooper shared Irving's inability to take seriously an American type. As he develops in the course of the book, however, his ridiculous appearance is forgotten, and he becomes a self-reliant individualist in rational rebellion against society and its rules, regulations, inflexibility, and waste. In *The Last of the Mohicans* he is a very glorification of the empiricist, the alert and accurate observer whose ready inferences are immediately translated into actions and whose self-reliant individualism is the salvation of those representatives of society who are in his charge; and in *The Prairie* he becomes the somewhat sentimentalized symbol of the past, the follower of a way of life which has no place in the modern world. It is only in the last two books that his intuitive qualities are greatly emphasized and the reader becomes acutely conscious of his natural goodness. The development of Natty Bumppo's character, in fact, parallels the development of American literature during the early part of the nineteenth century and provides a romanticized but rather extraordinary reflection of what the authors of the Declaration of Independence called "the American Mind."

It is for that reason, perhaps, that the character of Natty Bumppo has remained Cooper's crowning achievement in fiction despite the fact that he was to write richer and more thoughtful novels than any of the Leatherstocking Tales. In Europe he took offense at Scott's failure to deal with social progress in his historical novels and attempted to improve on his master in a trilogy—*The Bravo, The Heidenmauer,* and *The Headsman* (1831–33)—which presented an American democrat's view of the shortcomings of the Venetian republic, the effects of the reformation in Germany, and a fantastic survival of primogeniture in Switzerland. After his return to his own country in 1833 he found that his beloved democracy had changed character in the age of Andrew Jackson, and he became involved in bitter quarrels while devoting himself mostly to the social criticism of such novels as *Homeward Bound* and *Home as Found* (1838) and the instructive essays of *The American Democrat,* of the same year. Out of his antagonism toward the proletarian revolt of the early forties, which found expression in the reform movements, the breakup of political parties, and the rent wars of New York state, grew his finest novels of social history—particularly *Satanstoe* (1845), which provided the eighteenth-century background of the settlement described in *The Chain-*

bearer (1845) and brought the background up to date with the anti-rent violence in *The Redskins* (1846). He also wrote other novels of the American frontier, such as *Wyandotté* (1843), and dealt with the sea in many stories, of which *The Red Rover* (1828) and *Wing-and-Wing* (1842) are perhaps the best; and by the time his prolific career was brought to a close by his death in 1851 the American scene and the American past had become thoroughly absorbed in the main stream of American literature.

In his later years Cooper was joined by a host of writers who pursued similar themes in fiction. John Neal, in *Logan* (1822), had actually preceded him in an elaborate treatment of the Indian; and James K. Paulding's *Koningsmarke: the Long Finne* (1823) discovered the frontiersman simultaneously with *The Pioneers*. But it was not until the middle of the next decade that historical and frontier fiction began to flourish: Robert Montgomery Bird of Philadelphia created the most horrific of Indian fighters in *Nick of the Woods* (1837), and John Pendleton Kennedy of Baltimore turned from the nostalgic local color of *Swallow Barn* (1832) to an effective treatment of the Revolution in *Horse-Shoe Robinson* (1835). By the time Charles Fenno Hoffman produced *Greyslaer* and Daniel Pierce Thompson achieved a perennial popularity with *The Green Mountain Boys*, in 1839, novels and stories of the American past had become a fad.

Among the many writers in the new fashion, however, Cooper's only serious rival was the South Carolinian William Gilmore Simms. Beginning with *Guy Rivers* (1834) and *The Yemassee* (1835), Simms published a large number of exciting border tales, which included a series on the American Revolution running from *The Partisan* (1835) to *Eutaw* (1856) and the sensational *Beauchampe* (1842) based upon a recent Kentucky tragedy which Poe had tried to dramatize. But Simms's virtue was that of a storyteller rather than that of the serious artist whose driving compulsion is to make literary symbols come to terms with those inbred qualities of mind of which he might not be fully aware but upon which he depends for coherence and depth of communication. An ardent southerner who was never completely accepted by his native Charleston, Simms was sectional rather than national and somewhat superficially sectional at that. He neither created nor captured a national or a regional myth, and despite his success in creating exciting plots and vivid scenes his literary style is less vital than even Cooper's.

For James Fenimore Cooper, successful though he was in transferring the Romantic symbol of the past into the American forest, did not triumph over all the difficulties in the way of developing a national literature. His lesser symbols, his actual words, never achieved the life which attracts the sensibilities of later readers and stimulates them to search for deeper meanings than lie on the surface of literature. Although many of the faults which Mark Twain was later to list as his "literary offenses" were the faults of his time, Twain was right in his attribution of insensitivity to a man who did not, while writing, live his material, however much of it he may have drawn from his own past experience. What Cooper did—most evidently in the hero of the Leatherstocking Tales—was to incorporate in fiction the underlying and almost undefinable results of two centuries of American experience. He observed the law of organized society moving into a new land and focused the sympathies of his readers upon a representative American who followed the impulses of his own individuality. He gave his representative American a rare degree of reason in making him a complete observer, acute in his inferences, sound in his judgments, and inclined to follow intuition rather than argument in matters that could not be settled by sensory perception. And he represented him as the natural product of his own environment rather than as a borrowed type placed in a new setting. Such accomplishments represent successive stages in the trial of American literature to see whether it was ready for a genuinely independent development. But Cooper realized all this within the character of Natty Bumppo rather than within himself. It was not until the writer incorporated within himself the results of this slow growth of "the American mind" that his verbal symbols became alive and American literature reached its period of triumph.

PART TWO

The Achievement
1829–1867

CHAPTER FOUR

The Empirical Attitude

I

IF any single author epitomizes the American literary experience of the second quarter of the nineteenth century he is Edgar Allan Poe. Born in Boston of strolling players, he was orphaned at the age of three and taken into the home of John Allan in Richmond, Virginia, and educated in private schools in England and Richmond in preparation for the University of Virginia. After a financially catastrophic year at the university he quarreled with his foster father and ran away to his native Boston where, at the age of eighteen, he enlisted under an assumed name as a private in the United States Army and left with a printer his first volume of verse, *Tamerlane and Other Poems,* which appeared in 1827 with no other signature than "By a Bostonian" on its title page. When a year and a half of successful soldiering found him stationed near Richmond, he renewed his relationships with John Allan and gained his assistance in getting a discharge from the ranks and an appointment to the United

States Military Academy at West Point. He was not again accepted into the Allan household, however, and while awaiting his long-delayed appointment sought out his paternal relatives in Baltimore, where he made his home with his inadequately pensioned grandfather, his aunt, Maria Clemm, and her small daughter Virginia. There he published a second volume of *Poems* in 1829, under his own name, and entered the academy in the autumn of 1830. He had been a good enlisted man, but he was now writing poetry and was rebellious against the discipline used to turn him into an officer and gentleman. As a result, he tried in vain to get an honorable discharge, committed a record number of disciplinary offenses, and left for New York with the permission of the authorities, who court-martialed and officially dismissed him *in absentia*. He took with him enough manuscripts to justify a new edition of his *Poems* and enough subscriptions from his fellow cadets to enable him to print it a few months later in 1831.

This brief personal history is important because it helps explain why Poe, in four short years, made his own peculiar way through the whole literary experience of the preceding generation. He was a socially displaced person—a man who called himself a Bostonian in Virginia accents, who had been reared as an orphan in a city which judged a person by his family background, and brought up to be a gentleman without the funds to sustain his gentility. Both proud and weak, he had no sustaining background which he could proudly call his own; and in his weakness, as his poems show, he was inclined to project himself by his imagination into other backgrounds and take on the protective coloring he found there. His experience resembled that of the earlier generation because he borrowed the symbols of English Romanticism, but it was peculiar in that Poe's symbols were not so much the major subjects and themes of the Romantics as the personalities of the Romantic poets themselves. He apparently tried to be—not simply to write like—Lord Byron and Samuel Taylor Coleridge and, to a lesser extent, John Keats and Percy Bysshe Shelley.

Poe's deeper inclination toward personal rather than toward thematic symbols was not the result of indifference toward the latter. For the title poem of his first volume, *Tamerlane*, was a consciously associationist poem dealing with the influence of nature upon the human spirit in terms of the psychological theories of David Hartley. Under the influence of his natural surroundings its hero developed ideas of sensation, imagination, ambition, and self-interest, and was seduced by a "fickle star within" himself to leave his native mountains and conquer the world before he acquired the higher and more complex ideas of sympathy, God, and morality, for which he eventually returned. But the returned hero is Byronic—old in deeds but not in years, the proud outlaw of his own dark mind, self-exiled from his own success—and attention is focused so intensely, through the device of the confessional monologue, upon the character of the hero that the theme of the poem is generally overlooked. Writing in the first person with many suggestions of self-revelation, Poe identified himself with the Byron of the later *Childe Harold* and *Manfred* and confirmed

the identification in his revisions of the poem by ex-
cising some of the associationist language and trans-
forming the "fickle star" which led him astray into a
Byronic inner "fire."

Such Byronism was not at all unusual, of course, in
a time when a majority of young American poets were
adopting a "pale but interesting" pose, and it seems
natural enough to discover it in "Dreams," "Spirits of
the Dead," "Stanzas," and various other poems in the
1827 volume. The peculiar quality of Poe's imagination only becomes evident when he abandoned his
Byronism and adopted the personality of Keats for his
"Sonnet—To Science" in 1829 and to a certain extent
for "Al Aaraaf" in the same volume. In 1831 he became Shelley for a while in his Platonic conception of
"Israfel," and both Shelley and Byron entered for a
moment into the composition of the otherwise Cole-
ridgean poem "The Sleeper." He had evidently discovered and been captivated by the Galignani pirated
edition of Coleridge, Shelley, and Keats; and of the
three the personality of Coleridge made the deepest
impression upon him. It was to last for a long time,
but among his early writings it is most apparent in
"The City in the Sea" (1831), where he followed the
dreamy imagination of the author of "Kubla Khan"
down through the "caverns measureless to man into a
sunless sea," where he found a city which may have
been designed for pleasure but was inhabited by
Death.

The literary evidences of a tendency toward borrowed personality are hard to separate from evidences
of imitation and even parody, and Poe's first ventures

into prose fiction, in his plan for a collection of "Tales of the Folio Club," show that he actually depended upon imitation and parody for his literary inspiration. The only practical distinction between the two processes, perhaps, must be made in terms of depth. When Poe wrote "The Scythe of Time" (later called "The Predicament"), for example, he was obviously writing a parody of the kind of magazine fiction he had satirized in "How to Write a Blackwood Article"; but when he used the same formula and the same conceit of the scythe of time in "The Pit and the Pendulum" he gave the impression of a personal sense of terror rather than that of the commercialized sensationalism which he had once satirized. Poe's success in creating this sort of illusion was first evident in the early horror story "Berenice," which he sent to the editor of the *Southern Literary Messenger* in 1834 with a letter of apology and explanation. The story might be considered a violation of good taste, he wrote, but it was of the kind that increased the circulation of the popular British magazines; and he cited numerous examples, including the serialized *Confessions of an English Opium Eater,* which was then thought to be the composition of Coleridge. The knowing references to opium dreams and other dissipations in such successive stories as "Ligeia" and "The Fall of the House of Usher" show that Poe was building his own Romantic personality out of elements of Coleridge and Byron and, as a writer at least, living this role convincingly.

This Romantic personality reached its most perfect development in "The Raven" in 1845, in which the Byronic hero was struggling, like Coleridge in the "Ode to Dejection," to find surcease from sorrow by abstruse research in strange and curious volumes of forgotten lore; and in the recitations he delivered as "the author of 'The Raven'" Poe seems to have played this role to the limit by making the most of his pale but interesting countenance and his threadbare suggestion of a proud past. But the role could have been satisfactory to him only in occasional creative moments. For Poe's normal life was anything but romantic. He had married his cousin Virginia when she had reached the age of thirteen, and by doing so had acquired a mother in Mrs. Clemm and the obligation to support a family in the hard world of commerical journalism. As editor of the *Southern Literary Messenger*, Burton's *Gentleman's Magazine*, and *Graham's*, as free-lance writer and eventually as proprietor of his own *Broadway Journal*, he fought off poverty from 1835 to 1845 with copyreading, criticism, reviewing, and creative work in a profession where competition was stiff and ruthless and he himself was handicapped by susceptibility to alcohol. To survive and maintain his pathetic pride in such an environment he had to play an empirical as well as a Romantic role.

His earliest approaches to commercial fiction were in themselves indicative of an empirical strain of mind, and this strain found a public outlet in his early criticism. But this anti-Romantic attitude became a role about 1841 when he began to write such calculated "tales of ratiocination" as "The Murders in the Rue Morgue," "A Descent into the Maelström," "The Mystery of Marie Rogêt," and "The Gold Bug." At about the same time, in 1842, he systematized his critical formula for the short story in a review of Nathaniel Hawthorne's *Twice-Told Tales* which stressed the need for "unity of effect" through an appeal to some single intellectual faculty comparable to faculties identified by the pseudoscientific theories of phrenology. In his detailed account of M. Dupin's methods of observation and inference in "The Murders in the Rue Morgue" Poe had identified and described the sort of ratiocination used in these stories and in much of his criticism, but he did not lay claim to it as the dominant quality of his own mind until he published "The Philosophy of Composition" (1846) in a gesture of rebellion against any identification of himself with the hero of "The Raven." For the hero of this fantastic account of how he wrote the poem is the complete opposite of the Romantic—a coldly calculating emotional engineer whose approach to poetry is rational rather than emotional, empirical rather than intuitive —a kind of Benjamin Franklin among poets who could pass himself off as a Byron whenever he put his mind to it. The personal implications of the poem and the essay are almost schizophrenic.

But Poe, however morbid he might appear in the pages of biographers who were overimpressed by his Romantic past, was not a mental case. He was an American, striving to find a successful way to adapt borrowed literary symbols to an inbred attitude of mind. He had obscurely felt, as Cooper had not, that the adaptation should be made within himself; and his unfortunate personal circumstances had enabled him first to project himself into his symbols. But his whole cultural environment was against this experiment, and he reacted by professing to be a sort of architect of composition who was as practical and materialistic as the world in which he moved. Yet he knew that his reaction was extreme, and even before writing "The Philosophy of Composition" he had sought a middle ground of intellectuality on which he could stand firmly. He defined it in a revised characterization of M. Dupin in "The Purloined Letter" of 1845. In this story Dupin developed into a man of intuition as well as a man of reasoning, a poet as well as a mathematician, whose imagination provided him with a hypothesis, whose reason controlled its application in terms of probability, and whose observation merely verified it. He reversed the procedure he had followed in "The Murders in the Rue Morgue" and "The Mystery of Marie Rogêt" by first solving the mystery and then looking over the situation. In the language of eighteenth-century American intellectual history, he followed "an intellectual light within him" when the "light of sense" (as represented by such a highly trained observer as the prefect of police) had failed.

This was the intellectual pattern that Poe himself, in his later years, was determined to follow and by which he was to reconcile the two extremes of his affected personalities. He was to write like the introspective hero of "The Raven" in such later poems as "Ulalume" and "Annabel Lee," like the calculating author of "The Philosophy of Composition" in "The Bells," and perhaps like a combination of the two in the technically magnificent short story "The Cask of Amontillado"; but the work he took most seriously and by which he expected to be known to posterity was his prose poem *Eureka*, published in 1848, the year before his death. In it he attempted to solve the mystery of the universe, its creation and destruction, and he began by a grotesque satire upon traditional modes of reasoning and an intensely serious description of the intellectual path that he himself would pursue. The reasoning processes he satirized were the "creeping and crawling" methods of deductive logic from Aristotle to Immanuel Kant and of inductive logic from Francis Bacon to John Stuart Mill. The true advancement of learning, he maintained, came through leaps of intuition, which produced theories that could be called truths when they were corrected and cleared of their inconsistencies. By this method he developed his highly imaginative conception of a universe which had been created by an explosion of "unparticled matter" and which was falling rapidly toward its own center and would eventually collapse into the nothingness of unparticled matter again.

Such a grandiose theory, of course, was unlike M. Dupin's theory of the purloined letter in that it could not be verified by observation; and Poe's last mad gesture of escape was to spurn all solid ground while allowing his imagination to take off into infinity under the exclusive control of his phrenological bump of comparison. Yet in his own peculiar way he discovered the method of bringing life into the verbal symbols of American literature by striving intensely within himself to bring into adjustment the larger symbols of popular communication in English and the basic attitude of mind absorbed from his American environment. He was pursuing what Nathaniel Hawthorne, in a favorite phrase, called "wisdom tested by the tenor of a life." The inadequacy and pretentiousness of his wisdom and the waywardness and perversity of his life limit his greatness but not his vitality. His words live to be read—with pleasure, fascination, and often distaste, but with an inner value that cannot be denied. With him American literature passed through its trial and entered its period of triumph.

II

The tenor of Nathaniel Hawthorne's life was as different from that of Poe's as was his background. For Hawthorne was a firmly settled New Englander, born and bred in the oldest of Massachusetts Bay towns, Salem, where until the age of thirty-four he lived with his widowed mother and older sisters with only such ventures abroad as were required by summer vacations, a college education in Bowdoin, and a brief interval of magazine editorship in Boston. Three years after his graduation from college he published his first novel, *Fanshawe* (1828), which started out as an imitation and ended up as a synopsis of the manner of Sir Walter Scott—a performance which evidently shocked its author as soon as he saw it in print, for he immediately withdrew it from circulation and attempted to destroy the existing copies. When he recovered he began the slow process of learning to write, and the rest of his life was devoted to the two severely practical activities of writing and earning a living. He rarely mixed the two—never, after his first early experience, attempted to become a journalist like Poe. He earned very little from his short stories, and before he became a novelist he lived by working in the Boston Customs House from 1838 to 1840, by acting as the unpaid treasurer for Brook Farm (in the vain hope of finding in that Transcendental community a place to live cheaply, write, and bring his wife-to-be during the following year), and by serving as surveyor of customs in his native Salem from 1847 to 1849. Eight years later he was appointed American consul in Liverpool by a classmate who had been elected president of the United States, and after four fairly remunerative years he turned again to writing, in Italy and England, before coming home to die in 1863.

From intensive reading in the secluded atmosphere of old Salem and from the folklore he picked up on his vacations, Hawthorne acquired a richer knowledge of the New England past than was possessed by most writers of his generation, and he was closely associated with it through the traditions of his own family, which included a judge in the notorious Salem witchcraft trials of the seventeenth century and the popular hero of a Revolutionary sea ballad. *Fanshawe,* though its scene was a college town very much like the one he knew, had shown how much he had been attracted by the historical romance; and it was only natural, when he began to write more seriously, that he should have accepted the popular symbol of the past as his medium of communication. He was also attracted, like Poe, by the Gothic element in English Romanticism and was to make frequent use of the supernatural and the occult. He was not, however, a sensationalist by nature or by affectation. By cultural tradition he was a moralist and by disposition an observer, and his creative imagination was compact of Romantic symbols and realistic observations leading to some moral conclusion. The tenor of his own life was detached, matter-of-fact almost to the point of skepticism, and judicious; and the wisdom which passed its test was mildly speculative and largely empirical.

The story of Hawthorne's development as a literary artist is the story of a growing firmness of confidence in his own wisdom and of a gradual shift of emphasis from symbol to substance until Romantic material became a flexible medium of realistic self-expression. One of the earliest of his published short stories, a mere sketch called "The Hollow of the Three Hills" (1830), is interesting chiefly as an illustration of his starting point. Its time is the colonial period, its setting something like Poe's later "misty mid-region of Wier," and its characters a witch and her client who wants a supernatural vision of the effects of her elopement upon her abandoned husband and family. She learns that the effects have been devastating and dies in an illustration of the moral, so conventional to the triangle story in sentimental fiction, that the wages of sin is death. From such an unpromising beginning Hawthorne developed a richness of intellectual and artistic interests which can only be sampled in terms of certain questions which he posed to himself and answered as he grew in assurance. The most important of these, perhaps, concerned the validity of empirical observations—the trustworthiness of those appearances from which the senses collected material for judgment.

Hawthorne posed the question in the story of "Young Goodman Brown" (1835) who either attended or dreamed that he had attended a witches' Sabbath and saw there all the good people of his seventeenth-century New England village. Was his experience real or imaginary? Were the good people hiding hearts of evil or were they what they seemed? Young Goodman Brown was never allowed to know because Hawthorne himself had not yet made up his mind. He offered a tentative opinion almost immediately in the allegory of "The Minister's Black Veil" (1836) in which the veil was a symbol of the minister's conviction that every man's heart was obscure to his fellows, but it was not until 1843, in "Egotism, or The Bosom Serpent" that he expressed his own belief in the ubiquity of secret sin. The questioning skepticism apparent in these stories, however, was a permanent quality of his mind.

Such skepticism posed another question for the artist who had to deal in appearances but had to go beneath them in order to avoid the superficial and the commonplace. Could he do so? He could, Hawthorne decided, but only at a cost to himself. If he dug into his material with an inner wisdom, Hawthorne suggested in "Drowne's Wooden Image" (1844), he might, in "a brief period of excitement, kindled by love," find the touch of genius necessary to the life of his own images. But the price, he added in "The Artist of the Beautiful" (published in the same month), was isolation from the common affairs of humanity through a predominating "sense of moral cold," which placed ordinary human love in competition with his art. Even if he succeeded in the supreme act of creation, the practical attitude of the world might rob his work of its life, or carelessness might destroy it. The artist was a lonely man whose greatest accomplishment had to be realized entirely within himself.

Most of Hawthorne's American contemporaries felt that the writer's place was on the world's great field of battle—that he should be up and doing—and Hawthorne himself found a resemblance between the isolation of the poet and that of such active types as the prophet, the reformer, and the criminal. So, in the years of his development, he had to face a final question concerning the responsibilities of a man whose pursuits placed him "either in advance of mankind, or apart from it." He had already expressed the opinion, in "Dr. Heidegger's Experiment" (1837), that it was vain to interfere with the normal course of natural events, and in "The Birth Mark" (1843) he concluded that the effort to do so would lead only to tragedy. His world was the everyday world, and his role in it was that of a penetrating observer who brought forth wisdom and expressed it in a form designed for delight. Such was the wisdom he had tested by the tenor of his own life and brought to literary perfection in the last and finest of his short stories from this period— "Rappaccini's Daughter" (1844), the Gothic folk tale of a poison maiden whose beautiful appearance concealed the death within and whose innocent love affair demonstrated the tragedy of cold-blooded interference with the course of nature. Hawthorne's use of Romantic material to express his realistic view of the world reached its climax in that story.

But he was to continue to develop as an artist, and the short stories also reveal the influence of his intellect upon his art. For Hawthorne's compulsion to observe beneath the surface of human appearances pushed him into the realm of psychology. An impulse in that direction may be seen in one of the earliest of his tales, "Roger Malvin's Burial" (1832), in which he shows an interest in the effects of a broken promise upon a young man's later life and his tragic release from its burden. The impulse is stronger in "Young Goodman Brown," where the question of the actuality of Brown's experience is irrelevant to the author's concern with the question raised by its effect upon him. "The Minister's Black Veil" often puzzles readers by its subtitle "A Parable" because the parable is in the minister's act of donning the veil and the story is mostly about the psychological effects of the act upon the puzzled parishioners. What was happening in these and other stories was that Hawthorne's artistic interest was developing in two directions—one the direction of meditating upon the questions posed in his tales and eventually expressing his opinions in the form of conclusive moral allegories, and the other the direction of pursuing his answers through the minds of his characters. "Rappaccini's Daughter" owes much of its effectiveness to the fact that it avoided these extremes and is neither a psychological story nor an allegory but a fantasy which includes motive and meaning, and it was in this state of balance between two artistic directions that Hawthorne escaped from the pressure of constant writing and gathered his forces for a return to the longer form of fiction.

In the two decades after *Fanshawe* Hawthorne's total publication amounted to only three volumes of short stories: *Twice-Told Tales* in 1837, a second edition with an added volume in 1842, and *Mosses from an Old Manse* in 1846. The last took its title from the house in Concord, Massachusetts, to which he had taken his bride, Sophia Peabody, and in which he lived until his savings were exhausted and he was in desperate need to stop writing and work for a living. A new political administration enabled him to receive an appointment as surveyor of customs in Salem, and he laid aside his pen and returned home in 1847. He was approaching the peak of his creative development, however, and his major intellectual preoccupations with secret sin and the evils of interfering with nature seem to have been pushing him toward some story which would be longer and more clearly moral than "Rappaccini's Daughter." What was going on in his mind and in the privacy of his office or study is not a matter of record, but we can infer from the results that he was at the crossroads of his development. He could either invent a story which had a meaning and thus continue with his parables or moral allegories, or he could make a story out of his own search for its meaning by exploring the effects of some significant action upon the inner lives of his characters and thus become a psychological novelist. Although he could not have seen his alternatives so clearly, it is probable that he considered the novel as an art form and rejected it because he did not trust himself to deal with the common affairs of everyday life as he thought a formal novelist must. Instead he settled upon the "romance"—something off the beaten paths of normal existence—which would give him the freedom of intellectual realism without the restraints of actuality. But his dilemma existed even within the bounds of this compromise.

The result, in 1849, was the "fragment" of an "abortive" moral romance and a completed historical one. The first was published in the *Boston Magazine* for January of the following year under the title "Ethan Brand." It took its origin from a suggestion contained in "Egotism, or The Bosom Serpent" that there was some wanderer abroad in the world whose secret sin was worse than egotism, and it identified this "unpardonable sin" as an abstract "hardness of heart." But a reference within the published story was more specific; for Ethan Brand, in his wandering search for the unpardonable sin, had at one time performed a "psychological experiment upon a young girl," and this violation of another personality was his most severe offense against human sympathy. The published story was another Gothic fantasy, but back of it lay some of Hawthorne's very real preoccupations and worries— his feeling that an artist's inquisitive observations estranged him from humanity, his agitated fears concerning his wife's interest in mesmerism as a possible psychological cure for her frequent headaches, his conscience-ridden notion that his own professional curiosity about the human mind somehow identified him with hypnotic charlatans of the stage and couch and categorized artists as passive brethren of criminals and reformers.

But Hawthorne was finding human beings too complex to be presented as figures in moral allegory. He had read the psychological writings of his old college professor Thomas Upham and had found in Upham's simplified theories a framework for analyzing individuals without risking the pitfalls of actuality. His finished romance, in consequence, was analytic rather than allegorical in its conception, deterministic rather than parabolic in its plot. *The Scarlet Letter* (1850) was a story of the three major characters in a conventional triangle plot: Hester Prynne, who was married to an elderly physician, Roger Chillingworth, and her lover, the brilliant young Puritan minister, Arthur Dimmesdale. The hackneyed love story so familiar to readers of the sentimental novel, however, was entirely in the background. Hawthorne began his tale with Hester's release from the colonial New England prison, where she had served the first part of her sentence for adultery; she was beginning her additional sentence, to wear forever in public the scarlet letter "A" as a sign of her sin. He could not have written the book had not two decades of observation, since "The Hollow of the Three Hills," taught him that the wages of sin might be life instead of death. For the story was about Hester's growth and her lover's and husband's decay —a growth and decay determined by the effects of her adultery upon three characters of distinctly different psychological composition.

In the terms used by Upham for his threefold analysis of personality—intellect, affections, and will—all three characters were of high intellectual capacity, although Hester's capacities were undeveloped. Her primary characteristic at the beginning of the story is the strength of will which enables her to endure her punishment, remain in her own community with her illegitimate child, and wear her symbol of adultery boldly while stubbornly concealing the identity of her lover. The first part of the book deals with her intellectual growth until "her life had turned, in a great measure, from passion and feeling, to thought," and she had assumed "a freedom of speculation" almost unknown in colonial America. But "the scarlet letter," Hawthorne said, "had not yet done its office." Her passion and feeling had been self-centered, and the remaining part of the story reveals the development of her social affections as her peculiar circumstances brought her into broader sympathy with humankind. She became, at the end, a completely developed person. In contrast, Roger Chillingworth's lack of sympathy destroyed him. Rich in his intellectual endowments, strong in will, he devoted himself to the purpose of discovering and destroying the man who had wronged him. His was the hardness of heart attributed to Ethan Brand, and he demonstrated it by the psychological experiment he performed on Arthur Dimmesdale while serving as a physician to his body as he tried to destroy his soul. What he actually accomplished was his own spiritual destruction. Between the two stood Arthur Dimmesdale, intellectual and compassionate, who was too weak to confess and pay the social penalty for his crime and whose weakness made him the battleground for the conflicting wills of Hester and Roger. He died physically of the strain but was saved spiritually when, with Hester's assistance, he found the strength of will necessary to gasp out his confession. This psychological plot was worked out in little more than outline, for Hawthorne was an expositor rather than an illustrator of the inner lives of his characters; but this was the plot determined by that "dark necessity" of which Roger Chillingworth spoke with "gloomy sternness" when he referred to "fate" in terms of a chain of causation beginning with Hester's first sin.

The Scarlet Letter is thus the first deterministic novel in English, but Hawthorne was a moralist rather than a logician, and the intellectual substance of the story is to be found in its anti-Puritan morality rather than in the Edwardsian or Cartesian logic of its plot. Unlike Alfred Tennyson in the contemporary *Idylls of the King*, Hawthorne had looked at the world rather than its conventions for the truth he would express in his art. He had discovered that empirical truth and proverbial morality did not always correspond and had merely chosen to rationalize his empirical observations in terms of psychological determinism. That his deterministic method was an artistic device rather than a serious intellectual quality is revealed by his next book, *The House of the Seven Gables* (1851), in which the determinism was purely romantic and the morality conventional—the working out of an old curse which visited the sins of the fathers upon the children of several generations. He came closer to the conventional novel in this story of contemporary Salem, which included among its characters a leading politician of the town, than he ever came in his other books; but he reversed his usual method by making the plot romantic and its trappings real and sacrificed his greatest strength in the change.

For Hawthorne's peculiar attraction for critics who are too sophisticated for the sensationalism of Poe is to be found in his use of Romantic symbols to express the thoughtful conclusions of a realistic mind. From that came the quality of ambiguity, ambivalence, or irony which many critics love faithfully despite their inconstant terminology; and the weakness of his later novels came from his efforts to escape or subordinate the Romantic symbols he had learned to use so well. His next book, *The Blithedale Romance* (1852), had as its working title the name of its central character, Hollingsworth, and was evidently designed as a realistic case study of a type prevalent on the American scene —the reformer, a man so obsessed with philanthropy that his natural human sympathies were perverted to the brink of madness. Its setting was partly in a Transcendental community like Brook Farm, which was "a little removed from the highway of ordinary travel," he said in the Preface, and was therefore a theater in which his characters could act out their parts "without exposing them to too close a comparison with the actual events of real lives." But he seems to have felt insecure without his Gothic symbols and so introduced into the book an unnecessary secondary villain, the mesmerist Westervelt, who performed a psychological experiment upon a young girl and brought with him an atmosphere of mystery but made no real contribution to the major plot. This was to be Hawthorne's last work of fiction for eight years. It represented a broadening of his psychological interests from the individuals he had examined in *The Scarlet Letter* to the types he had approached in *The House of the Seven Gables* and handled more firmly here. But it also represented a tendency toward speculative psychology which took him off the solid ground of observation, weakened his control over Romantic symbols, and made him use them for sensational rather than intellectual effects.

When Hawthorne had written his campaign biography of Franklin Pierce, served out his consular appointment at Liverpool, traveled in Italy, and returned to fiction with *The Marble Faun* (1860) his tendency toward speculation had increased and his interests broadened from the psychology of types to the philosophy of human nature. This was his most ambitious novel, for in it he attempted to sketch the Italy of monuments, art galleries, and expatriate Americans and to deal with the philosophical problem of evil as he had dealt with the individual problem in *The Scarlet Letter*. Its central character was the faunlike Donatello, Count of Monte Beni, who has the natural innocence and graceful simplicity of an animal until he commits a murder at the subtle instigation of a female character and is brought by punishment and remorse to a state of moral consciousness which makes him human. The story is a modern version of the Garden of Eden with the Miltonic thesis of the fortunate Fall through which humankind can be elevated to a new and greater estate than that of innocence. An American sculptor, Kenyon, makes its implications specific when he confesses to his "perplexity": "Sin has educated Donatello, and elevated him. Is sin, then,—

which we deem such a dreadful blackness in the universe,—is it, like sorrow, merely an element of human education, through which we struggle to a higher and purer state than we could otherwise have attained? Did Adam fall, that we might ultimately rise to a far loftier paradise than his?" With Hester Prynne, Hawthorne had been able to give a clearly affirmative answer to a comparable question because he had seen enough of the world to imagine an individual who could be improved by experiencing sin and suffering its consequences. Logically he could extend his imagination backward to the realization of such a character in a state of innocence comparable to that of the original Adam. But did he have any empirical evidence for the universal application of his particular observations? Could the Baconian method support a great philosophical truth?

In Hawthorne's mind it could not. The sculptor could only ask forgiveness of the shocked Hilda who protested that his speculations made mockery "not only of all religious sentiments, but of moral law." Hawthorne himself had the same limitations as Matthew Arnold in "Dover Beach"; he could merely say, in effect, "Ah, love, let us be true to one another," as the sea of his empirical wisdom withdrew over the drear and naked shingles of a world beyond his powers of observation. His wisdom was that of his own life— observant, questioning, perceptive, and assured only when his speculations could be supported by his individual perceptions. Like Poe, he was tempted to speculate beyond the limits of his individual wisdom; but, unlike the wayward author of *Eureka*, he held onto the light of the senses rather than discard it in favor of some intellectual light within. In doing so he sacrificed breadth and failed to master the great philosophical theme with which his fancy played in *The Marble Faun,* but he brought the symbols of Romanticism down to American earth and in *The Scarlet Letter* completely mastered them. He and Poe each illustrates in his own way the lesson that the American writer had been obliged to learn—that he had to find within himself the means of adapting the popular materials of a literature in English to the attitudes of mind characteristic of people who were not English but who were sharing with the English a cultural heritage which had begun to diverge into separate ways. He differed from Poe in that his life and mind were more firmly rooted in the prevailing empiricism of the American tradition, and in that difference lay Hawthorne's greatest strength and his greatest limitation.

III

The lesson illustrated by Poe and Hawthorne is one that American writers found hard to learn, and the external forces that encouraged a talented man to take the easy way of avoiding it are best revealed in the career of Henry Wadsworth Longfellow. A younger classmate of Hawthorne's at Bowdoin College, Longfellow was a more brilliant man to whom success came early. At the time of his graduation at the age of seventeen he was offered a position as instructor in modern languages at his college and went abroad to improve his knowledge of French, Spanish, and Ital-

ian. By the time he reached the age at which Hawthorne began his apprenticeship to the art of the short
story, Longfellow had proved himself a competent
poet and essayist and so able a teacher and scholar
that he was offered the Smith Professorship of Modern
Languages at Harvard on condition that he make another trip abroad in order to perfect himself in "the
German." On this trip his young wife died in Rotter-
dam, and the bereaved husband threw himself into the
study of modern German literature, escaping, somewhat as Poe did, into symbols created by other writers
and especially by the young Johann Wolfgang von
Goethe. He also met the stately young Frances Ap-
pleton, daughter of a prominent Boston banker, and
spelled his grief by long private periods of Romantic
passion.

When he returned to take up his duties at Harvard,
he continued to pursue Frances, proposed marriage
and was rejected, and exposed his pursuit and passion
most romantically in two books published in 1839—
Hyperion: A Romance, strongly influenced by Goethe's *The Sorrows of Young Werther,* and a volume of
poems appropriately called *Voices of the Night.* The
two books revealed enough to contemporary Boston to
cause something of a scandal, and the second reveals
enough to the historian to show that Longfellow had
learned early and consciously the lesson that Poe and
Hawthorne illustrate. For the collection of poems included some of his early nature verse in the manner of
English Romanticism, and in the "Proem" to the volume he referred to them and declared that he should
put aside such childish things and look into his heart

and write. He resolved to do so, expressing his passionate distress in such verses as those of the title poem and indicating his determination to overcome it in "The Psalm of Life," which he had written to illustrate and grasp the mature wisdom of the Goethe who composed the articles of indenture for the conclusion of *Wilhelm Meister's Apprenticeship*. But the public reaction to his attempt to wear a German heart on a Boston sleeve evidently made him review his lesson and discard it. Instead of developing a greater emotional maturity in his verse, he suppressed the dictates of his heart, produced a collection of popular *Ballads and Other Poems* in 1842, and never again exposed his inner life to the public although he worried himself to the verge of a nervous breakdown and made another trip abroad to recover.

The rewards for his discretion were many and great. He quickly became the most popular and most highly paid magazine poet in America, Frances married him in 1843, and he settled down to a widely admired family life in Craigie House as a scholar-poet whose adaptations of foreign meters to English words made him one of the most versatile poetic technicians in the language. The shorter poems collected in such volumes as *The Belfrey of Bruges and Other Poems* (1846) and *The Seaside and the Fireside* (1850), the narrative *Tales of a Wayside Inn* (1863, 1872, 1873), and the long single poems *Evangeline* (1847), *Hiawatha* (1855), and *The Courtship of Miles Standish* (1858) were all enormously popular and made him the best known of all American writers abroad. But he had his secret disappointments. The posthumously published sonnet, "Mezzo Cammin," written on his thirty-fifth birthday during his third trip abroad, reflects his regret at having spent half his life without accomplishing some great work; and he evidently tried to force such an accomplishment by finding some great subject. He experimented unsuccessfully with the major reform movement of his time in some *Poems on Slavery* (1842) but eventually settled upon a poetic history of Christianity in the form of a dramatic trilogy. He began with a considerable amount of energy by a treatment of Christianity in the Middle Ages in *The Golden Legend* (1851) but had to force himself to the continuation in *The New England Tragedies* (1868)—one of them, *John Endicott*, actually written in prose and translated into blank verse—and to the first drama of the trilogy, *The Divine Tragedy* (1871). Published all together as *Christus: A Mystery*, they sold well but represented no great literary achievement: Longfellow never succeeded in erecting that "lofty parapet of song" of which he dreamed in his youth.

Yet running through the great amount of his work is a thin strain of memorable poetry which stands out in impressive contrast to the wordy hexameters of the sentimental *Evangeline* and the even wordier trochees of the Indian epic *Hiawatha*. And most of it shows that he had ignored rather than forgotten the lesson summarized in the "Proem" for his first collection of verse. For Longfellow's best poems were formed by the union of some detached image with a deep emotion which he was able only obliquely to express. "The Arsenal at Springfield" (1844) is a magnificent exercise in metaphor comparing the massed guns to an organ, but it is vitalized by a passion for peace under the threat of imminent war; and "The Building of the Ship" (1849) gathers force from the concluding intensity of the poet's demand for union at a time when the sentiment for disunion was strong in New England. Such poems as "My Lost Youth" (which adapted Johann von Herder's translation of a Lapland song to Longfellow's nostalgia for Portland, Maine) or "Jugurtha" and other poems on old age may be exceptions to the rule in that they are direct expressions of conventional emotions, but Longfellow's finest poetic achievement was a direct outgrowth of his deepest and most carefully controlled feeling.

The six sonnets of the "Divina Commèdia" sequence were written and used as introductions and conclusions to Longfellow's translation of the three parts of Dante Alighieri's poem. But they bear reference to the tragic occasion which forced him into the labor of translation—the death of Frances, by fire from an exploding lamp, in the spring of 1861. As he had done after the death of his first wife, Longfellow sought to escape from personal sorrow by entering into another literature in another language; but this time he was able to blend his greater grief with a work of art more intellectually and emotionally mature than the products of German Romanticism. The first sonnet, used to introduce the *Inferno*, is the most directly personal. In it Longfellow compares Dante's "medieval miracle of song" to a great Gothic cathedral into which he can enter, "not ashamed to pray," and escape "the loud reverberations of the street" while "the eternal ages watch and wait." The allusion, however, is to the turmoil accompanying the outbreak of the American Civil War in that year, and it is only by indirection that the reader can follow the author in this and successive sonnets through the stages of his private grief for which the stages of Dante's poem serve as a device which some modern critics would call an "objective correlative." Yet the fifth sonnet, introducing the *Paradiso*, is deeply moving in its imagery of Beatrice "clothed in a garment as of flame" and of the rose; and the sixth, with its great tribute to the poet whose words provided "the pathway of thought for all Italy," may have acquired dignity from the author's own determination to continue building, almost immediately, his own lofty parapet of song. Longfellow was to pay fine and discriminating tribute to other poets in other sonnets during the years that followed, and he may have been at his best in recognizing in others those qualities that he had not been able to achieve.

In some respects the most happy of American writers were those who faced the conditions faced by Longfellow—the rich rewards of conformity to the public taste and the condemnation of all deviation into European manners—and found within themselves the qualities which a superficial public liked. Such a person, at any rate, was Oliver Wendell Holmes—a wit and man of sentiment who blended his two characteristics into a light charm from which he rarely deviated in his poems or essays. From the time he brought together the sentiment of "Old Ironsides" and the wit and humor of "The Ballad of the Oysterman" in "The Last Leaf" (1831) to the time he composed "Dorothy Q" (1871) in his declining years, he preserved an astonishing unity of poetic tone which is perhaps best exemplified in the perfection of "On Lending a Punch Bowl" (1849). The secret of his success, perhaps, may be found in his earliest essays written for the *New England Magazine* in 1832, for they are obvious imitations of Laurence Sterne and readily caught the fancy of a public which had a long and happy acquaintance with Shandyism. Yet Holmes was his own Yorick and his own Mr. Shandy, and when he began his essays again, after a twenty-five year interruption, for the *Atlantic* in 1857, "The Autocrat of the Breakfast Table" could no longer be classed as an imitator of anybody. His sentiments and his prejudices, his wit and his passion for punning (which he humorously denounced as a form of "verbicide") had become so characteristically Holmesian that he could sustain them through a long series of "breakfast table" papers attributed to "the Autocrat," "the Poet," and "the Professor" until he moved them into the twilight of "Over the Teacups" (1890) at the age of eighty-one.

As a scientist, surgeon, and distinguished physician, he was profoundly serious about some things—carelessness and quackery in his own profession, which he attacked in such essays as "The Contagiousness of Puerperal Fever" (1843) and "Homoeopathy and Its Kindred Delusions"; the notion of conflict between science and religion, which he denied implicitly in "The Chambered Nautilus" (1858) and explicitly in "The Secret of the Stars"; and the Calvinistic dogma of predestination, which he bitterly opposed in his essay "Jonathan Edwards" (1880) and in the first of his "medicated novels" *Elsie Venner* (1861). But he was at his best when he was taking even serious matters lightly, as in the veiled satire on the logic of Jonathan Edwards in "The Deacon's Masterpiece; or, The Wonderful 'One-Hoss Shay'" among the verses included in the *Autocrat of the Breakfast Table* (1858). Rarely in his literary writings did he lose his temper—as he did when he felt pushed around by too many reformers and wrote the biting verses of "The Moral Bully" (1862)—but, instead, kept the equanimity of a man who was sure of himself within a small but popularly acceptable range of feeling and who was therefore one of the most consistently successful minor writers of his time.

These men—Poe, Hawthorne, Longfellow, and Holmes—represent the empirical strain in American literature of the mid-nineteenth century. They indulged in various fancies and experienced varying degrees of emotion, but they followed reason in the Baconian sense of what John Locke had called the "human understanding" and tested wisdom by the tenor of individual lives that fell within the two patterns set by the flighty Poe and the solid Hawthorne. None of them (except Poe, perhaps, in his last mad fling) tried to magnify the intuitive light within them into an absolute guiding principle, and none of them, in consequence, brought the whole pattern of American thought to bear on the problem of literature. Their shortcomings left a vacuum into which another school of writers, usually called Transcendentalists, were all too eager to rush.

CHAPTER FIVE

Transcendentalism

I

RALPH WALDO EMERSON received an extraordinarily good if completely uncalculated training to become the leader of the Transcendental movement in America. Like Hawthorne, he lost his father at an early age, but he was not brought up in the atmosphere of seclusion which characterized the Hawthorne home. Mrs. William Emerson had four sons to rear, practically no financial resources, and a rugged sister-in-law who was determined that the boys would not only be reared but educated in the expectation that some if not all of them would enter the Congregational or at the worst the Unitarian ministry in which their father had been prominent. So the boys were brought up in the penny-pinching atmosphere of a boardinghouse—many boardinghouses, in fact, for Mrs. Emerson rarely made enough from her boarders to keep up with her rent—while the boys struggled through preparatory school and helped themselves and each other through Harvard College. Waldo graduated in 1821, made a trip south for his health, taught school for a while, passed through the Harvard Divinity School, and in 1829 was ordained as the assistant to the pastor of his father's old church in Boston. He was married in the same year to Ellen Tucker, who died in 1832.

Such an early background would normally tend to keep a young man's feet on the ground and turn him into a plodder after he achieved a position of security. But within it Emerson found certain impulses toward the clouds. In the first place, he possessed a considerable amount of private literary ambition, which found expression in the copious verses he was scribbling throughout his youth. In the second, he had instilled in him a driving self-reliance by the determination of his aunt, Mary Moody Emerson, and by the obstacles he had to overcome in his efforts to get an education. And in the third, he was caught by a rising tide of ideas that carried him forward on its crest. The tide had risen on the other side of the Atlantic and consisted of a body of intellectual symbols which were as important to the development of American literature as were the material symbols of Romanticism. They were ideas which were supposed to transcend those that John Locke attributed to sensation and reflection and were therefore eventually to be called Transcendental.

They began to elevate Emerson's mind so unobtrusively that he could hardly have thought of himself as doing more than drifting along on the stream of conformity. For Harvard College had developed in the American tradition and continued to reflect the prevailing American attitudes of mind. It placed great emphasis upon the philosophical training of its students and brought their training to a climax in their senior year by careful instruction in the empirical philosophy of Locke's *Essay on the Human Understanding*. But its authorities, like the good Americans they were, distrusted the elaborately rationalistic empiricists who followed Locke—Bishop George Berkeley, whose reasoning cast doubt on one's ability to know the real existence of the physical universe; David Hume, whose skepticism extended to ideas themselves; David Hartley, whose psychological theories were wholly material; and Bishop William Paley, whose observations and reflections had led him to a cold-blooded utilitarian morality and whose rationalism had to be balanced by the analogical reasoning of Bishop Butler before his religious theories could be made fit for undergraduates. Accordingly, every student who was tutored on the *Human Understanding* was formally required to write an essay criticizing Locke with respect to "certain controverted points."

The most essential of these points was Locke's use of the *tabula rasa*, or blank tablet on which ideas were engraved by experience and reflection, as an image of the human mind and its implicit denial of the existence of innate ideas. It violated the well-established American belief in self-evident truths, and Harvard would have none of it as an absolute principle. The hard-headed New Englanders were quite willing to assume that the external world was self-evidently real, most of them were quite willing to accept God on the same basis, and they had found a school of kindred souls in Scotland who were willing to assert as much in an aggressive philosophical system. Under the leadership of Thomas Reid, they had been called the Scottish "Common-Sense" school of philosophy because they insisted that all human beings, in all times and places, had a common sense of reality, morality, and beauty. They had modernized the residual Platonism in Puritan thought, put it in opposition to the empiricism of Locke, and used it to attack the new skepticism. The Harvard students of Emerson's generation were required to study Reid's *Inquiry into the Human Mind* before they were allowed to approach Locke. At the personal suggestion of Harvard's president, Emerson also read Dugald Stewart, Reid's most important follower, and prepared an undergraduate prize essay which showed his acquaintance with the Scottish modifications of empiricism.

These modifications, however, were not very exciting to a young mind. They simply loosened the grip that Locke might otherwise have held on it. The excitement came when Emerson read Coleridge's *Aids to Reflection* in the edition issued by President James Marsh, of the University of Vermont, in 1829. There he found a dramatic distinction between Locke's ordinary human "understanding" and the transcendent intuitive "reason" as well as an exposition of the importance of the latter. He had been finding support for an anti-empirical theory of knowledge in his other reading, he had found no inspiration in the Divinity School, and he was perhaps already dissatisfied with the "pale negations of Unitarianism." At any rate, he was ready for a wave of inspiration to look within himself for some sort of guidance that he had not received from the forces that beat upon him from outside. In his first sermon, three years before his ordination, he had announced that man was the architect of his own fortunes and that his spiritual guide was his inner conscience—and after three years of formal ministry he found his conscience, now a rational faculty which transcended the ordinary "understanding"—at variance with his material fortunes. He resigned his pulpit in 1832 and, a lonely widower threatened with tuberculosis, set sail for the Mediterranean. In the course of his travels through Italy and back by England he met the great men of English literature, Walter Savage Landor, William Wordsworth, and Samuel Taylor Coleridge, and was disappointed by them all. Traveling itself had no intellectual appeal for him, and by the time he reached Scotland and drove out to Craigenputtock to see Thomas Carlyle he was ready for a new wave of influence.

He got it with a rush from a man who was lonelier than himself and with whom he spent a night in order to talk and lay the foundation for a lifelong friendship. He returned home to Concord, Massachusetts, where he had decided to settle, with an agreement to reprint the first volume of Carlyle's *Miscellanies* and to publish the strange novel *Sartor Resartus,* which was then running serially in *Frazer's Magazine*. The latter, at once hard-bitten and intensely inspirational, had a powerful effect upon him. Germanic rather than native in its background, it detached the lingering elements of Scottish philosophy from the defense of material reality (to which Emerson was indifferent) and devoted its enormous energy to an attack on empiricism which was sardonic, evangelical, autobiographical, and as moving as some great moral force. To Carlyle, the whole material universe and time itself was either an emblem or a means of concealing some nonmaterial reality—a "garment of the Spirit," he said in the figure of speech around which the book was constructed—and the question of its absolute existence was relatively unimportant. What did matter was that man should recognize the existence of spiritual force, accept it as the ultimate good, and follow its dictates at the expense of all material desires. He was a lay preacher, whose doctrine Emerson could accept as an expression of his own independent ethical impulses but with whose dogmas he could disagree because they were personal rather than authoritative. The Scot's words and ideas were to echo long in the American's mind as he took to the lecture platform for his pulpit and living and as he sat down in his study to write.

But Emerson did not become a slavish follower of Carlyle. The aristocratic social pattern into which Carlyle unconsciously fitted his thought, the excessive self-abnegation of an arrogant spirit, the harshness of phrase and the bitter humor—all these were foreign to Emerson's make-up. And he had learned the lesson of the American writer before he began to write: "Every man's condition is a solution in hieroglyphic," he said in the Introduction to his first book, "to those inquiries he would put. He acts it as life, before he apprehends it as truth." He had to look within himself and find a solution for various inquiries before he could become an effective evangelist for what he had already begun to call "human culture." Furthermore, despite his intense interest in the new symbols of an intellectual Romanticism, he was as fully exposed as any of his contemporaries to the older symbols of Romantic material. His first and most important problem was a reconciliation of their conflicting claims. His first and most important inquiry would be into the hieroglyphic of "nature"—the material world of "not me." Why is it? What is it? Where did it come from? To what will it lead? These were the questions—undreamed of in Hawthorne's philosophy—which Emerson felt obliged to put.

The most important of these inquiries was the first: Why is nature? For Emerson, despite what he was to say in his lecture on "The Transcendentalist" in 1841, was never a philosophical idealist except in occasional moments of poetic fancy. The universe he set out to explore in the little book called *Nature* (1836) was clearly a dualistic one, consisting of matter and spirit with man standing between the two, composed of both, and having direct knowledge of the material world through his human "understanding" and of the world of spirit through his Transcendental "reason." One value of the material world Emerson derived directly from the tradition of English literary Romanticism: The open air and unspoiled landscape put one in tune with the infinite—"In the woods, we return to reason and faith. . . . all mean egotism vanishes . . . the currents of Universal Being circulate through me; I am part or parcel of God." Another value was commonplace: Nature provided the commodities required to sustain life and work. A third, beauty, was more complex, for Emerson conceived of beauty in a threefold sense: natural beauty, perceptible to the sense; spiritual beauty, made evident to the understanding by acts of heroism and virtue; and, finally, beauty as an "object of the intellect," which "searches out the absolute order of things as they stand in the mind of God" and attempts to re-create it through the active powers in the forms of art. "Thus is Art," he said, "a nature passed through the alembic of man." And in this final concept of beauty may be found the distinctive doctrine of American Transcendentalism—a gospel of practical activity based upon an intuitive perception of ideal order, a perception which was and must be that of each individual person. The alembic of one man's genius could do no more than distill something which would stimulate the perceptions of others, and the responsibility of the American Transcendentalist was not to command but to inspire.

At the time he was writing *Nature*, however, Emerson was not prepared to develop the implications of his distinctive point of view. He was still forming his ideas, reading his inner hieroglyphic; and the influence of Carlyle was still strong upon him. His fourth justification for the existence of the material world, in the chapter on "language," seems to have been directly inspired by Carlyle's notion of the emblematic nature of the universe; and his fifth, in terms of "Discipline," is a gentler version of Carlyle's stern inspirationalism. Nature disciplines the understanding to the material world and also disciplines the reason by an emblematic verification of its premonitions. The contrast between brute nature and the potentialities of mankind suggests the final reason for the existence of unconscious matter—to make injured, marred, and defective human beings realize that they "all rest like fountain-pipes on the unfathomed sea of thought and virtue whereto they alone, of all organizations, are the entrances."

After his creative and inspirational justification of the existence of nature, Emerson was relatively indifferent to the philosophical question of what it was, whether it was a reality or an illusion. "Idealism" was "a noble doubt" of the outward existence of nature, he said in his chapter on that subject, for which he found certain empirical justifications but which he rejected out of an intuition which hardly seems to be more than pure sentiment. The origin of the material world was of even less concern, for in a discursive chapter on "Spirit," he did no more than offer casually the Miltonic notion that it was the "remoter and inferior incarnation of God, a projection of God in the unconscious" —an affirmation which denied the popular pantheism of William Cullen Bryant and casts more light upon Emerson's theology than upon his philosophical inquisitiveness. His own interests were primarily ethical and were revealed in the enthusiasm of his final chapter, "Prospects." His inquiry into nature had demonstrated the inadequacy of the understanding and had so excited him over the value of reason that he could declare "that a dream may let us deeper into the secret of nature than a hundred concerted experiments." "At present, man applies to nature but half his force. . . . his power over it is through the understanding, as by manure; the economic use of fire, wind, water, and the mariner's needle; steam, coal, chemical agriculture; the repairs of the human body by the dentist and the surgeon. This is such a resumption of power as if a banished king should buy his territories inch by inch, instead of vaulting at once into his throne." His own call was clear. He would teach man to use his entire force, his reason as well as his understanding, and trust that the march of the intellect toward a universal perception of absolute order would produce its own genius for other types of action. In any event, he would have nothing to do with inch by inch reforms: "The problem of restoring to the world original and eternal beauty is solved by the redemption of the soul."

At the time that Emerson was writing *Nature* the United States was entering into an era of passionate reforms, which ranged from violent attacks on Negro slavery to the advocacy of Graham's whole-wheat bread as a moral substitute for meat. Emerson himself had been subject to successful pressure to raise his voice against the removal of American Indians to western reservations and to a much more intense but so far unsuccessful pressure to join the abolitionist movement. His own inbred compulsion to minister to the ills of the world made him sensitive to the spirit of the times, and for that reason perhaps the most significant inquiry he made in *Nature* was not an explicit one but rather the implicit search he made within himself for his proper place in the America of his day—for a wisdom of speech and action which conformed to the tenor of his own life. His decision to preach inspiration made him seem slightly mad to even so good a friend as Hawthorne (who distrusted all reformers but was particularly sardonic about a man who, like Hollingsworth in *The Blithedale Romance*, undertook a "grand project" of "reforming criminals by appealing to their higher instincts") and a laggard or skulker to the many good people for whom the evils of slavery were more vivid than the vision of "original and eternal beauty." But he had found in his own condition the only adjustment possible between the foreign symbols of a new intellectual Romanticism and the prevailing attitudes of mind in his own country, and the words with which he expressed this adjustment were so vitally alive that they made him the most controversial and the most important American literary figure in the first half of the nineteenth century.

II

The literary importance of Emerson is to be seen less in his individual and rather chaotic philosophy than in the way he expressed it in comparison with America's two other leading Transcendentalists—Amos Bronson Alcott and Henry David Thoreau. Alcott was Emerson's older contemporary, his Concord friend and neighbor, and to a certain extent his mentor. Without a formal education, he had formed his Transcendental ideas out of his efforts to digest his miscellaneous reading under the probable influence of doctrines of the mystical "inner light" taught by the Society of Friends, or Quakers, for he had been exposed to them during his wanderings as a Yankee peddler in North Carolina. While Emerson was forming his ideas, Alcott was in Boston spreading his by formal "conversations" with adults on Friday evenings and Sunday mornings and with the children of the Temple School from whose unspoiled intuitions he hoped to derive a new harmony of the Gospels. Although nominally an Episcopalian, Alcott was a radical in religion who went far beyond the Unitarians in denying the peculiar divinity of Jesus and in insisting upon the divine nature of all mankind. He was also interested in the progress of literature and the arts, and for their encouragement he instigated, in the autumn of 1836, a plan for less formal conversations among the intellectual leaders of Boston and its environs. Ralph Waldo Emerson, George Ripley, Frederick H. Hedge, James Freeman Clarke, Orestes A. Brownson, Convers Francis, Theodore Parker, John Sullivan Dwight, C. A. Bartol, W. H. Channing, Henry David Thoreau, Elizabeth Peabody, and Margaret Fuller were among those who eventually participated in these gatherings of what came to be called the Transcendental Club, and through them the influence of the new movement spread from Maine to New York and as far west as Cincinnati, Ohio.

But Alcott was a thoroughly impractical man. The publication of his *Conversations on the Gospel* with the Temple School children brought down the wrath of Boston upon his head and almost provoked a riot against his person. Yet he never learned discretion. When the group of Transcendentalists established their ideal community at Brook Farm (1840–44) with its relatively sound attempts at profit sharing and production and its progressive experiments in education and the encouragement of music and literature, Alcott was not a participant. Instead he sowed his own extravagant crop of "Transcendental wild oats" (as his daughter, Louisa, put it) at Fruitlands, where he not only undertook to keep his group of "Pythagoreans" free from all animal matter in food and dress but limited them to "aspiring" vegetables whose fruits grew upward and forbade them cotton because it was produced by slaves. Pure linen and beans, however, offered a poor defense against the rigors of a New England winter, and the experiment failed. His "Orphic Sayings," published in the Transcendental periodical *The Dial* (1840–44), had none of the inspirational quality which people seem to have found in his conversations; and, although he was to live long and in his old age preside over the Concord School of Philosophy, his achievement survives as a fantastic story rather than a substantial record. Emerson may have had him in mind when he asked the question: "Of what use is genius, if the organ is too convex or too concave and cannot find a focal distance within the actual horizon of human life?"

At any rate, Emerson kept the focal point of his own genius upon everyday human life. Most of his writings represent a practical application of the ideas he had developed in *Nature*. His first major opportunity occurred in 1837 when he was invited to address the Phi Beta Kappa society at Harvard to whose undergraduate membership he had not been entitled by his own academic record. Taking as his subject "The American Scholar," he spoke formally on education by nature, books, and action. But his plea was for the young scholar to vault into his intellectual throne by making use of that universal reason which the understanding too often corrupts into eccentricity. With reference to books, this called for "creative reading"—the bold rejection of scholarly and literary authority unless the reader's own heart flamed with awareness of "the authentic utterances of the oracles." For "in yourself," he concluded, "slumbers the whole of Reason; it is for you to know all; it is for you to dare all." Such a line of discourse was enormously stimulating to young men who for years had been "meek young men in libraries" and were now ready to strike out for themselves without quite knowing what problems they would face. But when Emerson used it again the following year in his Divinity School Address he ran into trouble. Even the most liberal of theological professors could not allow him to attack the authority of historical revelation and advise each fledgling minister: "Yourself a newborn bard of the Holy Ghost, cast behind you all conformity, and acquaint men at first hand with Deity." This "latest form of infidelity," as it was called in a pamphlet issued by Professor Andrews Norton, aroused a storm of opposition which kept Emerson off the Harvard lecture platform for almost three decades.

But the lyceum platform welcomed him all over the United States, and out of his various lectures he composed the aphoristic *Essays* (first series), which he published in 1841. They ranged in subject from "History" to "Art" and included practical applications of the ideas developed in *Nature* to such matters as "Compensation," "Friendship," "Prudence," and "Heroism." Two of them, however, were of especial importance. His essay on "Self-Reliance" is the best epitome of his philosophy. Inclinations toward social conformity and intellectual consistency were the greatest obstacles to self-reliance, he declared, and the major faults of the age were its reliance upon such props as a belief in an external God, upon the "superstition of Travelling," upon faith in the cultural influence of literature and art, and upon the hope for social progress and reform. "Whoso would be a man, must be a nonconformist," he exclaimed. "Nothing is at last sacred but the integrity of your own mind." This integrity depended upon absolute allegiance to "the aboriginal Self on which a universal reliance may be founded"—an "immense intelligence" in which all men lie and from which they receive intuitions of truth and justice. In another essay, "The Over-Soul," he tried to define this intelligence, or at least separate it from all the anthropomorphic connotations of God, by identifying it with such terms as Platonic "unity," the Quaker "light," the metaphysical "divine mind," mystic "fire," and psychological "energy." He seems to have been almost completely indifferent to the theoretical identification of the source of knowledge so long as it was recognized as knowledge which transcended that gained from the experience of the senses and the ordinary reflections of the mind.

These early addresses and essays reveal Emerson's Transcendental gospel at its evangelical height. In the *Essays, Second Series* (1844) he brought the oversoul into closer contact with the earth, writing on more specific subjects ranging from "The Poet" to "New-England Reformers" and including discussions of "Character," "Manners," "Gifts," "Nature," "Nominalist and Realist," and "Politics." The most significant essay in this series is perhaps that on "Experience" in which he divided "the Lords of Life"—the intellectual inclinations by which men lived—into two equal groups, transcendental and empirical, and identified them with moods of varying value according to each individual's temperament. "The mid-world is best," he wrote, returning to his concept of intellectual beauty, which combined the genius for intuitive perception with that for practical expression, a balance between "power and form." In a series of lectures composed shortly afterward and published in 1850 under the title *Representative Men*, he preserved this ideal of the balanced intellect, standing apart from the extremes of the mystic as represented by Emanuel Swedenborg and the man of the world as represented by Napoleon Bonaparte. His ideal philosopher was Plato because he was "a balanced soul" who combined the intuitive genius of the East with the empirical genius of the West and "could see two sides of a thing." In *Representative Men*, too, he demonstrated the basic difference between the democratic individualism of his own pattern of thought and the aristocratic absolutism of Carlyle's. For although his choice of a subject was obviously influenced by Carlyle's *Heroes and Hero-Worship*, Emerson did not present his great men as the godlike embodiments of some social ideal which captured the best instincts of the masses. His great men were representative of types, not of an archetype, and greatness itself was a kind of eyewash —"a collyrium," he said in his lecture on "The Uses of Great Men," "to clear our eyes from egotism, and enable us to see other people and their works." Yet "every hero becomes a bore at last," for "no man, in all the procession of famous men, is reason or illumination, or that essence we were looking for; but is an exhibition, in some quarter, of new possibilities."

Emerson was to depart from his democratic inspirationalism in his use of popular racial ideas in his otherwise shrewd analysis of *English Traits* (1856). But in general he was to preserve rather than modify or develop these basic attitudes in the essays collected in *The Conduct of Life* (1860), *Society and Solitude* (1870), and *Letters and Social Aims* (1876) before his death in 1882. The secret of his literary success lay not in the consistency of his ideas, however, but in his ability to deny worldly values in the language of worldly wisdom. His stylistic method was the opposite of Hawthorne's. For while Hawthorne was a man who used Romantic symbols to express the conclusions of a realistic mind, Emerson made his intellectual Romanticism sound like Franklin's Poor Richard leading people along "The Way to Wealth." Few of his readers and even fewer of his hearers understood the philosophical implications of his theory of the universe or of knowledge, but all could thrill to the words of his essay on "Self-Reliance." "To believe your own thought, to believe that what is true for you in your private heart is true for all men—that is genius" is an observation which might be variously interpreted, but in any interpretation it is one which appealed strongly to the attitude of mind that had become characteristic of Americans during the eighteenth century; and so was the suggestion that we are often "forced with shame to take our own opinion from another." The notion that "society everywhere is in conspiracy against the manhood of every one of its members" probably lurked in the mind of the worst failure ever driven to make a desperate new start on the frontier, and the lowest of stay-at-home rebels would agree that "the only right is what is after my constitution; the only wrong what is against it." Everyone can at some time or another take consolation from the belief that "a foolish consistency is the hobgoblin of little minds," just as every weary way-worn wanderer is sometimes prepared to agree that "travelling is a fool's paradise." The verbal garment of Emerson's Transcendental spirit was of traditional homespun.

This homespun quality of Emerson's aphorisms was the essence of what his admirers called his "wit," and it was often cryptic. "Art is a nature passed through the alembic of man," "Books are for a scholar's idle times," "Men descend to meet," "Poetry was all written before time was," "Let us treat men and women . . . as if they were real; perhaps they are"—such remarks as these contain the essence of all Emerson had to say, but their meaning is rarely obvious. Wit of this sort is especially characteristic of his poetry, which is often more cryptic, searching, and intimate than his prose, and is generally more admired by sophisticated modern readers. Written at various times and collected in two small volumes, *Poems* (1847) and *May-Day and Other Poems* (1867), it contains the record of profound personal experience and philosophical speculation which is controlled by the sort of wry humor and personal modesty that brought Emerson's intellectual pretentiousness down to earth and enabled him to dwell on common ground instead of in Alcott's clouds. "The Problem" analyzes his attitude toward the pulpit, "Uriel" is a light allegory giving his version of the Divinity School Address and its aftermath, and the "Ode" to W. H. Channing is a wry but soul-searching response to the pressure brought to bear upon him by the abolitionists. The basic personal explanation for the change in tone between the first and second series of *Essays* may perhaps be found in the reference to the loss of his "larger" optimism in his "less" grief found in the "Threnody" on the death of his son Waldo in 1842, and the popular little poem "Days" is his personal apology for not having been a better follower of his own doctrines.

His speculative poems are generally bolder and more searching than his prose. Although "Each and All" and "Give All to Love" are relatively simple, the light summary verses with which he frequently prefaced his essays suggest deeper thought than do the essays themselves—particularly in the case of "Compensation" and "Experience." But the most haunting of all his verses are those in which he attempted to express philosophical doctrines which fascinated him without gaining his acquiescence. "Hamatreya," asserting the permanence of the earth and the mortality of man, stands at one extreme among these; and "Brahma," denying the reality of the material world and of Lockean ideas, stands at the other. But perhaps the most teasing of all is "The Sphinx," which he wrote for the Transcendental periodical *The Dial* and insisted, to the distress of his friends and the discouragement of his readers, upon using as the introduction to all his collections of poems. In it he gave, through the person of "the poet," his customary answer to the question of what was wrong with man—a summary of his prose evangel, on the platform and through the press—and then denied it all in terms of the philosophical idealism he had specifically rejected in *Nature*. It provides the ultimate evidence of his refusal to take himself solemnly—of the focus of his genius in a life whose intellectual activities could transcend the understanding but whose sympathies were with it.

III

By the middle of the nineteenth century the American attitude toward European literary symbols—the insistence upon modifying them until they made sense in terms of the individual's own experience—had become so deeply rooted that it was ready to flower into some sort of symbolic expression of its own; and, among the Transcendentalists, Henry David Thoreau was the writer who gave it this sort of expression. Like Emerson, he had been prepared for the new thought before he was exposed to German philosophy, either directly or at second hand through Coleridge and Carlyle, and before he developed a fancy for Oriental literature. But his preparation had been more indigenous and radical, for he was brought up in a Concord household which was devoted to the doctrines of radical abolitionism—the doctrines of William Lloyd Garrison and his followers who believed in the moral obligation of the individual to follow the dictates of an intuitively perceived, ideal, and absolute moral law. He seems to have been not greatly influenced by his studies at Harvard, from which he was a rebellious graduate in the class of 1837, but he was prepared to be affected by Emerson's *Nature* when he received an advance copy of that little book a few days before its formal publication. Accordingly, when he returned home to Concord he was ready for a meeting of minds with his older neighbor, which resulted in a relationship of mutual influence rather than that of teacher and disciple.

In Concord, Thoreau was as much a rebel as he had been in Harvard. A sometime schoolteacher, pencil maker, and surveyor, he was primarily an independent Yankee odd-jobs man who could do Emerson's household chores for hire without having his judgment in any way affected by his menial position when he collaborated in the editorship of *The Dial*. He wrote poetry and published some of the best of it in *The Dial*, and, like so many of his contemporaries, he kept a copious private Journal. From his Journal, his verse manuscripts, and even from his college essays came his first book, *A Week on the Concord and Merrimac Rivers* (1849), which was a miscellany of observations on abstract subjects and external nature, given a semblance of form by the incidents of a trip that he had made with his brother John. Its reception was discouraging, for he was obliged to publish it at his own expense, and about four-fifths of the edition was returned to him unsold. In the same year he also published, in Elizabeth Peabody's collection of *Aesthetic Papers*, his famous essay "On the Duty of Civil Disobedience"; but that, too, left the contemporary public cold because it seemed to be little more than a belated expression of the antigovernment sentiment

which the radical abolitionists had made commonplace five years before. With the help of America's
foremost newspaper editor, Horace Greeley, and with
the loyal support of the editors of *Putnam's Magazine*,
he was more successful in the periodicals and published accounts of various walking trips under the
titles of "The Maine Woods," "Cape Cod," and "A
Yankee in Canada," which appeared in book form after
his death. Posthumous collections were also made from
his Journals and published under the titles *Excursions*
(1863), *Early Spring in Massachusetts* (1881), *Summer* (1884), *Winter* (1888), and *Autumn* (1892);
and his *Collected Poems* appeared in 1943. But the
only book after the *Week* which he himself prepared
for the press was the gradually evolved *Walden*
(1854), which purportedly deals with his personal experiences as a hermit on the shores of Walden Pond
from July 4, 1845, to September 6, 1847, but is actually
a symbolic expression of his whole life.

Thoreau went into retirement for the same reasons
that had led several of his friends to find huts in the
woods and many of his contemporaries to join in the
establishment of such Utopian colonies as Brook Farm.
He wanted to live economically, escape distractions,
and find leisure to read and think and perhaps to
write. The experience was by no means unique, but
the book which grew out of it was. For *Walden* is not
a simple record of life in the woods. It is a testimonial
of what that episode in life had come to mean to him
after almost a decade of reflection during which the
original manuscript record grew greatly in size and
deepened in implication. His purpose is suggested in

a sentence near the beginning of the book: "When one man has reduced a fact of the imagination to be a fact to his understanding," he wrote, "I foresee that all men will at length establish their lives on that basis." Like Emerson, he wanted to reform the world by opening men's eyes to their own potentialities rather than by changing social conditions; but his method was by example rather than by evangelism. He had a less sublime faith in the currents of Universal Being, comparing them to the vegetable juices or sap of a plant, and believed that the mass of men could escape the quiet desperation of their lives more readily by the light of common understanding than by that of Transcendental reason. He was trying to bring the oversoul down to earth by action rather than by words, an empirical Transcendentalist who wanted to make his own life a factual emblem of the imaginative doctrines of "Self-Reliance."

The result was a book which in some respects succeeded better than anything Emerson ever wrote in adapting the Transcendental theory of knowledge to the pattern of logic that had already formed a characteristically American attitude of mind. It was practical in that it was a report on an experiment designed to show that the economic problems of living could be easily solved by a simplification of life and that man was a self-sufficient creature who could find infinite entertainment in the solitude of the woods. It admitted the importance of intuitive knowledge and insisted that, in times of crisis, a man had to stand on his principles even if he went to jail for them; but its stress was upon the material activities of daily living.

Man could live by higher laws, Thoreau maintained, but could not change the animal nature within him— although, upon second thought, he recognized a moral obligation to overcome it. This high-minded approach to practical life—or the practical approach to the high-minded life—produced some of the most luminous prose in nineteenth-century literature, and especially in the sections dealing with his observations, such as "Brute Neighbors" and "The Pond in Winter," Thoreau wrote with a clarity and suggestiveness which none of his American contemporaries could rival.

Yet *Walden* was not nearly so well adapted to contemporary readers as were Emerson's essays. For Emerson addressed himself to readers who still felt that they could assert their individual manhood within the framework of society however much it might be in conspiracy against them. Thoreau seems to have assumed that the conspiracy had succeeded—that he could maintain the integrity of his own soul only by withdrawal, either in spirit or body or both. "Civil Disobedience" had been his testament of spiritual withdrawal, a declaration that "I, Henry Thoreau, do not wish to be regarded as a member of any incorporated society which I have not joined" and "am not responsible for the successful working of the machinery of society." In *Walden* he simply withdrew a little bit further into the symbol of the hermitage. The withdrawal itself was to become a successful revolutionary tactic with Mahatma Gandhi and his Indian followers—and "Civil Disobedience" was to be used to advocate it—but first the symbol had to acquire a new emotional value in later generations, when the conflict between the individual and society became more pronounced. For Thoreau's sensitivity was ahead of his times, and it took the form of excessive aggressiveness. He revealed it in his own version of what had now become the American writer's conventional scheme of reference within himself: "I should not talk so much about myself," he announced in the second paragraph of *Walden*, "if there were anybody else whom I knew so well." Such an attitude is indicative of something more than an advanced sensitivity, and Thoreau's writing often suggests personal frustration by giving the impression that he would rather show up the world than improve it. His early poems had revealed a tendency toward hero worship which was to continue through and perhaps partially explain his later essays on John Brown, and it may be that he was always affected by a personal ambition to play the hero in patched breeches. At any rate, he addressed *Walden* particularly to "poor students" and to such other readers as would "accept such portions as apply to them." Whatever he may have been when he went into the woods, rebel, escapist, or genuine experimenter, he used himself in his book as Emerson said a great man should be used—as a "collyrium" to clear men's eyes and suggest to them their own potentialities if they would follow the bent of their individual geniuses. The hero of *Walden* is a "representative" common man.

Such a contemporary as James Russell Lowell was utterly incapable of understanding this role. For Lowell, although only two years younger and a year behind Thoreau at Harvard, was the product of a different intellectual atmosphere. Born a member of what Oliver Wendell Holmes was to call "the Brahmin caste of New England," Lowell had had a well-established place in society and a tendency to accept a considerable amount of responsibility for the successful operation of its machinery. Furthermore, the academic influences upon his mind were different from those which supported Emerson and Thoreau. An age of sentiment was approaching in America, dominated in popular literature by women and women's magazines; and Harvard, as usual, had its corporate ear to the ground. Had Lowell completed his studies with his class he might have escaped some of its worst effects, but he was a careless student who was "rusticated" to Concord for a summer of new philosophical study before he was allowed to take his degree. Harvard's new philosophy, as presented in a textbook by Sir James Mackintosh, resembled the old in that it was opposed to Locke's empiricism, but it based its opposition upon a belief in innate sentiments rather than innate ideas. A basic moral feeling frequently referred to as "sympathy" was common to all mankind in all ages, it held, and out of this active and universal sentiment all moral ideas were formed. As a young man Lowell was almost as wayward and impressionable as Poe, and, although he resented Harvard, his alma mater's endorsement of feeling as a guide to thought and action enabled him in later years to justify his erratic and sometimes violent literary career on moral grounds.

Lowell's anger at being sent to Concord kept him from becoming closely associated with the Transcendentalists there, and, although he published in *The Dial* and the Brook Farm *Harbinger,* he was never to admit any formal allegiance with that school. Yet he fell under direct Transcendental influence through the person of Maria White, the young woman he married in 1844, who taught him to admire Carlyle and see physical objects as the emblems of some spiritual reality. Through Maria, too, he came in contact with the radical abolitionist thought which had helped prepare Thoreau for Transcendentalism and with the Platonism in which she took refuge from her fear of sensual experience. The result was that a person of intense emotional disposition refused to conceal his emotion, as did Longfellow, but forced it outward toward all humanity. "That love for one, from which there doth not spring Wide love for all," he wrote in the best of the sonnets to Maria published in *A Year's Life* (1841), "is but a worthless thing"; and his whole early attitude was that his personal emotion should bear the "goodly fruit" of humanitarianism. Accordingly he became active in every reform movement into which Maria directed him, especially the abolitionist movement with which her family was associated and which provided Lowell, after their marriage, with employment on the editorial staffs of the *Pennsylvania Freeman* and the *National Anti-Slavery Standard.*

Yet Lowell was not, by temperament, the insensitive and violent radical that many of his antislavery poems and most of his editorials suggest. He considered himself primarily a poet, and in an early "Ode" (originally published in 1842 and revised for the 1844 *Poems*) he attempted to define the role of the poet in the modern world as an old-fashioned prophet and teacher brought up-to-date by a feeling of love and kinship for common humanity. But he was not a man of action, as Lowell made clear in "An Incident in a Railway Car," which described the effect of Burns's poetry upon a group: the poet might be something of a philosopher in his effort to translate feeling into thought, but his proper function was to translate this thought into words sufficiently stirring to make ordinary men conscious of their basic moral feelings. His own problem, since he was committed to exclusive reliance upon some aboriginal self of intellectually undirected feeling, was that of remaining stable long enough to find and be himself—for he was as firmly convinced as any of his contemporaries that a man's writings were closely identified with his own individuality. The problem was one he never solved. He was a man of natural wit who strove earnestly for high seriousness. His impulses were convivial and social, but he was involved in the bitterest controversy of his generation. He had a sensuous interest in material objects and an almost Keatsian genius for expressing it, but he had been persuaded by Maria and Poe (under whose editorial influence he fell for a time) that the proper aim of poetry was a vague "ideality." All his qualities and commitments were, in the emotional sense of the word, honest. But they could be neither reconciled nor accepted as the momentarily inconsistent dictates of a wise oversoul. As a result, he worried and never acquired much vital assurance except in occasional moments of escape from self-consciousness.

In these moments, however, he produced some of
the most brilliant verse of his time. He was freest when
he wrote under the pseudonym of the shrewd but
semiliterate Yankee, Hosea Biglow, and the first of the
Biglow "papers" is not only a fine example of Lowell's
wit but the best succinct summary of radical abolitionist sentiment—for its earthy shrewdness, nagging irritability, humanitarian faith, and political disunion-
ism—to be found in American literature. The collected
first series of *Biglow Papers* (1848) reveal the inconsistency of Lowell's political thought (for some of
them were as conservatively Whig as others were
radical), but Hosea remained the best part of Lowell
as a poet, and the happiest combination of his sensu-
ousness and his wit is the quietly personal "Sunthin'
in the Pastoral Line" in the *Biglow Papers, Second
Series* of 1867. His wit also broke through his cultivated seriousness in the anonymous poem *A Fable for
Critics* (1848), which was an extraordinarily clever
and generally acute survey of contemporary American
writers, including himself with his "bale of isms,"
vainly attempting to climb Parnassus. But to balance
and perhaps compensate for these he published, in
the same year, *The Vision of Sir Launfal* as an exhibition of the vague "ideality" which was his most
consistent aim and his greatest curse. In later years he
was to display his remarkable technical virtuosity in
the Harvard "Commemoration Ode" (1865) for the
Civil War dead and his capacity for meditative verse
in *The Cathedral* (1870), but he was never able to
direct all his powers into a single channel. His talents
were greater and more varied than those of most of

his contemporaries, but he failed as a poet because he could not find in the tenor of his own life a sound test for his wisdom. His inner light was too flickering to read by with steady vision.

When Lowell faced the fact that his poetic ambitions were vain he settled down as a literary critic, and his later reputation was based upon the essays written while he was Smith Professor of Modern Languages at Harvard and editor of the *Atlantic Monthly* and the *North American Review* and the addresses he gave while serving as the American minister to Great Britain. Collected under such titles as *Fireside Travels* (1864), *Among My Books* (1870, 1876), *My Study Windows* (1871), *Democracy and Other Addresses* (1887), and *Political Essays* (1888), they reveal a mind which could range widely over literature with a capacity for meticulous observation and an intuitive perception which found something fresh and new in the most hackneyed subject. He had been forced, while delivering a series of Lowell Institute Lectures in Boston in 1855, to work out a series of categories or commonplaces—ranging from a Transcendental imagination to a sound understanding —through which he sought out the essential characteristic of an author and his work; and this system served him, as a scholarly critic, instead of the character he failed to achieve as a poet. In one of his essays he called Thoreau "a skulker" for taking his high-mindedness into the woods rather than onto the battlefield and exercising his sympathetic imagination upon fish rather than directing it toward mankind. Despite all his acumen he could not learn that a writer—at least an American writer—must achieve lasting respect by individual integrity rather than by good intentions or by good social works. Nor could he guess that posterity would accept almost any system of professed values in literature provided they were focused in the depths of a coherent personality, which he himself lacked but which is required to give words a vital relationship that makes them endure and perhaps say more to one generation than they do to another.

CHAPTER SIX

The Time of Tension

I

AT the halfway point in the nineteenth century there was no American writer who could be considered fully "representative" of that intangible generality which may be called, with purely figurative succinctness, the American mind. Authors had learned that they could not borrow literary symbols without giving them a life from within themselves which had some relationship to the prevailing attitudes of life around them. But none had captured completely within himself the prevailing attitude of mind which had developed during the eighteenth century. Poe had shown an impulse to do so but had abandoned the solid ground of American thought in the desperate egotism of *Eureka*. Hawthorne was holding the empirical line in *The Scarlet Letter* after having satirized Transcendentalism in various short stories which anticipated the attitude he was to display in *The Blithedale Romance*. Emerson's early addresses and essays were providing an evangelical complement to the empiricism of Haw-

thorne and his fellows but were extravagantly over-
estimating the power of Transcendental reason, while
Thoreau was in the process of struggling to achieve
a balance upon an instrument too sensitive for its task,
and Lowell was illustrating the vagaries of something
like a Transcendental impulse which was outwardly
directed. The period was one of tension and conflict
between the forces of empiricism and Transcendentalism, skepticism and faith, foreshadowing the later
conflict between the symbols of science and religion.
America had not yet developed, in short, a theory of
knowledge which would fit into its well-established
pattern of logic.

It was perhaps too early to expect any single author to absorb—much less to reconcile—the conflicts of
American thought which were securely within the
tradition of literature. For, after all, the major problem of the new American literature had been that of
finding its own national character within such a great
and firmly established tradition of writing in English
that it might well have been overwhelming. A literary
American had to absorb a great deal of the conscious
thought of Great Britain and the Continent before he
could absorb that of his own country, and, from one
point of view, it was triumph enough that one generation could be sufficiently united by the undercurrents
of national thought to find a characteristically American way of handling the international substance of
literature and give it a subtly independent tone. In
any case, the writers of the mid-century who most
nearly caught the tensions of the whole country were
all self-educated, relatively unaffected by academic

ties with Europe and the esthetic allegiance that accompanied these, and therefore as free to be influenced by American writing as by that from abroad.

The youngest of these at the time of his greatest success was Herman Melville. Born in New York City, he was one of eight children left by their father's early death without means for much formal education, and he grew up during a financial depression which gave him a strong feeling of responsibility for his family's support. After various attempts at employment in commerce and engineering he shipped as a common sailor across the Atlantic in the summer of 1839, returned to a poorly paid job as a schoolteacher, and tried his fortunes in western Illinois before becoming desperate enough to sign up for a Pacific whaling voyage at Christmastime in 1840. The whaling ship, he was to say later, became his Yale and his Harvard. It and other kinds of ships certainly provided him with the material for his writing and made him independent of most of the literary symbols with which his contemporaries were compelled to deal. He deserted his first ship, the *Acushnet* of New Bedford, in the Marquesas in the summer of 1842, spent a month as a nervous refugee among the cannibal tribe of native Typees, and was rescued by an Australian whaler on which conditions were so bad that he refused service in the harbor of Tahiti and spent some time under arrest in the local open-air calaboose. After escaping to the neighboring island of Morea, he was on the beach for a couple of weeks before finding another whaler which would take him on for a voyage and discharge him in the Hawaiian Islands. There he obtained a job with a respectable but antimissionary merchant and planned to stay for at least a year. But he became homesick and enlisted in the United States Navy for transportation back to Boston, which did not materialize until he had spent fourteen months at sea, mostly off the coast of South America, where he was bored by inaction and upset by the severity of naval discipline. Eventually he received his discharge in October 1844 and made his way back home to the village of Lansingburgh on the upper Hudson River, where he began to tell the tales that formed the substance of his first book.

He called the book *Typee, or a Peep at Polynesian Life* (1846), and it was a titillating narrative of hardship and escape, fears of being eaten, fascination with primitive life, and friendly relations with dusky maidens. It was first published in England, however, as one of a series of travel books guaranteed to be factually true but as exciting as fiction; and to satisfy his publisher Melville may have included in it more anthropological detail than he otherwise might have thought of—more than he could remember, anyway, for *Typee* marked the beginning of his lifelong practice of telling a story and amplifying it with technical and circumstantial details based upon later research. The book was a popular success both in England and in his own country, and he followed it immediately with an account of his adventures in Tahiti, which he called *Omoo* (1847). It was not as exciting as *Typee*, but it contained more humor and a greater air of authenticity; and its success persuaded Melville that he was so well launched as an author that he could propose mar-

riage to Elizabeth Shaw, daughter of the Chief Justice
of Massachusetts, and move with his whole family
(his mother, four sisters, and two younger brothers)
to the better literary atmosphere of New York City.
His next book would be a continuation of his adventures, but this time in his imagination rather than in
fact—a work of fiction rather than semifictionalized
autobiography. He began it before his marriage and
removal.

The elements of external autobiography in his first
two books, however, had made it unnecessary for him
to learn the lesson that had been compulsory for other
American writers of his generation—that art was no
substitute for integrity, that even a work of pure fiction
had to come to a focus within an author's individual
experience in order to acquire form and life. And
Melville's experience had hitherto been of the body
and not the mind. Furthermore, in New York his mind
was in a chaos of belated stimulation. He was discovering the literature of the Renaissance and of the
English seventeenth century in the rich library of his
new friends, Evert and George Duyckinck, and was
enormously stimulated by the robust vigor of François
Rabelais, the allegorical meanings of Edmund Spenser, the eccentricities of Robert Burton, and the
rhetoric of Sir Thomas Browne. He may have given
some thought to the differences between formality
and essential belief as he made the transition from the
Dutch Reformed church in which he had been reared
into the Episcopal church favored by Elizabeth. He
was learning about politics at a time when the old
parties were breaking up under the pressure of the

antislavery and other reform movements and tensions were particularly great in the Democratic circles in which he moved. Under those influences his book kept changing character. It changed from an adventure story to a pilgrimage of talkers and storytellers who found themselves on a quest which resembled the Rabelaisian quest for the Holy Bottle modified by the softness of Spenserian allegory and the sentimentality of Victorian flower symbolism.

Mardi, as it was called when it was published in March 1849, was purportedly a satiric allegory of a voyage through the world, but actually there was little intellectual coherence in it except in those chapters which were introduced as an afterthought—after Melville had become interested in the French Revolution of 1848, brought together his political ideas, and expressed them in an easily interpreted commentary on revolution in Europe, imperialism and reform in England, and social conditions in the United States. He took a strong stand against slavery, satirized American democracy, and attributed the individual freedom of Americans to the existence of an open frontier rather than to the democratic institutions which had existed and passed away in other countries in earlier days. Although the chapters of religious allegory in *Mardi* indicate a belief in some intuitive light within and an inclination to identify "reason" with it, the dominant intellectual tone of the book is empirical, skeptical, and often sardonic; and it concluded with the suggestion that although some men may accept religion or resignation as a substitute for happiness, the hero must pursue it and be pursued by fate forever and in vain. The book failed both at home and in England, but it had opened Melville's mind to a new sensitivity and a new growth. When economic pressures forced him to the hasty composition of books based upon the tried method of exploiting personal experiences—*Red-burn* (1849), dealing with his first voyage on a merchant vessel, and *White-Jacket* (1850), describing his life on a man-of-war with a combination of humor and bitterness—he was more contemptuous of them than they deserved. For they both reflected a remarkable development in literary art—in the power to focus the thoughts and emotions of the moment upon his recollections of the past and, by doing so, re-create characters with an imagination that made them more real in fiction than they may have appeared to be in fact. Without realizing it, Melville became a novelist.

If it had not been for the experience of imagining and writing these two books, Melville could not have produced *Moby Dick*, which came into being almost unplanned during the year and nine months which followed a trip abroad in the winter of 1849–50. He wrote one version of it rapidly—"a romantic and fanciful account of the whale fishery," as it was described by a friend in early August 1850—but the published book was painfully composed during the prolonged process of revision which normally required only the insertion of technical details. And back of the pain lay a major struggle with the conflicts of American thought—the influence of Emerson, Coleridge, and Carlyle as opposed to that of Hawthorne and Melville's own intellectual predilections as revealed in his earlier books, passionate enthusiasm as opposed to everyday common sense. It was a struggle intensified on paper by Melville's own ambition, curiously acquired during the summer of 1850, to prove that the dramatic heights of Shakespeare could be reached in an American novel. Out of the struggle and the ambition came Captain Ahab, the grandest tragic hero in American fiction, the sensible First Mate Starbuck, the meditative narrator Ishmael, and the strange members of a crew which included four pagan harpooners whose primitive souls were easily stirred by passion. Ahab and Starbuck might easily be taken as representing enthusiasm and common sense, and Melville may have originally based his plot on their antagonism. But the final struggle is not between them, for Starbuck is too easily subdued, and as the revision of the book progressed, Melville increasingly referred to it as a story of "the whale," rather than "the whale fishery," indicating his growing interest in the great white whale—Moby Dick himself—as Ahab's more than worthy antagonist.

In a narrative and dramatic sense, the obvious struggle was between Ahab and the whale, a fabulous whale whose teeth had sheared off Ahab's leg in a previous encounter and to whose discovery and destruction Ahab had dedicated all his calculating cunning and fierce passion. The whale is the only character in the book known to have been drawn directly from life, and to the account of his systematic pursuit Melville brings to bear all the realistic knowledge of whaling he had gained from experience and research. The human actors in the drama—with the exception of the Parsi crew of Ahab's boat—are all individual examples of real types, however fancifully gathered together in a single ship; and the book as a whole might be described as a literary effort to balance romance and reality, enrich both with allusiveness and symbolism, and bring a novel to the high pitch of intensity found in tragic drama. The composition of it was, for Melville, a genuine catharsis. "I have written a wicked book," he told Hawthorne, to whom it was dedicated, "and I feel as innocent as a lamb."

Yet for all its suggestiveness and symbolism, there is a gross underestimation of the final depth and power of *Moby Dick* implicit in the common tendency to make the two antagonists, the captain and the whale, symbolic of anything in Melville's own mind. He conceived of them as realities and, as a dramatist, gave them emblematic qualities only in the minds of others. The "part and parcel allegoricalness of the whole" book, which Hawthorne immediately recognized and Melville admitted with some surprise, is a result of the fact that its tragic plot was essentially a fable so deeply moving to the author that it apparently colored his unconscious imagination and gave the story an uncalculated emotional and intellectual coherence. The literal fable may be easily followed by any reader who will keep his own quirks of personality out of the book and assume that Melville was a deeply imaginative creator rather than a craftsman, crank, or critic: Ahab was a man who arbitrarily assumed that a single brute creature was the emblem of all the evil and malice of the universe and made a heroic but tragic attempt to destroy it by striking at and through its mask. Its essential meaning is to be found in the fact that the drama is a tragedy and that Melville constantly reminds his readers of his hero's biblical prototype—King Ahab of old who had "done evil in the sight of the Lord" and was led by "a lying spirit" to a bad but somewhat accidental end. No one can err greatly in his interpretation of *Moby Dick* if he simply recognizes Ahab as a tragic hero whose arbitrary assumption is his tragic flaw.

A great tragedy, however, has the seductive power of inducing readers to identify themselves with its hero, and the existence of this power in Melville's book has produced innumerable "interpretations" by critics who have made the white whale emblematic of their own frustrations rather than of Ahab's and have attributed their own obsessions to the author of the fable. Melville invites this, to be sure, by his dramatic sympathy for Ahab and his admiration for the captain's intensity, power, and defiant spirit. Yet this sort of emotional relationship to a character of one's own creation does not imply intellectual approval of his attitudes or actions, and the calculated meaning of the fable is fairly plain in the light of its literary relationships. For Ahab's emblematic theory of the universe—his conviction that "all visible objects" were but "pasteboard masks" for some spiritual reality—is strikingly like the Transcendentalism of Carlyle, and Ahab bears a close resemblance to the hero of *Sartor Resartus* in his defiant state of what Carlyle called "the Everlasting No." The implications of the fable, though, suggest the intellectual attitude of the empirical Hawthorne in whose stories Melville had recently discovered what he called the "black" truth that illusion led

to destruction, and evil was engendered by the heart
of man.

Melville's psychological analysis of Ahab, through
the narrator Ishmael, is therefore his most rational expression of opinion concerning the philosophical theories of his own day. Crazy Ahab was suffering from
an obsession which caused him to transfer his inner
frustrations to some outer object, and his vision of
Transcendental reality was actually but a morbid disease. Yet Ishmael's meditations on evidences of non-
empirical knowledge, in the chapter on "The Whiteness
of the Whale," suggest that Melville was not entirely
convinced that his rational fable was a genuinely true
one; and much of the tension found in the book comes
from the intellectual reservations of Melville's ration-
ality as well as from the conflict between the emotional sympathy and the intellectual disapproval he
displays toward his hero. All of this, complex though
it may be, is a reflection of the prevailing attitude of
mind in mid-nineteenth-century America—a rational
commitment to empiricism as a philosophy but with
enough doubts and reservations to admit the possibility of intuition and inspiration and permit admiration
for those bold spirits who, like Emerson and Thoreau
in literature, would follow their own genius to whatever crazy lengths it might lead. Melville was the first
American author to realize within himself his whole
intellectual heritage and give it expression in the underlying pattern which controlled the composition of
a single book. *Moby Dick* is the "representative"
American novel of its time, and it is a great novel because it brings a broad cultural heritage to focus within

a single individual's capacity for realization and thus transmits it, with a new emotional power, to posterity.

II

The greatness of a book like *Moby Dick*—at least, in what we broadly call a "Romantic" era in literature —is the product of a deep and largely unconscious sensitivity rather than of deliberate planning, and most of the writers of Melville's generation possessed a sensitivity which reflected the dominant moods of the times. Melville himself, in his later writings, was more restricted than he had been in *Moby Dick*. The novel which immediately followed, *Pierre; or, The Ambiguities* (1852), seems to have been planned as a lighter handling of the same theme, in which a younger and less heroic hero than Ahab would be allowed to follow his own inexpedient notions of absolute morality while the author dwelt upon the ambiguities of human actions and motives. The action, however, turned into that of a grotesque tragedy as Melville subordinated any concern for plausibility of plot to his increasing concern for the plausibility of motives— exploring "the cavern of man," as he put it, to its inmost depths in an effort to distinguish between intuitive impulse and hidden neurosis. Because the suggested neurosis, in this case, was incestuous the book was a failure in its own day and attracted favorable attention only after the spread of Freudian theories enabled the public to realize that Melville was actually pioneering the psychoanalytical novel.

But Melville of course could neither realize the

artistic significance of his pioneering nor resist the public pressure always exerted upon a writer who uses his pen as a means of support. Consequently he turned to the ready market for magazine fiction and the discreet judgment of its editors, producing the short stories collected in the *Piazza Tales* (1856) and *The Apple-Tree Table and Other Stories* (1922) and the novel *Israel Potter* (1855). One group of his stories and sketches, "The Encantadas" (1853), may have formed the basis for a planned novel on tortoise hunting in the Galápagos Islands for which he had signed a contract shortly before his publishing house was destroyed by fire in 1853; and the most haunting of his longer stories, "Benito Cereno," may have actually been an abortive novel which was discouraged by the injudicious caution of a magazine editor. Both of them, like such complete short stories as "Bartleby the Scrivener" (1853) and "The Bell Tower" (1855), are rich in suggestiveness and in the revelation of a meditative imagination profoundly at work, but none has the far-ranging implications of *Moby Dick* or the psychological depths of *Pierre*. The nearest Melville came to recapturing his earlier breadth and depth during this period was in *The Confidence Man* (1857), a loosely constructed fantasy based upon his experiences on a Mississippi River steamer, in which he satirized both the gullibility and lack of faith found in mankind. It was the least coherent of all Melville's novels, however, and he had difficulty in arranging for its publication before he left home in 1856 on a new voyage of sight-seeing and refreshment, physical and spiritual, to Europe, Egypt, and the Holy Land.

After his return in 1857 he turned to public lecturing for three seasons and to poetry, giving up fiction entirely for more than thirty years. Throughout the bitter American Civil War, from 1861 to 1865, he followed the action in verse and in 1866 published his first collection of poems under the title *Battle Pieces and Aspects of the War.* A position as inspector in the New York Customs House freed him from the financial compulsion to write, and his only publication during that period was a long philosophical poem, *Clarel, A Poem and Pilgrimage to the Holy Land,* published in two volumes in 1876. It was his most ambitious single work, for within its narrative framework he attempted a descriptive survey of Palestine, a summary of most of the religious attitudes current in the nineteenth century, and an account of a young man's effort to restore his religious faith under the influence of holy places, in an atmosphere of religious debate, and in spite of severe emotional strain. The octosyllabic verse he adopted (perhaps in imitation of the narrative poems of Scott), however, was not equal to the serious demands he made upon it; and the poem as a whole, though picturesque in many of its details, vivid in its characterizations, and moving in some of its scenes, is difficult to follow. Perhaps the major reason for this is that Melville's interest was by now more centered upon people than upon philosophy, and the old conflict between Transcendentalism and empiricism—here expressed in the post-Darwinian symbols of religious belief versus scientific doubt—was of less concern to him than the individuals who were by temperament or conditioning inclined to one side of the controversy or the other. At any rate, many of the characters in the poem were finely and sympathetically drawn, while the philosophical problem was left unresolved by Clarel's bitter disappointment and by the author's advice, in an Epilogue, that he should nevertheless keep his faith. Once again Melville had found himself incapable of committing himself without reservations to a rational empiricism, but this time the tensions, once inherent in this attitude of mind, were reduced by his awareness of the enormous diversity of human beings and their individual attitudes of mind.

Near the end of his life Melville was to publish two more volumes of poems, *John Marr and Other Sailors* (1888) and *Timoleon and Other Poems* (1891), both mostly concerned with individual people in peculiarly individual circumstances and both printed in limited editions of twenty-five copies for his close friends. He was also to leave a considerable amount of verse for posthumous publication, but the most impressive work of his later years was to be the short novel *Billy Budd*, written between 1888 and 1891 and left unprepared for printing. The story is in part one of conflict between good and evil, innocence and sophistication, exemplified by the handsome sailor Billy Budd and a malignant master-at-arms Claggert who falsely accuses Billy of plotting mutiny and is struck and killed in Billy's outburst of speechless indignation. But the focus of attention is upon Captain Vere, who directs the court-martial which orders Billy to be hanged from the yardarm despite every one's realization that he is morally innocent of any crime. Its basic theme is that of conflict between individual and social morality or between principles of justice based upon the judge's responsibility to the individual or to the society of which he is a small part. Melville represents Captain Vere as a perceptive, sympathetic, and conscientious man who is acutely aware of Billy's personal innocence but chooses to sacrifice the sailor's life and his own ease of conscience to the necessity of preserving discipline in a navy upon which his country depends for its existence at that crucial moment. It is not a happy story but it is a vital one in its indication of Melville's awareness, in his old age, that he must face the facts of life in a society grown too complex to tolerate the tragic heroism of a Captain Ahab or the reckless naïveté of a Pierre Glendinning.

The transition of Melville's concern from principles to people and their problems in society is characteristic of American literature as a whole during the latter part of the nineteenth century, and it is perhaps most evident in those writers who were more obviously and superficially involved in the tensions of the prewar period and found an easier means of release afterward. Such a one was John Greenleaf Whittier, the most important of the abolitionist poets, who showed an extraordinary capacity for devoting almost thirty years of his life to aggressive reform and then, the reform accomplished, settling down to an equally long period of peaceful productivity. Whittier was a New England Quaker farm boy and apprentice shoemaker who had little formal education but was inspired to write poetry by the example of Robert Burns. One of his poems attracted the attention of William Lloyd Garrison, who encouraged him to pursue a career of poetry and journalism while also recruiting him to what Whittier eventually called the "Moral Warfare" against "the folly of an evil time"—that is, Negro slavery. His first important prose work, a pamphlet entitled "Justice and Expediency" (1833), clearly sets forth the principle on which he based his reforming activities and, incidentally, provides an interesting contrast to the attitude Melville was to display many years later in *Billy Budd*. Whittier, like the somewhat Transcendental Garrison, believed in absolute moral justice intuitively perceived by the Quaker "inner light." He was sternly opposed to what he considered the immoral expediency of utilitarian social morality based upon an empirical estimate of "the greatest good for the greatest number." For him slavery was a violation of the absolute principle of freedom, and the enforcement of the fugitive slave law, however expedient in terms of national union, provoked the powerful indignation of "Massachusetts to Virginia" (1843); and when Senator Daniel Webster, in the interest of national unity, supported the Compromise of 1850, Whittier poured forth upon him the scorn of "Ichabod." These were the strongest poems written in support of the abolitionist cause and they bear witness to the ringing power of Whittier's feeling.

When President Abraham Lincoln issued his Emancipation Proclamation in the midst of the Civil War, Whittier felt that his cause was won and celebrated the victory in the equally strong phrases of "Laus Deo" and turned to quieter things. He had always been interested in New England history, people, and customs (as illustrated in the beautifully restrained and sensitive "Telling the Bees" of 1860); and "Snowbound" (1866), the best of his long poems, is a fine idyll of country life, filled with sensitive and sympathetic human understanding and touched by a humorous appreciation of the eccentricities of thought and behavior. It also suggests that Whittier, as he approached the age of sixty, was experiencing the feeling so common among the English Romantic poets in their youth—that of the passing of some emotional glory from life and the necessity of taking refuge in the strength of a philosophic mind. He revealed the attitude from which he drew his own strength in "Abraham Davenport" (1867), a poem based upon an incident in colonial history when the legislature of Connecticut fell into a panic because it believed that an eclipse of the sun marked the beginning of doomsday. But Davenport, the presiding officer, remained calm. "Let God do his work, we will see to ours," he ordered as the darkness thickened: "Bring in the candles." Whittier's own inner light burned with less heat as it became less concerned with God's justice than with human foibles, but it never went out.

An abolitionist of a different sort but with a similar career was Harriet Beecher Stowe. Her attack upon slavery was based more upon sentiment than upon any informing principle, yet, perhaps for that reason, her *Uncle Tom's Cabin* (1852) was the most widely read American novel of the nineteenth century and the most influential work of literature inspired by the antislavery cause. Mrs. Stowe was careful to direct her attack against the institution of slavery rather than against the South or its slaveholders, and she was exaggeratedly kind toward her southern characters while making her most notorious villain, Simon Legree, a New Englander by birth. Yet she crowded her book with all the abuses she could discover by hearsay and research and made the old Negro Tom the most saintly character ever canonized by sentiment. To the extremes of characterization she added almost all the other ingredients of popular fiction—pathos and humor, the misfortunes of chance, the excitement of the chase, and the melodrama of violence—and it was successfully dramatized both as a serious propaganda play and as a new variation on the Negro minstrel show. When its popularity provoked challenges from the South she published a *Key* documenting the abuses it portrayed and attempted to duplicate its success in *Dred: A Tale of the Great Dismal Swamp* (1856). But she had exhausted her effectiveness and on the eve of the Civil War turned, perhaps with some relief, in *The Minister's Wooing* (1859) to the quieter subject of New England village life, which she was to pursue most successfully after the war in *Oldtown Folks* (1869), a book which made an influential contribution to the local-color movement.

Mrs. Stowe was a writer of considerable perceptiveness but no considerable depth, and her work is a popular symptom of the literary drift of the times—a drift, at least temporarily, toward the surface of everyday life and away from intellectual commitments, social passions, and artistic involvement with one's materials. The intemperate passions which preceded the Civil War, the long and bitter conflict itself, and the

natural reaction which followed all tended to disturb
the tenor of the individual life by which the American
writer had learned to test his wisdom. The tradition
of an American way of thinking, of assaying literary
symbols, and of writing had grown up during the second quarter of the nineteenth century. The question,
in the third quarter, was whether it could be defined
and preserved before it was lost in the tumult of social
and political change.

III

Literary history is a complicated affair because—as
we have already observed—it is concerned with the
large symbols of communication which have value at
a particular time, with the intangible patterns of tacit
belief and ways of thinking which are in the process
of creating new symbols, and with language, which
acquires its own symbolic or suggestive value when it
becomes informed with both thought and the power of
communication. Herman Melville is a crucial figure in
American literary history because he absorbed the full
strength of the prevailing pattern of thought, expressed it in terms of old symbols which still retained
their power of communication, and found in the combination a vitality of language which gave *Moby Dick*
a suggestive quality beyond the power of any author's
calculated achievement, Walt Whitman is equally crucial but in an entirely different way. He translated
the existing pattern of thought into a new large symbolism which defined it, adapted it to a new idiom of
expression, and made it available to a new generation

which was being subjected to changes in both conscious and tacit belief.

There was less in Whitman's early background than in Melville's to suggest the role he was going to play. Two months older than Melville and a native of the same region, he also left school at the age of thirteen and got his education from reading and experience. His early reading, however, was less Romantic and less literary; for the Whitman household were followers of the rationalistic Quaker, Elias Hicks, and young Walt seems to have been strongly impressed by the sermons of Hicks, by the political and religious writings of Tom Paine, and by the visions which the French Count Constantin de Volney had of mankind progressing toward some ideal state of nature and allegiance to its laws. He was apprenticed as a printer and moved from printing to journalism, free-lance writing in New York City, and eventually to the editorship of the Brooklyn *Eagle*—a position which he gave up when he became something of an abolitionist in 1847 and the paper remained conservatively Democratic. His serious concern for moral and social issues was rather late in developing, for his early contributions to magazines and newspapers, although they included a temperance novel and a short story attacking corporal punishment in the schoolroom, were superficial and perhaps even cynical in their use of popular reform sentiment for literary journalism. After leaving the *Eagle* he made a trip through the South, lived for a while in New Orleans, and returned to take charge of an antislavery newspaper, the *Freeman*, and continue the independent experiments in verse which were to culminate in the first edition of *Leaves of Grass* in 1855.

Leaves of Grass was an astonishing volume of verse, shockingly new in form, tone, and idiom. The form was free verse, influenced by the lyrical sections of the King James Bible, the irregular ode, and the popular Martin Farquhar Tupper, but not unaffected by the oratory of the Shakespearean stage and the rhythms of the sea, which Whitman heard as he recited his experimental verses on its shores. The clue to its unique tone was given in a sentence in its Preface in which the author described his book as being mainly an attempt "to put *a Person*, a human being (myself, in the latter half of the Nineteenth Century, in America) freely, fully, and truly on record"; and the new idiom is that of a person, as he saw himself or wanted himself to be seen by the public—rude and unconstrained, rebellious against the affectations of society, inclusive in his acceptance of the whole of life, and aggressive in identifying himself with all mankind while maintaining his own peculiar individuality. Emerson greeted him as a living essay in self-reliance, at "the beginning of a great career," and Thoreau saw him as a wild American buffalo breaking through the conventions from which he himself had withdrawn. The person revealed in *Leaves of Grass* was a representative American man.

The revelation was, in fact, not only extraordinarily comprehensive but remarkably subtle, perhaps more so than Whitman knew. The catalogues of human types, the displays of different attitudes, and the descriptive allusions by which he attempted to "tally"

America were all self-conscious exhibitions of his desire for "inclusiveness"—for absorbing his country, as he put it in the Preface, completely and affectionately —and they give his longest and most ambitious poem, later entitled the "Song of Myself," a panoramic quality rarely found in literature outside the novel. And his method of presenting his all-inclusive panorama was an equally self-conscious representation of the method Emerson and Hawthorne had found necessary for the American writer: Whitman was finding within himself a solution in hieroglyphics for the questions he would put and loudly professing a wisdom tested by the tenor of his own life. Beneath this was also a fairly well-balanced reflection of the prevailing American philosophy. The poem later called "There Was a Child Went Forth" is probably the best expression of Locke's empirical theory of knowledge that can be found in verse, yet in the "Song of Myself" Whitman professed to be not only the poet of the body but the poet of the soul and hinted of an intuitive and almost mystical experience by which he had achieved vision. Despite this note of Transcendentalism, however, the poems in this edition and in that of the enlarged edition of 1856 were predominantly poems of sensory perception and experience; and it is indicative of Whitman's attitude of mind at this time that his most striking poem in the third person was that on the philosophically conceived child who went forth every day and always would go forth to form his mind by sensation and reflection. While trying to capture the tangible fact of America for his book, Whitman had also managed to capture its intangible pattern of thought, and *Leaves of Grass* would be far more representative than *Moby Dick* as a reflection of the time were it not for one basic difference: Melville's individualism was in the creative depths from which his book was drawn; Whitman's was entirely on the surface. The author of *Leaves of Grass* discovered the wellspring of creative energy in American literature, but instead of tapping its force he made it gush.

The result was a writer who reveals none of the tensions which made Melville so suggestive and gave suggestive power to Hawthorne, Poe, Emerson, and Thoreau. Instead, in Whitman, the tension was released in reaction against the struggle to control literary material. "Walt, you contain enough, why don't you let it out then?" is the line from the "Song of Myself" which best reveals his own attitude toward his writing. The nineteenth-century American "person" in *Leaves of Grass* is not a coherent individual who adapts literary symbols to his individuality but rather an incoherent one whose individuality itself consists of a multiplicity of symbols. Consequently Whitman is most comprehensible when seen as a symbolic poet whose major literary symbol is the first personal pronoun and whose own changing attitudes may be followed through the shifting meanings he attached to the words "I," "me," and "myself."

These meanings at first were not carefully calculated; for Whitman was never a precise thinker, and the first Preface to *Leaves of Grass* stressed the virtues of a style which would suggest instead of define the poet's vision. Yet by the time he wrote "The Mystic Trumpeter" in 1872 he was sufficiently aware of this

quality in his work to describe his poetic development
in clearly symbolic terms, and in later editions of
Leaves of Grass he revised the opening section of the
"Song of Myself" until it defined, with reasonable
clarity, the four most distinct ways in which he thought
of himself as a person. The first of these and the one
of which he was most completely conscious at the beginning of his career was that of the representative
man—an "I" which included the entire population of
America in all of its social conditions and with all its
heritage of experience and history. The second was the
"natural," as opposed to the civilized, man who loafed
and invited his soul, who felt inclined to lie down with
the animals because they lived by instinct rather than
thought, and who sounded his barbaric yawp over the
roof of the world like the wild hawk. The third was the
unique individual poet who appeared here and there
in all of Whitman's verses but without achieving a
dominant role until after the Civil War. And the fourth
was an "I" symbolizing the biological race of man, not
very clearly defined in the opening section of the
"Song of Myself" and never extensively used although
it dominated the magnificent Section 44 of the poem
which represented humanity as "the acme of things
accomplished" in a long evolutionary process.

There can be little doubt that Whitman's greatest
appeal to his readers was in his second symbolic role—
that of the natural man, the free-spirited rebel against
conventions, who appeared frequently in the "Song of
Myself" and dominated the new poems of the 1856
edition of *Leaves of Grass,* where he appeared at his
best in the "Song of the Open Road" and caused the

most trouble in the poems grouped in the section later called "Children of Adam." It was time perhaps for the rebellion against Victorian conventions, which Swinburne was conducting in his own way in England, and from which Whitman's way differed in that it invoked a wider range of sensuous feeling, was more firmly based upon a philosophical tradition, and was expressed in a more modern and realistic idiom. For Whitman's most distinctive poetic achievement was that of taking the old philosophical concept of an ideal "state of nature" as he had found it in the eighteenth-century rationalists, particularly Volney, and translating it from the old language of abstract intellectuality into a new language of realistic adventure which appealed strongly to a lingering Romantic individualism. "Afoot and light-hearted," he took the open road to physical and spiritual freedom, finding his good fortune within himself, testing all philosophies by the feel of the morning dew, and inviting all men to accompany him on equal terms. He was the Declaration of Independence in the flesh—enjoying life, liberty, and the pursuit of happiness while accepting the doctrine of equality. He was a foot-loose Thoreau whose Walden was everywhere. He made the physical universe his oversoul. He transformed himself into a believable symbol of the union for which Melville yearned—a union between the free spirit of Transcendentalism and the undeniable reality of empirical experience.

Stimulating and inspiring though the role of the natural man was, Whitman could not maintain it for long and formally renounced it in the second half of

"Give Me the Splendid Silent Sun" (1865). For the demands of institutionalized society were pressing in upon the individual, and Whitman believed that individual freedom was possible only under the institution of political democracy, which he saw exemplified in the American Union. And the Union, in the late fifties, was being threatened by sectional differences, talk of southern secession, and the imminent likelihood of civil war. Misled perhaps by a peculiar psychological bias of his own, Whitman tried in the third edition of *Leaves of Grass* (1860) to meet this threat in individualistic terms rather than by the exercise of social force. The new poems in the "Calamus" section of this volume preached the gospel of "adhesiveness"—a phrenological term for comradeship or the affection of a person for others of his own sex—as a means of holding the Union together but did so with a naïve candor which was more shocking than persuasive to a public which had been unable to face the implications of Melville's *Pierre*. In any case, the Civil War was by then inevitable, and Whitman followed its developments from Washington, where he was a government employee in the Department of the Interior and a volunteer nurse in the military hospitals. There he collected material for the prose paragraphs of his *Specimen Days* and the poems incorporated in the *Leaves* under the title "Drum-Taps." There too he first attracted widespread public attention when he was discharged by a puritanical Secretary of the Interior (who found a copy of the 1860 *Leaves of Grass* on Whitman's desk), reemployed by the Attorney General, and defended by a group of young journalists including John Burroughs and William Douglas O'Connor, whose pamphlet, *The Good Gray Poet*, gave the prematurely grizzled Whitman a permanent label.

The triumphant conclusion of the war was to Whitman proof of the lasting strength of American democracy, and some of his patriotic exaltation seems to have entered his verse, for some of the poems in "Drum-Taps" and "Memories of President Lincoln"—especially "Pioneers! O Pioneers!" "O Captain! My Captain!" and "When Lilacs Last in the Dooryard Bloom'd"—share with the earlier "Out of the Cradle Endlessly Rocking" the distinction of being his most lyrical verses. But this note of sadness and triumph was not to last. Postwar America, at least as represented by political Washington, went morally to pieces in the materialistic corruption of what was to be called "the gilded age." In a series of prose essays, *Democratic Vistas* (1871), originally begun in answer to Carlyle's criticisms of America, Whitman was forced to admit that the spectacle was "appalling." Cynicism and corruption abounded on every side, and there was immediate need for a program of reform designed to restore human dignity and decency. Matthew Arnold's gospel of "culture" would not suffice, for it tended to produce a race of "supercilious infidels" instead of men of the robust natural dignity which lingered as an ideal in Whitman's mind from the time he had written the "Song of the Open Road." For the first time, in *Democratic Vistas*, he approached society rather than the individual from a philosophical point of view.

His approach was symptomatic of the new era in that it was based upon a theory of social evolution.

American society, as Whitman surveyed it, had to pass through three evolutionary stages. The first had already been completed in the achievement of political democracy on a permanent basis. The second—material growth and economic prosperity—was in the process of being achieved in contemporary activities which he morally deplored. The third stage would be that of greater individualism based upon a new awareness of spiritual values; and his new role, as the prophet and seer he had always thought of himself as being, would be that of hastening his country toward the climax of this evolutionary process by helping create "a new Literature, perhaps a new Metaphysics, certainly a new Poetry" which would be the support for a new American "Religious Democracy." His highest, final theme, he announced in "The Mystic Trumpeter," would be that of "a reborn race" and "a perfect world."

Unfortunately, the first of several paralytic attacks, occurring at about the time of this announcement, limited his energy and prevented the full development of this theme; and the most distinctive characteristic of his later poems is that they were almost all written from the point of view of the individual poet who had abandoned his symbolic role. Consequently it is difficult to interpret such poems as "Passage to India" (1870) and the "Prayer of Columbus" (1874). The first, written to celebrate the completion of the Suez Canal and the Union Pacific Railroad the year before, actually rejoices in the passage of the "soul" to an India conceived as a source of religious thought; and both strongly suggest that the poet had experienced some sort of ecstatic mystical vision. But it seems impossible to determine whether a genuine religious experience led Whitman to his personal interpretation of social evolution or whether his notions of social evolution led him to assume the role of mystic as a means of creating the new poetry of a religious democracy. His growing desire to emphasize the religious element in his verse, however, is clearly indicated by such later prefaces to *Leaves of Grass* as "Two Rivulets" (1876) and "A Backward Glance O'er Travel'd Roads" (1888) in which his critical retrospection found a stronger strain of spirituality in his early poems than would have been apparent to contemporary readers.

As a whole, Whitman's writings in verse and prose represent a verbalization or symbolization of an older tacit belief in the individual as a center of reference in estimating the value of intellectual systems and literary material. He was more self-conscious, artificial, and affected than the writers of the first half of the century and, for that reason, reflects a decadence of the creative spirit which brought American literature to its period of triumph over its inevitable borrowings from abroad. Yet the transmission of an attitude of mind from one generation to another must be substantially on a conscious level, and if the spring of individualism had not gushed in mid-century—not only in Whitman but in political, economic, and other non-literary manifestations—it might not have attained the place it did in the American tradition.

PART THREE

The Tradition
1868–1929

CHAPTER SEVEN

The Search for Reality

I

THE externalization of American individuality in Whitman's early work marked the climax of an attitude of mind which for a generation had been working its way toward self-consciousness. It was also symptomatic of a new age in which writers were to search for literary inspiration from without rather than from within, were to reject European literary fashions in favor of material they found around them, and were to attempt to control their work by external observation rather than by some inner wisdom. The word for the new approach was "realism," but it was a realism of appearances rather than of depths and its guides were the eye and ear rather than the mind. What Hawthorne had called "the truth of the human heart" was passed over lightly in terms of the clichés of sentiment and sentiments. When it was still associated with the intellectuality of the older generation, as in the later writings of Melville, it displayed a genuine concern for the characters of people who could hold certain opinions. When it was highly intelligent, as in the novels of John William De Forest, it explored the social scene and the backgrounds of prejudice with considerable skill. When it was simply popular, as in the publications of a host of magazine writers, it was primarily photographic, with an emphasis upon unusual settings or new angles of viewing the commonplace. The authors of the new literature, in general, tried to maintain something of a photographer's detachment from their material except for the display of such expected emotions as sympathy, humor, or, in a few cases, irony.

The only writers who remained unaffected by this prevailing literary climate were those who were out of touch with the main currents of public interest, and the finest of these was Emily Dickinson, who came to poetic maturity during the early years of the Civil War and remained relatively unaffected by external events as she continued to write, without publishing, in the seclusion of the little New England college town of Amherst. Like Whitman, she rebelled against the conventional demands for smoothness in meter and perfection in rhyme; but her rebellion took the form of going her own succinct way within the basic patterns of conventional verse rather than that of a verbose attempt to overwhelm them. For she was as quiet as Whitman was boisterous, and the first personal pronoun in her poems is the "I" of a self-sufficient private individual rather than that of an exhibitionist. Her verse often contains, in fact, the same suggestion of private communication that is to be found in the English metaphysical poets of the seventeenth century and certain English and American poets of the twen-

tieth, but it is more feminine, intimate, and delicate
in its emotional transitions, suggesting a thoughtful
passion which is deep and sometimes tragic but made
endurable by a strict refusal to be solemn.

The result is a rare quality of irony in her verse,
whether she is writing lightly or with deep feeling,
gently or sardonically. She could be a sophisticated
child describing how "A bird came down the walk,"
show a tough New England response to tragedy in
describing "The bustle in a house" after a death, display a tender grief for a child "Taken from men this
morning," or reveal casual scorn in damning a minister
when she realized that "He preached upon 'breadth'
till it argued him narrow." The subtlety of her poetic
inspiration was sometimes extraordinary, as when she
wrote that "A thought went up my mind" and tried to
capture its fleeting but unidentifiable familiarity; but,
on the other hand, she was capable of putting her
deepest personal tragedies into the little poem "I never
lost as much but twice," suggesting the depth of her
feeling in the equally short "Pain has an element of
blank," and mocking her own greatest disappointment
in the whimsey of "I asked no other thing." Nothing
could altogether escape her nimble-witted perceptiveness. She could agree wholeheartedly with the Transcendentalist Emerson in denouncing conformity with
the assertion that "Much madness is divinest sense"
and then tease her master for the solemnity of his essay
on "The Poet" by making fun of his Wordsworthian
advocacy of plain living and high thinking in "I taste
a liquor never brewed." Always succinct and often
cryptic, she addressed herself to the world on her own

terms, even though it meant the disappointment of her tentative impulse toward publication and a gradual complete retirement to her garden and her manuscripts.

At the other extreme from Emily Dickinson were the southern poets, who were estranged from the main currents of American literature by the Civil War, the defeat of the South, and the consequent eleven-year period of military occupation and social upheaval known as "Reconstruction." Henry Timrod, whose intense love for his native region as shown in such poems as "The Cotton Boll" and "Ethnogenesis" (1861) earned him the title of "Poet Laureate of the Confederacy," died before the Reconstruction period was under way; but his friend and associate, Paul Hamilton Hayne, revealed in "The Pines" and in various sonnets the tendency toward escape which in the younger poet Sidney Lanier produced a genuine outburst of American Romanticism in the purest English vein. At the beginning of the Reconstruction period Lanier had seemed a poet of his times, concentrating his attention upon the people and problems of his own locality and presenting them with a realism of observation and dialect which was characteristic of the new "local color" school in fiction. But as time went on, Lanier, though still concerned with the economic problems of the South, escaped emotionally into the conventional channels of an earlier period—into a preoccupation with the past (in such poems as "The Revenge of Hamish" and in his popular books for boys) and into a devotion to external nature which was as passionate as Wordsworth's and as sensuous as Keats's. His contemplation of "The Marshes of Glynn" (1878) made his soul "suddenly free" from a wearier weight than any earlier American nature poet knew; and although he realized that beneath the escape symbol of the Marshes there was something darker than he could face, he almost deified nature, and in "A Ballad of Trees and the Master" (1880) gave it the healing power of the Divine Spirit.

Lanier's other medium of escape—and his most significant one, from the point of view of purely southern literary history—was through the deliberate glorification of emotion at the expense of reason. In part, as his novel *Tiger Lilies* (1867) had revealed, this was a product of an intellectual background like Lowell's, which derived moral principles from innate sentiments; and the sometimes puzzling conclusion to his finest poem, "The Symphony" (1875)—"Music is Love in search of a word"—reflects a theory of knowledge comparable to Lowell's in which the moral sentiments grope upward through various media of communication until they find their perfect expression in the words of the poet. But "The Symphony" is a more complex poem than anything Lowell wrote, for Lanier was not simply being philosophical in verses ingeniously contrived to suggest the instruments in an orchestra. He was in deep rebellion against a contemporary world devoted to the calculating materialism of commerce, and he identified "trade" with the intellectual activities of the "head," while setting in opposition to it the higher sentiments of the "heart" as exemplified in the love of nature, the chivalric love of woman, and the charitable love of one's fellow man as ordered by

Christian doctrine. These were the resources available to his own downtrodden, poverty-stricken South; and these were the ideals on which he and southern literature for the generation to follow took a last ditch stand against the onslaughts of realism.

But the larger literary world belonged to the realists —of one sort or another—and the sort who flourished in the popular magazines were the local colorists. The *Atlantic Monthly, Harper's,* and *Lippincott's* vied eagerly for new writers who could present pictures of new localities with the proper sound effects of dialect and idiom. They already had Harriet Beecher Stowe and Rose Terry Cook for New England and were to find Rebecca Harding Davis for the iron mills of the Pennsylvania and West Virginia border, George Washington Cable and Grace King for New Orleans and the bayou country, Charles Egbert Craddock (actually Mary Murfree) for the Tennessee mountains, Edward Eggleston for the midwestern Hoosiers, and Emily Dickinson's friend Helen Hunt Jackson for southern California. The *Atlantic's* greatest find was Bret Harte, of San Francisco, who had tried his hand at romantic stories of the West but had turned to a Dickensian treatment of gold digging in such tales as "The Luck of Roaring Camp," "Tennessee's Partner," and "The Outcasts of Poker Flat," (1868–69), which brought him fame through the *Overland Monthly* and an extravagant and highly publicized contract with the *Atlantic,* which stimulated the whole movement enormously but got little of value from the quickly exhausted Harte. In its later stages the movement was to produce such fine regional books as Sarah Orne Jewett's *The*

Country of the Pointed Firs (1896) and Kate Chopin's
The Awakening (1899), but, in retrospect, its early
importance seems to lie in the fact that it opened up
the field of ordinary life to literary exploitation and
seduced readers through the charms of novelty to appreciate the realism of the commonplace.

The broader effects of the new tendency, at its beginning, may be seen in the work of John William De
Forest, who turned away from his prewar romances
and travel books to write *Miss Ravenel's Conversion
from Secession to Loyalty* (1867)—a novel which
ranges in scene from New Haven to New Orleans,
deals boldly with such a variety of matters as military
action, political chicanery, and domestic and somewhat undomestic manners while presenting realistically the variety of characters involved in the southern
heroine's change of attitude toward her native region.
De Forest was for some years associated with the
Freedmen's Bureau in South Carolina and drew upon
his experiences for a number of short stories which
were equally free from sentimentality and comparably
broad in their comprehension of both individual character and social conditions. But he did not consistently
remain in the realistic vein, and although *Kate Beau-
mont* (1872) and *Honest John Vane* (1875) are
solidly based upon the realities of prewar life in South
Carolina and contemporary American politics, the
serious search for reality within the commonplace was
conducted by the younger novelist William Dean
Howells.

Howells was a magazine editor—of the *Atlantic* in
Boston from 1871 to 1881, and of *Harper's* in New York

from 1885 to his death in 1920—who came East from
Ohio after four years of service as American consul in
Venice. His experiences abroad had provided him with
material for two travel books and his first novel, *Their
Wedding Journey* (1872), but he was quickly con-
verted to the new realism which the *Atlantic* was encouraging and began searching for his own proper
medium of expression. A mawkishly sentimental or humorous realism was not acceptable to his genuine intelligence, and farcical humor, which he attempted
from time to time, was not suited to his talents. The
fictional technique of Ivan Turgenev appealed to him
more than did that of any other novelist, and in the
Russian master he found a detachment which did not
have to be disguised by any artificial pose and which
enabled him to transform his own sense of the ridiculous into stylistic irony. He was able to direct this
irony effectively upon spiritualism in the Shaker community of Vardley in *The Undiscovered Country*
(1880) and upon the rocking-chair society of a seaside hotel in *Dr. Breen's Practice* (1881), but it was at
its best in *A Modern Instance* (1882), which portrayed a possessive young woman, her enterprising but
weak journalist husband, and the shrewd Yankee lawyer who was her father. Although the book touched
upon the problem of divorce, which was not common
at the time, it was a fine example of commonplace
realism sustained and lightened by style.

Howells was not entirely content, however, with this
sort of empirical fiction, based upon skillful observation
and informed only by a surface intelligence. He was
looking for a deeper reality and, perhaps naturally

enough, looked for it first in the traditional American belief in an innate moral sense or intuition which was capable of rising to an occasion without any evident preparation or training; and in a characteristic gesture he uncovered it in the type of American who was so widely damned for lacking it—the successful, self-made businessman. The hero of *The Rise of Silas Lapham* (1885) was realistically portrayed as a Vermont farmer who had become a manufacturer of paint and achieved financial success by the shrewd management of his business, the ruthless elimination of his partner, and a willingness to splash the countryside with advertisements of his product. At the opening of the book he is ready to retire, build a big house on Beacon Hill, and introduce his daughters to the Boston society in which his wife expects them to find cultivated husbands. The situation was commonplace enough, and so were most of the incidents of the novel—the financial misfortunes of a man who is wise in business but an innocent on the stock exchange, the return of the ruined partner, the family conferences, and the tragicomedies acted out by the *nouveaux riches* amid an established aristocracy. But the real story is of Lapham's moral rise, and it reaches its climax when he displays an ethical sensibility which causes him to sacrifice an opportunity to recoup his own fortunes and to relieve his ordinary conscience by restoring those of his former partner. It is a sensibility which rises above anything in Silas' training, above the highest concepts of business morality, and above the perceptions of his wife, who normally served as his ethical guide; and it demanded not only self-sacrifice but the sacrifice of the greatest good for the greatest number to some Transcendental abstraction within the man's individual consciousness. The basic reality presented in this book was the essential goodness of man.

But Howells could not hold on to the Transcendental tradition. The America of his day was a country of increasing social conflicts, and when Howells moved to the larger world of New York in 1885, fresh from four years abroad, he became aware of them. His sympathies, as he himself observed, could not embrace two million people; and, influenced by the new doctrines of socialism as he had already been influenced by the literary theories of Hippolyte Taine, he began to see individuals as representatives of social and economic classes. When the Haymarket riots occurred in Chicago in 1886 Howells jeopardized his own position on *Harper's* to defend the arrested anarchists, and their eventual conviction and execution (for their opinions rather than their guilt) helped powerfully to convince him that social forces were more real than an innate moral sense. Accordingly, in *A Hazard of New Fortunes* (1890), the most comprehensive and impressive of all his novels, he turned to presentation of the conflicting points of view he found in the society around him. The framework of the book was autobiographical in that it dealt with the removal of the March family from Boston to New York, and the action centered around the New York streetcar strike which had occurred soon after Howells' arrival. The characters were mostly associated with the publishing world that the author knew so well, and through them —the capitalist Dryfoos and his liberal son Conrad, the self-centered Beaton, the radically reactionary Colonel Woodburn, and the socialist Lindau—Howells presented a variety of beliefs that all had a stronger operative power than any possessed by the sensitive and open-minded March. In this book the man of sensibility was relegated to the position of an observer of realities outside himself, too powerful for him to control.

And there he remained through all the later novels which provide significant indications of Howells' intellectual position. In his two discursive Utopian romances, *A Traveler from Altruria* (1894) and *Through the Eye of the Needle* (1907), the weak and intellectually ineffective characters are the novelist and the clergyman, who are professionally devoted to sensibility and the moral sense, whereas the banker and the lawyer are best equipped to understand the realities of an altruistic civilization. For the Altrurians did not arrive at their ideal state through abstract reason, intuition, or even the Christian principles to which they so closely conformed, but by a long process of empirical trial and error which taught them that socialism was the best form of government because if men knew enough they would rarely have to be forced to do unto others what they would have others do unto them. Howells' final view of reality was that the forces which controlled men were to be found in the social order rather than within the individual himself, and his belief in the innate goodness of man was translated into an optimistic prophecy of social evolution toward a state of human relationships in which altruism would be indistinguishable from enlightened self-interest.

His principles of morality never changed. In fact, they became more clearly defined as he decided that they were less absolute than expedient.

II

While William Dean Howells was finding his way to the respectable realism of the magazines, his contemporary and eventually his close friend Mark Twain was becoming involved in a different kind of realism in the newspapers. For it was in the weekly newspaper that the western tradition of storytelling flourished. It had attracted widespread attention for the first time in 1834 with the publication of David Crockett's *Autobiography,* the story of a ring-tailed roarer who had come to Congress from the Tennessee canebrakes and who could jump into the air, crack his heels together three times, crow like a rooster, and come down to lick his weight in wildcats or run like a streak of greased lightning. The book may have been ghostwritten in the first place, and it certainly was in later editions when Whig propagandists used Crockett to attack Andrew Jackson; but it brought before the public an authentic frontier hero who was wilder and more extravagant than Cooper's Natty Bumppo and, to some tastes, considerably more amusing. The almanacs created Mike Fink, king of the keelboats and hero of the Mississippi; and, in oral tradition, the sort of folklore was developing which was eventually to produce the tallest of tall-story heroes in the person of Paul Bunyan.

But the type of literary taleteller who put such

stories into print was best represented by Augustus Baldwin Longstreet, classically educated at Yale, whose *Georgia Scenes* (1835) exemplifies a type of local color which was not to be found in the respectable magazines but flourished in such books as Joseph G. Baldwin's *Flush Times in Alabama and Mississippi* (1853) and hundreds of newspaper stories by known and unknown contributors—so many, in fact, that in 1831 William Trotter Porter had founded a New York newspaper, *The Spirit of the Times,* to disseminate them throughout the country. The stories were both cruel and comic, and the most distinctive thing about them was the manner of their telling: no matter how brutal the incidents or how extravagant the comic fantasy, they were told with the straight unrevealing face that later vaudevillians were to call "the dead-pan technique." The best storyteller, orally or on paper, was the one who could maintain the most complete detachment and allow his audience to build up its own emotions without any clue to the expected response. Unlike the magazine writers, who put their readers at ease by affecting sentiment or humor, the frontier storytellers attempted to make their audiences uncomfortable by playing a cat-and-mouse game with their feelings until detachment itself became the art of arts.

Samuel Langhorne Clemens had been brought up within touch of the frontier in the small town of Hannibal, Missouri, where immigrants crossed the Mississippi on their way west to the Oregon settlements and eventually the gold mines of California. As a journeyman printer in his youth he had become professionally familiar with newspaper humor, and as the pilot of a

Mississippi River steamer before the Civil War he was in a position to exchange stories with the masters of the art. But it was not until he became a newspaper reporter in the western silver-mining town of Virginia City, Nevada, that he became notorious as the teller of such tall tales as that of the "Petrified Man" and took as his nom de plume the cry of the Mississippi River leadsman, "Mark Twain"—a name which became nationally known to connoisseurs of American humor after a New York newspaper published in 1865 "The Celebrated Jumping Frog of Calaveras County." He had by this time moved to California, and a trip to the Sandwich Islands provided him with material for his first successful appearance as a humorous lecturer in the autumn of 1866 and for a series of newspaper articles which he later was to revise for *Roughing It* (1872). His first great success, however, came in 1869 with *The Innocents Abroad,* a book in which he used the technique of frontier storytelling in an account of a grand cruise through the Mediterranean and to the Holy Land. Here he could solemnly assure his readers that there was no conflict in the claims of two rival monasteries for the skull of Adam because a difference in size indicated that one was the skull of Adam as a boy and the other that of Adam as a man; and by such an application of a new art to old material he could not only delight the western readers of the *Alta California* (which sent him on the expedition) but also the eastern clients of a religious publishing house that distributed the book with misgivings which were quickly overcome by its sales.

The success of *The Innocents Abroad* enabled Twain

to take an eastern wife and settle down as a western writer and lecturer in an eastern home. The western pose was the secret of his success as a comic writer or funnyman, for it enabled him to affect a crude detachment from the sentiments expected of the well bred and thereby keep his readers in a constant state of shock. He cultivated the manner in various anecdotal sketches he published from time to time and in the autobiographical narrative of *Roughing It*, and he transferred it to the novel in *The Gilded Age* (1873), which he undertook in collaboration with Charles Dudley Warner. Although primarily an attack upon the materialism, speculation, and corruption of the postwar period, especially well personalized by the grandiose Colonel Sellers and the cynical Senator Dilworthy, *The Gilded Age* also contained autobiographical elements in the experiences of the Hawkins family; and it may be that Twain's partial identification of himself with young Washington Hawkins turned his thoughts back to his Missouri boyhood and caused him to write *The Adventures of Tom Sawyer* (1876). At any rate, Tom Sawyer was strongly reminiscent of his own boyhood and effective in its influence upon his imagination because it opened his eyes to the possibility of a boy's view of the world as a means of relief from that of the western humorist. He remained western, however, in his next autobiographical books, *A Tramp Abroad* (1880) and *Life on the Mississippi* (1883), although he used the boy's approach in *The Prince and the Pauper* (1882)—a historical novel which grew out of a long-time plan to satirize English customs and institutions but was transformed into a children's book as he tried out his approach on his own family. But all the while he was trying a completely new role, that of a boy who was totally unlike the young Sam Clemens or the mature and somewhat hackneyed humorist and who therefore offered him a freedom of outlook he had never before possessed. The boy had strolled into *Tom Sawyer* swinging a dead cat, and his name was Huckleberry Finn.

The *Adventures of Huckleberry Finn* appeared in 1885 and brought to a peak the creative achievement of Mark Twain and the western tradition in which he developed. For in writing this book Twain found what every outward-looking novelist seeks—that "lucid moment of balance" in which he becomes freshly involved in the world while remaining artistically detached from it. The fresh involvement came through the point of view of a boy character for whom the author felt no social or personal responsibility, a "poor white" in a class-conscious village, but through whom he could recapture the past and release a store of memories and associations that sophistication had suppressed. The detachment was achieved by maintaining the fiction that Huck Finn was a fictitious character, the representative of an insensitive class whose dead-pan attitude toward the world gave the false impression that he had "no more morals than a mud turtle" and made him an ideal storyteller in the western tradition. And so Mark Twain could let him drift from adventure to adventure down the river, the great central highway of prewar America, and take a fresh look at the richly varied society which the author himself knew so well.

The book is as plotless and as anecdotal as any of Mark Twain's autobiographical writings but infinitely more natural, human, and, in a sense, intimate. The reader knows Huck Finn as he never gets to know Mark Twain, and in fact the best thing we know about Mark Twain is that he was able to create this boy who is one of the most completely and deeply imagined characters in literature.

The faults of the book (and they are many) came from the loss of balance, as a result of either the author's excessive involvement in Huck or his occasional efforts at self-conscious detachment. For Huck knew everything that his creator knew, and he sometimes displayed more learning than he could have acquired in character. When he struggled with the moral problem of freeing the Negro Jim, for instance, he knew from an inward humanity very close to a "moral sense" that the conventions of a slaveholding society were harsher than his own abstract notions of hell; but he knew this as a boy would know it, impulsively and irrationally, and we accept it more readily than we accept Mark Twain's arguments against the southern feudal system in *Life on the Mississippi*. But when he explained the abuses of royalty within the European feudal system, he revealed what Mark Twain had learned from his recent researches for *The Prince and the Pauper* and became implausible by reason of the same identification with his creator which generally makes him so convincingly human. The greatest flaw in the novel, however, is the conclusion, where the detachment implicit in Huck's point of view is lost and he becomes a substitute narrator for the author of *Tom*

Sawyer. Here the artificial detachment of the self-conscious storyteller reveals the hackneyed quality of a role Mark Twain had played too long and from which he had had the great good fortune, in the better part of his book, to escape.

Twain was subtly aware that the spontaneity had disappeared from his storytelling, and on the lecture platform he tried to introduce variety into his performances by placing them in contrast to those of an author whose manner and temperament were completely different from his own. It was George Washington Cable, serving this purpose for a season, who gave him Sir Thomas Malory's *Morte d'Arthur* to read and so provided the inspiration necessary to turn a fantasy in his notebook into *A Connecticut Yankee in King Arthur's Court* (1889). For this new book was the tallest of all Mark Twain's tall tales, based upon the notion of translating into the fifth century a man with the nineteenth-century genius for trading and manufacturing and then having him remake its civilization in the modern American image. It was also the best sustained of his tall tales, for both the romantic chivalry and the artificial language of Malory provided fresh material for burlesque. The notion on which it was based could be exploited in innumerable ways, and it enabled Twain to carry out his long-time plan to satirize English institutions—especially those relics of "feudalism" which offended his rationalistic mind, the aristocracy of class distinctions and privileges and the established church. Into it he could pour the thoughtful results of his reading which had been suppressed in *The Prince and the Pauper* and had been struggling for expression in

Huckleberry Finn. The *Connecticut Yankee* is a book
as rich in artificial invention as *Huckleberry Finn* is in
the re-creation of memories.

Yet *A Connecticut Yankee* is not an emotionally
coherent book. The impulses back of it were more varied than those in any of Mark Twain's other writings.
The prevailing impulse seems to have been that of
fantasy and burlesque, but the intellectually sustaining
one was undoubtedly that of satire. For Twain was
growing indignant about the world toward which he
had been, as a humorist, so professionally cynical. His
satire of institutions was from an eighteenth-century
rationalistic point of view, but he added, from the
point of view of disillusioned humanity, bitter attacks
upon insensitivity and cruelty; and, with a new pessimism, he attacked eighteenth-century rationalism itself
by denying the possibility of educating superstition out
of a people. The only touch of mellowness in the story
comes from the sort of personal nostalgia found in *Tom
Sawyer, Huckleberry Finn,* and the first half of *Life on
the Mississippi,* for in their tour of the country, King
Arthur and the Yankee Sir Boss slip into the characters
of Huck and Tom in a subtle indication of the author's
feeling that humanity was tolerable only when it was
childlike.

Mark Twain referred to *A Connecticut Yankee* as his
"swan song" and, although the feeling back of the reference may have been only a lack of energy, the book
actually does mark the climax of his career as a humorous storyteller and the beginning of emotional and
intellectual insecurity. He had felt a reality beneath
the surface of the life he observed so accurately and

had sought it in an individual point of view—that of a humorist and impressionistic satirist, that of a nostalgic man and the various boys who were products of his nostalgia, and that of a rational satirist who was also filled with humane indignation. But none of these points of view was stable. The humorist and casual satirist had grown tired, nostalgia was only an occasional means of escape, and reason itself seemed untrustworthy. Like the Emerson of "Experience" he was becoming aware that life was a string of moods, and temperament was the wire upon which they were strung, but like Poe his own temperament was that of an actor who had appeared in different moods without achieving a private intellectual stability. Unlike Melville, who experienced similar but more profound stresses, he could not settle into a limited scale of living. Money—the enormous sums of money he earned from his writing and threw away in speculative investments—meant too much to him. In his mid-fifties, as he approached the later stage of his career, he could do nothing but write according to his moods while at the same time searching for something he could accept as intellectual reality.

The mood he tried to sustain in the many potboilers of his later years was that of the comedian, but the one which moved him most deeply was that of indignation. He became violent on such subjects as copyright laws, the political organization of Tammany Hall, and certain capitalists and corporation executives; and he became the defender of the underdogs of history in his essay "In Defense of Harriet Shelley" and his *Personal Recollections of Joan of Arc* (1896), and of the Negro race in *Pudd'nhead Wilson* (1894). But amidst these outbursts of indignation he was seeking for some form of belief. He implicitly denied the existence of an internal, uncorruptible moral sense in his story "The Man That Corrupted Hadleyburg" (1899) and sought refuge in a form of mechanistic determinism in his essay "What is Man?" which he withheld from publication until 1906. The best and most revealing book of his later years, however, was his posthumous novel *The Mysterious Stranger* (1916). Written in the nostalgic mood which caused him to revive his boy characters in *Tom Sawyer Abroad* (1894) and other stories of the nineties, it tells of three boys in medieval Austria who were visited by an angel named Satan and taught by him, first, that living beings were the playthings of their creator, that the moral sense was a quality in man which made him lower than the brutes, that life was in the chain of necessity, and, finally, that all this and existence itself was nothing more than an illusion of the mind. Cynical in theme, it was astonishingly tender in tone, and it presented Mark Twain's search for reality ending in a sort of discouraged philosophical idealism.

This was not the real conclusion. The author stopped here because he could go no further, and his friend Howells persuaded him that he had reached a perfect artistic if not a satisfactory philosophical conclusion. Mark Twain was never able to accept the empirical realities to which Howells learned to conform, nor could he find within his own mind a philosophy which he could accept as something more real than the world that was too much with him. His search led to disillusionment and bitterness but to no belief—perhaps because he began it too late, after his role as a detached, uncouth western humorist had separated him for almost a generation from other seekers after a personal philosophical refuge from the overwhelming forces of society.

III

The intellectual guiding spirit behind these other seekers, whether they accepted the fact or not, was Herbert Spencer and his theory of social evolution. Two ideas from Spencer were particularly influential upon American literature after the publication of the *First Principles* in 1862. One was his general formula for the evolutionary process, which moved from the simple to the complex in terms of an increasing tendency toward the specialization of parts and a greater integration of these parts into a coherent whole. The other was contained in the famous phrase he contributed to the Darwinian theory of evolution, "the survival of the fittest" in this process of change. With reference to society, the first of these ideas implied movement away from a simple culture in which people were more or less alike and were independently engaged in similar activities to the development of a complex civilization in which individual activities were highly specialized and closely integrated with each other. The second implied competition, ruthlessness, and allowed some of Spencer's American followers to see Darwin's law of the jungle within the highest form of civilization. Spencer's notion that "the integration of matter" was accompanied by a "concomitant dissipation of motion" was also influential in its suggestion, to some people at least, of wasted energy in modern life. The peak of social evolution would be reached in a highly organized society of completely heterogeneous individuals, and the implication was that these individuals would be fiercely competitive for their places in the organization and enormously wasteful of energy.

The great contribution that Darwin made to the intellectual climate of the late nineteenth century was that of increasing men's confidence in empirical knowledge by showing that it could answer questions which writers like Hawthorne had found beyond the empirical range—questions involving creation itself, which had hitherto been questions of faith or speculative reason. Spencer, as the philosopher of the evolutionary movement, was therefore offering a new and more solid version of natural law, partially verifiable by every man's observation in accord with a method now proved practicable for such a large inquiry. It was eminently suited to the defense of such economic tendencies in America as the exploitation of natural resources, the rapid growth of industrialization, and the establishment of large corporations and trusts; but it was also eminently suited to create discomfort among those old-fashioned individualists whose concepts of natural law were ethical and intuitive, who valued morality above success, or who longed for the security of the absolute. It was a new philosophical reality, in short, which some people were eager and others felt obliged to accept; and the literary response to it reflected the difficulty of fitting it into the American cultural tradition.

The first response, by Walt Whitman, suggested no difficulty at all. For Whitman, though intellectual enough to seize upon the idea of social evolution as a means of explaining the faults of democracy, was either too optimistic or not alert enough to grasp the implications of the Darwinian theory; and in *Democratic Vistas,* as we have seen, he simply welcomed the forthcoming age of individualism and redirected his aims as a poet toward hurrying it up and improving its moral tone. But the impulse of the younger writers whose lives spanned the Civil War period was to escape. They could neither deny the new reality nor reconcile themselves to existence within it, and the simplest and most direct of the escapists was Lafcadio Hearn.

Hearn had been born of an Irish father and a Greek mother on the Aegean island for which he was named, reared in Britain and France, and impelled to come to America as a youthful Bohemian devoted "to the worship of the Odd, the Queer, the Strange, the Exotic, and the Monstrous" in such varied places as Cincinnati, New Orleans, and the French West Indies. He had expressed his devotion in such newspaper sketches as those later collected as *Fantastics and Other Fancies* (1914) and *Creole Sketches* (1924), in a colorful novel *Chita* (1889), and in an autobiographical *Two Years in the French West Indies* (1890); but he was a noncompetitive individualist, financially unsuccessful and out of place in the world of Spencerian evolution which he had intellectually accepted in his early newspaper pieces. In 1889 he read Percival Lowell's *The Soul of the Far East* (1888), which interpreted Japan in Spencerian terms, and there discovered a land in which he could worship his own peculiar gods and at the same time escape the turbulent evolutionary stream by settling into the quiet eddies of an older culture of stable values where "impersonality" rather than "personality" was the ideal. There for a while he found what he was seeking and made effective literary use of the strange and exotic aspects of old Japan in several volumes of ghost and fairy stories. But his two most serious books on his adopted country, *Glimpses of Unfamiliar Japan* (1894) and *Japan: An Attempt at Interpretation* (1904), show a distressed recognition of the fact that Japan would have to become industrial and commercial if it survived in the modern world, and the old system of stability and unselfish ethics was being lost in the evolutionary current. By the time of his death he was disillusioned about the possibility of escape and anxious to return to America.

Even less successful in his effort to escape the overwhelming forces of social evolution was Henry Adams. The great-grandson and the grandson of American presidents and the son of America's most influential minister to Great Britain, Adams seems to have identified himself early as one of the ablest members of his family and one of the least likely to succeed. The trouble was with the world, not with the Adams breed. For the Adamses were men of character and merit in a world whose standards of values had grown so poor that real merit was no longer recognized and a man of character could no longer be called from his plow to manage the ship of state. The political arena after the Civil War had become a place for wild beasts and wilder men, unfit for a Roman, and so Henry Adams became a man of letters—a journalist and editor of the *North American Review*, a historian of early nineteenth-century America, and an anonymous and pseudonymous novelist with *Democracy* (1879) and *Esther* (1884) when the continued attractions of politics induced him to move to Washington and attempt to be influential behind scenes. Protected by a thin wall of sardonic irony, he stood aside from the social forces of his own day and tried to understand them. But the protection broke under the severe emotional blow of his wife's suicide in 1885, and he made the same attempt to escape that Hearn was to make a few years later—first to Japan, where he was uncomfortable and ill at ease, and later to Tahiti, where he sought through the memories of old men to find the pre-evolutionary civilization which existed before the French came to the islands.

Although he traveled much, Adams' refuge was in the past. He published his monumental *History of the United States during the Administrations of Jefferson and Madison* (1884–89) in nine volumes and devoted the next fifteen years of his literary life to the meticulous reconstruction of a world he might have loved and the analysis of one he hated. His love was focused upon twelfth-century France, and he described it in *Mont-Saint-Michel and Chartres,* which was eventually published privately in 1904. There he partially found and partially created a homogeneous culture whose energy was not dissipated but was directed toward an end which could be readily symbolized by the worship of the Virgin and which was expressed in the magnificent cathedral at Chartres. It was a civilization more depersonalized than Hearn's Japan, and the anonymity of the architect of Chartres was, to Adams, one of the most significant facts in it. He loved it with the meditative passion of a weary man's dream of nirvana, and sacrificed his historical conscience to it as he re-created it as a sanctuary which would be tragically violated by the evolutionary processes which produced modern America. In contrast to it he placed the world of his own lifetime in *The Education of Henry Adams* (1907), where the man of character, an Adams, was lost in the rush toward heterogeneity and the undirected dissipation of power for which he found a symbol in the dynamo. The *Education* purported to be an autobiography, but, in actual fact, it skipped the most important period in Adams' life and, instead, revealed the state of mind of a man whose consciousness was haunted by evolutionary symbols—the Terebratula which had failed to survive or evolve, the Limulus or horseshoe crab which had survived unchanged from the Silurian period, the sharklike Pteraspis which was the first of the vertebrates and hence the ancestor of man, and the Cunard liner which was the symbol of social man's most spectacular dissipation of power. Evolution was a reality he was forced to accept, but he hated it with an intensity which made him long for the period of dissolution which would inevitably follow; and the last activity of his sardonic mind was the composition of two essays (posthumously published by his brother Brooks as *The Degradation of the Democratic*

Dogma) in which he attempted to find a mechanistic formula for dissolution in the second law of thermodynamics and apply his brother's "rule of phase" to the evolutionary process in a way that might hurry it to an end within his own lifetime.

Another reluctant Spencerian of Adams' generation was Ambrose Bierce, who served in the Civil War, began his career as a journalist in San Francisco, and went to London in 1872, where he cultivated the rather grim and ghastly humor which led him during the nineties into a cynicism as bitter as that of Mark Twain. Less a seeker than an escapist, however, he expressed his cynicism in his column of "Prattle" for the San Francisco *Examiner* and in the form of artificially constructed short stories of the sort perfected by Edgar Allan Poe, cultivated by Rudyard Kipling, and brought to a state of decadence in America by the popular O. Henry. But Bierce's cynicism was not the stuff for popular publishers, and his best collection of stories, *Tales of Soldiers and Civilians* (1891), owed its existence to the generosity of a San Francisco merchant and did not appear commercially until seven years later and then under the title *In the Midst of Life*. This, with another collection of stories, *Can Such Things Be?* (1893), and a collection of epigrams, first called *The Cynic's Word Book* (1906) and later *The Devil's Dictionary*, formed the basis for his reputation as one of the leading eccentrics of the era, who dramatized his reputation by disappearing into Mexico at the age of seventy-one to join the army of the insurgent Pancho Villa and removing himself permanently from the civilization he so despised.

The younger American writers who were born into the age of Spencer and Darwin were less rebellious than Hearn, Adams, and Bierce and more willing to accept the principle of evolution as a natural law under which they must live and to assume a certain amount of individual freedom within the framework of social necessity. Some of the more humane and optimistic souls, in fact, were able to turn their backs on Darwin, ignore Spencer's theory of the dissipation of motion as society became more coherent, and hope that social evolution would eventually result in a civilization of finer individuals who were freed from their animal impulses by the perfection of their communal organizations. Howells was to fall into this group in *A Traveller from Altruria,* but by far the most popular and influential of these Utopians was Edward Bellamy, whose *Looking Backward, 2000–1887* (1888) pictured a society in which abundance had been achieved by the intelligent direction of the power of the machine, selfishness and material competition had disappeared, and something like Whitman's "re-born race" of superior persons had been developed. The book's achievement of a tremendous popularity bore witness to a widespread belief that social evolution was not something to escape but to control, and the first problem of the realists who shared this belief was that of indicating what needed to be controlled.

In an age of large fortunes and abject poverty, exploitation and the abuse of privilege, the greatest need for control seemed to be within the economic system; and of the later realists young Hamlin Garland was the most acutely conscious of the economic forces which made life, as he had known it, on the western plains, so drab. An ardent Spencerian, he had moved to Boston and attempted a history of American literature on evolutionary principles; but as he turned to more creative work in the short stories of *Main-Travelled Roads* (1891) and *Prairie Folks* (1893), he devoted himself to the impressionistic use of his own early experiences in a way which suggested the need for reform before any development could occur in the direction that another of his literary heroes, Whitman, had foretold. He had already found the means of reform in the single-tax system advocated by Henry George in *Progress and Poverty* (1879), and the economic bias of his stories was against landlords and mortgage holders who profited by the increased value of land at the expense of its users. There was a vividness of realistic detail in these stories, like that of such earlier books from the Middle West as Edgar Watson Howe's *The Story of a Country Town* (1883) and Joseph Kirkland's *Zury* (1887), but there was no great power in Garland's thought, and he was easily diverted to the artificial romances which became popular at the end of the century.

The strongest and most effective writers of this group, in fact, were those who exhibited the intellectual detachment claimed by Émile Zola for naturalism and the experimental novel. Although probably not influenced by the French naturalists, Stephen Crane was of their temper in his desire to present the brutal facts of life that needed public attention and to do so with a power which invited reform without attempting to direct it. Crane was a minister's son and a rebel against his upbringing whose two volumes of free verse, *The Black Riders* (1895) and *War Is Kind* (1899), reveal a young man who was almost the calculated opposite of the hero Christian in John Bunyan's *Pilgrim's Progress;* and he sent a copy of his first novel, *Maggie, A Girl of the Streets* (1892), to a clergyman with a note to the effect that it tried to show how tremendous a thing environment was in the shaping of lives. His most successful book, *The Red Badge of Courage* (1895), owes its effectiveness to Crane's imaginative feat in capturing the private soldier's environment during a military action and making him subject to it. The same quality is to be found in the best of his short stories published in *The Open Boat* (1898), and one story, "The Blue Hotel," concludes with a brief comment upon crime and causation which is purely naturalistic in its implication.

Crane's contemporary, Frank Norris, was an avowed naturalist who had studied art in Paris and perhaps learned there about the new school of writers whose principles he adopted while in a writing course at Harvard where he wrote the posthumously published novel *Vandover and the Brute* (1914) and partially wrote his most famous novel *McTeague* (1899). Before completing the latter, however, he tried his hand at two kinds of popular romance in *Moran of the Lady Letty* (1898) and *Blix* (1899); and he experimented again with an adventure story of the Far North in *A Man's Woman* (1900) before deciding that the naturalistic method was the most desirable one to use for the epic trilogy of wheat which was left uncompleted at the time of his early death. *McTeague* is a memorably detailed story of simple people driven to destruction by chance, circumstance, and the primitive passion of greed; and, despite its moments of western melodrama, it is the best example of French naturalism in nineteenth-century American literature. It lacks the feeling for the power of social and natural forces, however, which is evident in *The Octopus* (1901), the first of the wheat trilogy, in which Norris throws the California ranchers of the San Joaquin Valley into conflict with the corporate railroad octopus and allows them to be destroyed. More powerful than the economic organization with all its political ramifications, though, is the power of nature as symbolized by the wheat which flows through this book and into the next, *The Pit* (1903), as a stream which can neither be dammed nor controlled by all the efforts of human ingenuity exercised on the Chicago grain exchange. It is not clear whether Norris really felt the power of nature or was merely using it for dramatic purposes, but it is clear from these books that he thought of the strongest, most intelligent, and most heroically determined individuals as being subject to forces over which they had no control. Reality for him, as for most of his contemporaries, was something outside himself; and, in common with many of them, he was inclined to see it as some onward-moving, irresistible natural force.

CHAPTER EIGHT

Society and the Individual

I

WITH so strong a feeling for external reality dominating late nineteenth-century America, it is perhaps not surprising that the writer who best preserved the traditional confidence in the individual human spirit was the expatriate Henry James. For James had been educated mostly abroad by a father who gave an international exhibition of the sort of individualistic, eccentric Transcendentalism that Thoreau had displayed at Walden Pond; and the effect of this education was to give the future novelist external familiarity with international society and the internal detachment of an observer who studied social conventions without allowing himself to be dominated by them. To James these conventions represented social reality, and he observed them acutely and with what must have become a fascinated interest in their subtlety. He knew little or nothing of the commonplace middle-class life which was so real to Howells, he could not realize (even by a calculated act of the imagination, as in his novel *The*

Princess Casamassima) the economic and class conflicts which obsessed so many of his contemporaries,
and he was completely indifferent to the theory of
social evolution. The grandson of an Irish immigrant
who had made a fortune in the new world, he did not
feel with Henry Adams that he had inherited a judicious position at the center of the universe, nor did he
have Mark Twain's compulsion to strike an outsider's
pose. He felt free to choose his own world and adapt
himself to it, and in 1876 he chose London because he
preferred it as a center of operation for a man of letters
who, at the age of thirty-three, had published two
novels, some twenty-five short stories, and twice as
many reviews but was just beginning his serious career
as an artist.

The primary aim of the elder Henry James in educating his four sons had been to give them freedom—
freedom to pick and choose not only among countries
but among occupations, ideas, and religions—and he
was successful enough to affect the minds of all of them
as they reached maturity. In young Henry it seems also
to have affected his literary style in the earliest of his
short stories by causing him to hesitate over an observation as he was later to hesitate over his choice of
residence, displaying an anxiety to pick and a reluctance to choose which gave him a tendency to see everything through the eyes of fictitious observers rather
than commit himself directly to paper. Like the insecure Poe and the escapist author of *Huckleberry Finn*,
he found his best release from constrictive self-consciousness by pretending to be somebody else; but,
with James, the pretense never became a role that the

author obviously played. Instead, it was incorporated so early into his technique of storytelling that it became the very basis of his art and the source of his greatest strength and greatest weakness. For as he matured and his choosing became more firm, his picking developed into a mannerism which made some of the most imaginative novels in American literature intolerable to many readers.

There were certain choices, however, that James as a writer had to make fairly early, and one was of the general area of his interest or the major symbols with which he would deal. He began to make it in several of his early stories, most notably "The Passionate Pilgrim" (1871), and confirmed it in the second of his two early novels, *Roderick Hudson* (1876); it would be the impact of European society, which so evidently fascinated him, upon the stranger within its gates who had been "prepared for culture" (as he thought that he himself had been) by an American background. In *Roderick Hudson* he could only find the impact overwhelming, and he concluded his story with Roderick's suicide. But such a conclusion was essentially unrealistic in view of his own decision to live as an American abroad and also impractical in the restrictions it placed upon him as a novelist interested in this theme. Accordingly he was forced, perhaps without fully being aware of it, to the second major choice in his literary life—that of a belief in some reality which would enable a man to survive, as an independent human being, the social pressures to which he was exposed. For a basically shy person of James's upbringing, the choice was probably inevitable; and he made it in *The Ameri-*

can (1877), which told the story of an American appropriately named Christopher Newman who went to Paris, fell in love with the daughter of an aristocratic French family, was rejected by family pressure which sent the girl into a convent, and finally found evidence of a crime which put the family under his complete control. As a matter of course he destroyed it, sacrificing his own feelings and perhaps those of the girl who loved him to some internal moral sense which was superior to all ordinary standards of tolerable self-interest and conventional justice. Like Howells in *The Rise of Silas Lapham* a few years later, James found his highest reality in the American tradition of Emerson, Thoreau, and his own father.

The difference between the two friends and literary rivals was that James held onto the tradition, refining the concept of morality and removing it from its more sanctimonious implications by identifying it with innocence, goodness, perceptiveness, and artistic sensibility. The much-misunderstood and consequently greatly denounced *Daisy Miller* (1879) showed the vicious potentiality of conventions in their effect upon unprotected innocence, but the finest of his early novels, *The Portrait of a Lady* (1881), presented Isabel Archer as another American girl abroad whose innate goodness triumphed over disillusionment and gave her, it would seem, moral control over a situation which within a system of values other than James's would be tragic. James had published a biography of Hawthorne only two years before, and there may have been a bit of Hester Prynne as well as a good deal of his cousin Mary Temple in the character of Isabel; but when she returned to her husband she returned with a strength of character which had been revealed rather than developed by suffering, for James believed in the spirit rather than in the will, the emotions, or the intellect.

For a long while after *The Portrait of a Lady* James made little use of what may be called, in retrospect, his greatest theme—that of an individual, usually American, with a moral sense in a European society without it. He had already attempted a wholly American novel in *Washington Square* (1881) and was to do another in *The Bostonians* (1886); and he was to write, with unusual suspense, of a slum-bred revolutionary's growing awareness of the amenities of upper-class life in *The Princess Casamassima* (1886) and of the rebellion of the artist against these amenities in *The Tragic Muse* (1890). But such popularity as he had enjoyed through his early books was on the wane, and he was turning to the essay, the short story, and the drama. The most notable of his essays during this period was "The Art of Fiction" (1884), in which he defended the novel as a serious esthetic form, based its appeal upon the author's individual "sense of reality" and identified its quality in terms of the intelligence of the writer with particular reference to the "point at which the moral sense and the artistic sense lie very near together." The essay provides a significant indication of James's place in the American tradition, for its theme was that of Emerson's definition of art as "a nature"—that is, some chosen aspect of the external world —"passed through the alembic of man" and it contained the germ of the later novel in which James most clearly revealed his Emersonian concept of man.

The novel, *What Maisie Knew* (1897), was evidently James's attempt to do what the essay said Edmond de Goncourt had "failed deplorably" to do in *Chérie*—to trace "the development of the moral consciousness of a child"—and in it James struck a subtle blow against both the empirical naturalists and the affected morality of Victorian conventions. For he gave the child Maisie a thoroughly corrupt environment in the form of her parents and their associates, relieved it only by the person of the governess Mrs. Wix and her prattling "moral sense" of the proprieties, and allowed Maisie to develop within these surroundings the sort of sensitive perception of good and evil which was characteristic of the innate goodness he had portrayed in Isabel Archer. Maisie's "moral sense" was so delicate that some critics have refused to take it seriously, but if James had not clarified his belief in its innate quality in this book he might never have been able to assert its power in one of the finest of his mature novels, *The Wings of the Dove* (1902)—a book which resolved the ambiguity of the final sentences in *The Portrait of a Lady* by declaring, in dramatic terms, that individual goodness could not only face and perhaps endure the viciousness of a materialistic society but actually overcome it. Milly Theale in the later novel is another Isabel Archer, and Kate Croy and Merton Densher are closely related to Madame Merle and Gilbert Osmond; but the story is extended beyond that of *The Portrait of a Lady* when the "wings" of Milly's influence are transformed from the symbol of wealth to the symbol of unselfish generosity and their moral influence is spread as effectively over Kate and Densher at the end as their mercenary influence was at the beginning.

James's mature novels, however, were not merely the products of a growing assurance of belief—an increasing firmness of choice between the values of a society which fascinated him and those of the various individuals who could remain free from its worst influences. The maturity was also the result of a rare art which had been brought to perfection in the experimental short stories composed during his period of lost popularity and of disappointment with the drama. Some of these were experiments with themes that he was later to handle in longer works, as "The Pupil" (1891) anticipated the problem of the moral consciousness of a child in *What Maisie Knew* and was related to the influence of innate goodness asserted in *The Wings of the Dove* and to the portrayal of sophistication embarrassed by innocence in *The Awkward Age* (1899). Others such as "The Lesson of the Master" (1888), "The Real Thing" (1893), "The Death of the Lion" (1894), and "The Figure in the Carpet" (1896) affirmed with increasing sureness and subtlety the quality of creative intelligence which must belong to the true artist; and the last went so far as to suggest that it is beyond discovery, or at least definition, by the analytic or discursive intellect. In these stories James was, in effect, identifying the artistic intelligence with that refusal to commit himself which he had revealed in his own earliest style and of which his own mature imagination was certainly compact—an anxiety to pick the right detail or word which had become so pronounced that it disguised the fact that his choice was no longer hesitant but was firmly made for the artistic purpose of achieving suggestiveness on a higher level of consciousness than can be found in the ambiguities of Hawthorne, Melville, or any of his predecessors in American or English fiction. Consequently the most technically interesting of the short stories are those tours de force he used to test his range.

Several of them, like "The Jolly Corner" (1908) and the related fragment of a novel *The Sense of the Past* (1917), dealt with the supernatural; and of these the one which has proved most fascinating is "The Turn of the Screw" (1898), which used the governess of two small children as a means of narration and also as a means of avoiding commitment as to what happened in fact and what might have occurred only in the young woman's morbid imagination. The details were selected with a masterly teasing designed to bring the reader's own imagination into the story, and the several critics who have been seduced into rational expositions of it bear strong witness to James's claims for the superiority of "silken threads suspended in the chamber of consciousness" over discursive reason, even when the artistic mind is not, as he would have it be, "sincere." The critical inclination to look into James's personality rather than into his art for an explanation of his stories might perhaps be better applied to "The Beast in the Jungle" (1903), another tour de force in its creation of intolerable suspense without action. For John Marcher is what Henry James might have been had he not been a writer, and his fears are of the same stuff as that with which James created his fiction—anxiety and an "enormous sensibility," which, in Marcher's case, is not informed by the energy of creation.

But James's energy was as enormous as his sensibility, and in the decade from 1897 to 1907 it found expression in not only *What Maisie Knew* and *The Awkward Age* and a considerable number of shorter stories but in the perfect and ironic short novel, *The Spoils of Poynton* (1897), the less successful *The Sacred Fount* (1901), and in the great major novels of three successive years: *The Wings of the Dove* (1902), *The Ambassadors* (1903), and *The Golden Bowl* (1904). In addition he was able to produce a two-volume biography of *William Wetmore Story and his Friends* (1903) and (after a return to the United States at the age of sixty) a travel book full of the fresh immediacy of *The American Scene* (1907). It is in the three great novels that James's literary achievement reached its climax in a combination of artistic skill and firmness of belief. The refined Jamesian version of the moral sense, whose power he asserted in *The Wings of the Dove*, became identified with the artistic sense in *The Ambassadors* when Lambert Strether, an elderly businessman from Woollett, Massachusetts, achieved his emancipation from the conventional and vulgar American notions of Paris and learned to see things as they really were and appreciate a certain rightness in the atmosphere and relationships of a city from which he withdrew in evidence of his freedom even from its charm. *The Ambassadors* has been the most popular of James's last novels, perhaps because it revived the American-in-Europe theme most pointedly and effectively and perhaps because it is the most carefully controlled through the use of Strether's single point of view. But for the latter reason it is also less appealing than *The Golden Bowl* to the confirmed Jamesians, who prefer to capture their author's vision of life through the intellectual or perceptive montage which was the peculiar outgrowth of his style and the final flowering of his art. For in this queer quadrangular romance of Maggie Verver, her father, her friend and stepmother, and her husband and stepmother's lover, James weaves a web of relationships which captures "in the chamber of consciousness" a perception of *how* the combination of intelligence, sensitivity, and goodness which was his moral ideal could possess the strength he had so often attributed to it. The most tortured example of the mannered picking of his way through a narrative, it is also the surest evidence of his choice of spiritual freedom— freedom not only from materialism but from the demands of resentment and the protests of passion—as the main figure in his own slowly woven but at last complete literary carpet.

II

Against the background of the American tradition the pattern of Henry James's mind should be both familiar and clear. He was devoted to careful observation of the world around him, skillful in drawing inferences, indifferent to the prevailing rationalistic notions of necessity, and convinced that reason was choice and that individuals could freely choose to follow some supreme intellectual light within them. The significance of the reappearance of this pattern at the end of the nineteenth century, however, may be better realized if it is placed in contrast to that of his leading disciple, Edith Wharton, who thoroughly learned the lesson of the master without ever being able to follow the figure in his carpet. For Mrs. Wharton possessed to a greater or less degree many of the qualities James drew upon for his fiction—a more intimate knowledge of international and especially of American society, a comparable sensitivity to the nuances of human relationship, and an equal sympathy for the individual in society— without having his capacity for belief in the reality of freedom. As with James, her books tended to have as their central characters heroines rather than heroes, but hers were morally defeated rather than triumphant. In the best of her novels of contemporary society, *The House of Mirth* (1905) and *The Custom of the Country* (1913), Lily Bart and Undine Spragg jeopardized or sacrificed their integrity in vain efforts to hold and to gain places in a social order which rejected them for their lack of wealth or of cultivation; and in her finest full-length novel, a nostalgic recapturing of *The Age of Innocence* (1920), she told the story of two lovers whose deep, genuine, and lasting emotion could make no headway against the barriers of convention which kept them apart. Even in such stories of New England country life as the extraordinarily succinct and deeply moving *Ethan Frome* (1911) and *Summer* (1917) chance and circumstance exercised their control over rebels and kept them in their places.

There was, in short, a certain individual negativism or pessimism in Mrs. Wharton's sophisticated view of the world; and the struggle against this negativism is the most evident common characteristic of the less sophisticated writers of her generation who continued the search for reality within the framework of evolutionary theory and who did not have Mrs. Wharton's personal excuse for doubting an individual's power to resist the pressures of his social environment. Of these, the one who achieved the greatest stature was Theodore Dreiser, the hulking, awkward, self-conscious son of a severe moralist and a gentle mystic who learned a great deal about the struggle for existence as he worked his own way upward from the position of a common laborer to that of a newspaper reporter and magazine editor before he became a successful novelist. An early convert to the theory of social evolution, he was more impressed than most Spencerians by the concept of a mysterious life force, which the English philosopher had called "the Unknowable," and seems to have felt that the business of the literary artist was to find this life force in the raw materials of human life, as George Bellows and other members of the "Ash Can School" of painters had found it in the derelicts and alleys of the slums. Exposed at second hand to French naturalism through the writings of a fellow reporter, Robert H. Hazard, Dreiser was actually a more avid reader of Balzac than of Zola; but his background was more journalistic than literary, and his novels were generally based upon real incidents and people and involved detailed reporting informed by his own view of life.

He expressed the essence of this view in his first novel when he referred to contemporary civilization as being in "a middle stage" of evolution in which man was "far removed from the lairs of the jungles, his innate instincts dulled by too near an approach to free-will, his free-will not sufficiently developed to replace his instincts and afford him perfect guidance . . . even as a wisp in the wind, moved by every breath of passion, acting now by his will and now by his instincts, erring with one, only to retrieve by the other, falling by one, only to rise by the other—a creature of incalculable variability." And the novel itself, called *Sister Carrie* (1900) despite the temptation to change its title to *The Flesh and the Spirit*, was a story of the rise of Carrie and the fall of her lover, Hurstwood, without an attribution of a determining free will to either of them: they profit or lose by chance and circumstance as they are pushed onward by social forces over which they have no control. Yet it is obvious to the reader that although Carrie was the partial portrait of the author's own sister he realized the character of Hurstwood more effectively and believed more firmly in his reality and in the reality of his fate. Carrie the good and Carrie the fortunate had to be written out of his system in his second novel, *Jennie Gerhardt* (1911), whose heroine's goodness caused her to sacrifice her good fortune, before he could write the novels in which the real strength of his belief was expressed.

The first of these were the two parts of a trilogy, *The Financier* (1912) and *The Titan* (1914), completed by the publication of *The Stoic* (1947) after his death, in which Dreiser undertook to tell the story of a transportation magnate named Frank Cowperwood, who began his operations in Philadelphia in the first book and landed in jail but began anew in Chicago in the second and eventually gained control of the street railroad system. It was a story of the law of the jungle in modern civilization—of a magnetic personality whose sexual and financial ruthlessness made him "fit" to survive and whose magnetism is explained in chemical terms which would have allowed him to take no account of the goodness suggested in Carrie and portrayed in Jennie. Dreiser's world was a moral chaos to be mastered by animal energy and a willingness to meet society on its own terms, and his basic conviction that these terms were materialistic and economic is indicated by the comparative failure of his next novel, *The Genius* (1915), in which Eugene Witla displayed many of the qualities of Cowperwood but proved a weakling in his pursuit of art rather than financial power. These novels, however, revealed only one side of Dreiser's attitude toward the world. The other side was revealed in the tenderness and sentimentality of several autobiographical works, and in the sympathy amounting to an enormous pity for the misfits and the unfortunate most notably displayed in the unactable drama, *The Hand of the Potter* (1918), and the essays of *Hey, Rub-a-Dub-Dub* (1920), which was aptly subtitled *A Book of the Mystery and Terror of Life.* For life, even as he had found it interpreted by Herbert Spencer and the various scientists he had been reading since, remained a mystery to Dreiser; and his early belief that "it was not so much the business of the writer to indict as to interpret" was always modified by the notion that such a code was cruel unless the failure to indict society was compensated for by a display of pity for its victims.

Something of a balance between detachment and

sympathy may be found in the collections of short stories, *Free* (1918), *Twelve Men* (1919), *Chains* (1927), and *A Gallery of Women* (1929), but it was best achieved in his most carefully controlled and impressively detailed novel *An American Tragedy* (1925). The story of the weak but attractive son of two street evangelists, it presented in the person of Clyde Griffiths a young man who was the plaything of his environment. Forced by an automobile accident to abandon his employment as a hotel bellhop and leave town, he moved to a smaller city where he had wealthy relatives who provided him with employment in a factory. The breath of passion involved him with an attractive fellow worker, but he decided to abandon her for a wealthy marriage made possible by the social contacts provided by his relatives. Learning that she was pregnant, he made elaborate preparations to fake an accident which would get her out of the way, only to lose his nerve at the last moment and allow her to drown by the genuine accident of an overturned boat and his own panic. Suspicion was aroused, however, by his preparations; and he was arrested, convicted on circumstantial evidence by a politically inspired prosecuter, sentenced to death, and executed. *An American Tragedy* is one of the most powerful of twentieth-century American novels, and much of its power comes from the combination of Dreiser's sympathetic interpretation of Clyde as a "wisp in the wind of social forces" and his steadfast refusal to issue an explicit indictment against the society which tossed him to destruction. For the book is one to provoke an infinite amount of discussion of guilt and innocence, moral and social responsibility—a book of many ambiguities which are made to seem as real as life by the meticulous detail of Dreiser's reportorial technique and the lumbering, uncalculated, awkward honesty of its style.

By the time Dreiser wrote *An American Tragedy* he seems to have lost his belief in social evolution, for he gave his book a general implication by the use of the indefinite article in its title and by making its last scene a repetition of the first, with a younger boy taking the place of Clyde. And in the remaining two decades of his life he was to waver curiously in his search for a philosophy, leaning toward communism in a sympathetic book on Russia and toward Transcendentalism in a collection of social and political essays on Thoreau before he created, in the posthumous novel *The Bulwark* (1946), his last hero in the person of Solon Barnes, who was as sternly religious as the author's own father but more sympathetically comprehended as a member of the Society of Friends than as a Roman Catholic. The most consistently close to the naturalists of all major American novelists, Dreiser always revealed an undercurrent of rebellion, part intellectual and part emotional, against the biological and social determinism which he asserted as his major article of faith.

The other aspect of the struggle against negativism in the early twentieth century was more logical than that represented by Theodore Dreiser, more "rational" in what had come to be the Continental meaning of the word. Its exponents did not question the power of the social order to overwhelm the ordinary individual or the prevalence of the law of tooth and claw in the existing order. They simply reasoned that since human misery was a widespread product of the social organization, then society should be reorganized to promote happiness. This was the implication which lay back of the "muckraking" journalists of *McClure's Magazine*—Ida M. Tarbell, Ray Stannard Baker, and Lincoln Steffens (whose *Autobiography*, published in 1931, is the best account of the movement and its social philosophy)—and of such early novels as David Graham Phillips' *The Great God Success* (1901) and Robert Herrick's *The Common Lot* (1904). It was most succinctly expressed, however, in the poetry of William Vaughn Moody, whose "Ode in Time of Hesitation" (1900) and other poems of the Spanish-American War bear witness to the moral impulse back of his social consciousness and whose "The Menagerie" is the most amusing expression of evolutionary belief in American literature. For in "Gloucester Moors" Moody represented the earth as a "ship of souls" gallantly moving forward without knowing its port. As he saw it with some men in the cabin and some before the mast, with a noisome hold full of men kept down because "the ship sails faster thus," he thought it "better captainless" than brought to harbor by leaders who would break the souls of men rather than turn them into brotherly shipmates. The new suggestive implication of this imagery, like that of the muckraker's attacks on large fortunes, was social revolution.

Yet there were few American writers prepared to advocate revolutionary socialism as opposed to the optimistic Fabian dreams of William Dean Howells. Jack London, in fact, was the only one to be widely read at home and abroad; and the violence of his socialism was less impressive at home than the romantic love of violence which made him one of the most popular writers of his day. Sailor, laborer, hobo, and adventurer in the Far North and the South Seas, London began as a teller of tales and gained his greatest popular success with a dog story, *The Call of the Wild*, in 1903. In the same year he published his first attack upon contemporary society in *The People of the Abyss*, which grew out of his observations of the London slums; and the following years saw a strange alternation of popular adventure stories and books of social protest—*The Sea Wolf* (1904) and *War of the Classes* (1905), *White Fang* (1906) and *The Iron Heel* (1907), *Burning Daylight* (1910) and *Revolution* (1909)—with a tendency toward the end of his life to such troubled autobiographical novels as *Martin Eden* (1909) and *John Barleycorn* (1913). Where his heart lay may perhaps be seen in a comparison between the vitality he gave to the brutal Wolf Larsen in *The Sea Wolf* and the woodenness of the self-sacrificing hero of *The Iron Heel* and the remnants of life still to be found in the style of the first and the dull heaviness which pervades the second. An avowed Spencerian, London was eager for the help of Karl Marx in the direction of social evolution; but he was basically an escapist, a he-man Lafcadio Hearn or a Cro-Magnon Henry Adams, whose primary impulse was to go over the horizon or revert to primitivism because his hatred of the existing order was more real than his hope for changing it.

In the less violent area of political revolution, however, the socialist cause found a brilliant and single-

minded recruit in the prolific and well-bred young ro-
mancer Upton Sinclair whose novel *The Jungle* (1906)
displayed such extraordinary naturalistic power that
one critic was moved to complain of its propagandist
conclusion, with more bitterness than wit, that its author had "sold his birthright for a pot of message."
Growing out of Sinclair's own investigation of the
Chicago stockyards, *The Jungle* told the story of the
merciless exploitation of a Lithuanian immigrant family from the moment of their first hopeful settlement
in a home of their own in the new world until the
only survivor escaped the toils of capitalism and its
law and found refuge in the socialist party and new
hope in its belief that "the country will be ours." Its
description of the economic jungle and the helpless
human creatures who suffer in it is the most vivid
and convincing in American fiction, and the power of
its vividness, in fact, defeated its purpose. For, as Sinclair was to complain, it was an appeal to its readers'
heads and hearts which, instead, hit them in their
stomachs. Its casual but sickening accounts of the un-
sanitary conditions in the meat-packing industry set up
a public hue and cry which hurried the passage of the
federal Food and Drug Act and left its rationalistic
appeal for socialism almost unnoticed. Sinclair had
proved himself magnificently capable of achieving the
naturalists' aim of diagnosing the evils of society so
effectively that the legislators would be forced to find
a cure for them, and had he been content with this
aim he might have become America's greatest realistic
novelist.

But Sinclair proved to be the rarest type of American writer—the man of great individual talent who could not use it without the support of an orthodoxy. His own logic had provided him with socialism as the legislation needed, and his later investigations of social evils were not designed to demand some cure but to argue for his own cure. For two decades he vigorously attacked a great variety of capitalistic interests in such novels as *The Money-Changers* (1908), *King Coal* (1917), *Jimmie Higgins* (1919), *Oil!* (1927), and *Boston* (1928) and in such journalistic muckraking as *The Profits of Religion* (1918), *The Brass Check: A Study of American Journalism* (1919), *The Goose-Step: A Study of American Education* (1922), *The Goslings: A Study of American Schools* (1924), *Mammonart* (1925), and *Money Writes!* (1927). He was almost alone among American socialist writers to stick tenaciously to his principles after the party was almost destroyed by its pacifistic stand during the First World War, and it was not until he himself seriously entered practical politics in his unsuccessful California gubernatorial race in 1934 that he relaxed his rigid orthodoxy in a way which permitted him to turn in fiction to a representation of individual good works in the Lanny Budd series of novels which began with *World's End* in 1940. There is a certain fascination about the Lanny Budd novels, for their detailed effort to cover the whole of the contemporary world through the activity of a single man of good will suggests that Sinclair is doing more than trying to perpetuate his own view of modern history. He may be recapturing the true literary personality of a man who was always a behind-scenes romantic at heart and who had held too rigidly to his dogmatic principles because he did not know quite what to do without them.

III

Although the main stream of American fiction in the early twentieth century appears in retrospect to have been realistic and dominated by social consciousness, the popular fiction was a literature of escape into Romanticism and sentimentalism. The historical novel flourished under the temporary dominance of Winston Churchill, whose *Richard Carvel* (1899), *The Crisis* (1901), and *The Crossing* (1904) surveyed American history from the colonial period through the Civil War; and various writers who were to achieve greater literary stature contributed to the genre—Upton Sinclair with *Manassas* (1904) and Ellen Glasgow with *The Battle-Ground* (1902)—while others in a semihistorical vein tried to capture the color of the past as Joseph Hergesheimer did in *The Three Black Pennys* (1917) and *Java Head* (1919). Sentimentalism dominated the popular magazines and the widely read later writers of the local-color schools and was both used and mocked by the most complex of the Romanticists, James Branch Cabell, whose short stories collected in *The Line of Love* (1905) and whose medieval novel *The Soul of Melicent* (1913) were, in their original versions, highly sentimental but whose novels of contemporary life, leading up to *The Rivet in Grandfather's Neck* (1915) and *The Cream of the Jest* (1917) were increasingly inclined toward mockery. Cabell, however, was an unusually alert and sophisticated writer for this period, who tried to define certain historical attitudes of mind in the contrasting short stories of *Gallantry* (1907) and *Chivalry* (1909) and who dealt interpretively with historical figures in the stories of *The Certain Hour* (1916); and his maturity belongs to the period after the First World War when he himself realized the full implication of the tendencies displayed in his early work.

These implications were of the creative importance of a return to individual values rather than a turn to conventional Romanticism as a means of escape from the oppressive weight of social consciousness whether felt in terms of evolutionary theory or the need for reform; and this return was led not only by Henry James but by a new group of poets who found in poetry itself an escape from that shadow of social consciousness which had so darkened the realistic novel. And the earliest of these poets was Edwin Arlington Robinson, on whom the shadow of the world lay heavy but who was second only to the expatriate James in the persistence with which he followed his own intellectual "light" and attributed such a private illumination to a host of fictitious characters.

Educated for two years at Harvard and there exposed to the residual influences of Emersonian Transcendentalism, Robinson published his first public volume of verse in 1897 with the significant title *The Children of the Night*. Most of the individuals in this volume and in *Captain Craig* (1902), *The Town Down the River* (1910), and *The Man Against the Sky* (1916), too, were people who received no guidance from the shrouded world around them but were some-

how greater than they would have been had they simply made a "blind atomic pilgrimage" because their
brains and bones and cartilage would have it so. The
sex-ridden "John Evereldown," the gentlemanly suicide "Richard Corey," the broken "Annandale" who
"went out" by instrumentality of a kindly physician, the
drunken and romantic consumptive "Miniver Cheevy,"
the gracious beggar "Flammonde," and the mysteri-
ously secluded victim of "Eros Turannos"—these are
only a few of the many characters in Robinson's poems
who are in no way conventionally admirable but who
attract a sympathetic respect because they have a
quality of individual independence never given to the
characters in the novels of Edith Wharton, Theodore
Dreiser, or Upton Sinclair. If they are social misfits it
is because they have been created out of the poet's
own private preoccupation with the infinite variety of
the human impulse toward self-destruction which he
found even in the greatest of men and which enabled
him, in "Ben Jonson Entertains a Man from Stratford,"
to draw one of the most sympathetic portraits of Shakespeare in literature by allowing the plain-thinking
Jonson to meditate upon the significance of his friend's
new house in his native town.

In many of these early poems Robinson showed a
mastery of disciplined verse forms and an epigram-
matic wit which makes him one of the most quotable
of modern American poets, but his novelist's interest in
people was also accompanied by a tendency toward
verbosity which led him into a kind of colloquial verse
narrative that was effective in the carefully controlled
"Isaac and Archibald" (1902), in the earlier Arthu-

rian poems, *Merlin* (1917) and *Lancelot* (1920), and
in the somewhat melodramatic *Avon's Harvest* (1921),
and that became subtly magnificent in the restrained
passion of *Tristram* (1927). But this was a dangerous
tendency in the sort of person who could look outward
only when the larger world affected his own private
convenience (as the Prohibition amendment did when
he composed *Dionysus in Doubt* in 1925 and the economic depression did when he wrote the allegorical
King Jasper at the end of his life), and the bulk of his
later work from *Roman Bartholow* (1923) to *Ama-
ranth* (1934) was of an introspective flatness which
aroused enthusiasm only among his most confirmed
admirers.

Less prolific and less ambitious in range than Robinson, Robert Frost was also much less given to errors in
judgment and the mistakes of introspection; for there
is probably no twentieth-century American poet who
has been more firmly and soundly devoted to the principle that wisdom should be tested by the tenor of
one's own life or that literary symbols should make
sense in terms of one's own experience. Although he
was born in San Francisco and made his poetic reputation in England (with *A Boy's Will* in 1913 and *North
of Boston* in 1914), his work is more strongly marked
than Robinson's by the New England physical environment and by the New England tradition of Emerson,
Hawthorne, Thoreau, and Dickinson. The poems in
A Boy's Will are mostly lyric and those in *North of
Boston* dramatic, with both forms appearing in *Mountain Interval* (1916), and they are all packed with
thought and feeling realized in terms of simple per-

sonal experience. "Mending Wall," for example, is a meditation upon an annual spring chore undertaken with a neighbor which suggests more than the novelists of the time were able to say about the difficulty of impressing the conventional consciousness with an individual sense of values; but Frost records the difficulty with a serene humor which also suggests that he looks upon convention as a tolerable eccentricity rather than as a depressing weight. Similarly, "Birches" suggests a philosophy of aspiration and contentment with earth which explains why Frost was able to capture so much of the tragedy of the New England back country in these volumes without losing its humor or his own capacity for enjoying his "Good Hours" of intense awareness.

In *New Hampshire* (1923) and *West-Running Brook* (1928) he became somewhat more discursively philosophical (as in the title poem for each volume and the amusing verses on "The Bear" in the latter) but without losing the suggestiveness which makes "Stopping by Woods on a Snowy Evening" so haunting, the lyricism which makes "Spring Pools" so perfect, or the intensity of personal feeling which makes the sonnet to "A Soldier" so moving. In later volumes, composed in more pressing times, this reflective discursiveness was directed toward contemporary problems—labor in *A Further Range* (1936) and politics in *A Witness Tree* (1942) and *Steeple Bush* (1947)—and broadened into the larger issues of his verse dramas, *A Masque of Reason* (1945) and *A Masque of Mercy* (1947). Yet even when he showed signs of impatience and irritability with the contemporary world Frost maintained an attitude of wry humor which preserved the individuality of his own values and kept him in the position he has assigned to himself—that of one who "had a lover's quarrel with the world."

Compared with Frost and the best of Robinson, the prewar poets of the Middle West seem artificial and excessively self-conscious—as in fact they were, for they bore the same relationship to the revival of individualism that Whitman bore to its earlier triumph in that they paraded it and made it a symbol rather than a tacit attitude of mind. The oldest and the most flamboyant of them was Vachel Lindsay, the dreamy would-be artist son of a Campbellite minister who fed his dreams on Edgar Allan Poe, William Blake, and Emanuel Swedenborg in his native Springfield, Illinois, and eventually took to the open road in an effort to beat the economic "system" by trading rhymes for bread. His success, however, came with his acceptance of the system and his rebellion against the poetic conventions of his own early verse; and the title poem of *General William Booth Enters into Heaven* (1913) was written to the strong rhythm of a Salvation Army song with an indicated drum and brass accompaniment. Such a poem was written for reading before a mass audience, and Lindsay found a means of capturing audiences in the tom-tom beat of *The Congo* (1914), which enabled him to spend the next decade and a half in what he called "the higher vaudeville," reading these and such other poems as "The Ghosts of Buffaloes" and "The Santa Fé Trail" with a variety of sound effects ranging from the thin cadences of *The Chinese Nightingale* (1917) to the roaring and caterwauling of "The Calliope." Lindsay was a new kind of folk poet—with public-school teachers as his folk—who could be nostalgic in "The Building of Springfield" and tender in "Abraham Lincoln Walks at Midnight" but was probably at his best when capturing the gaudier aspects of the American scene and translating them into verses for ears primarily attuned to popular songs.

Carl Sandburg also looked upon himself as a people's poet, but he was, like Whitman, more the poet of the people than for the people. Like Whitman, too, he was devoted to the long lines of free verse, but he was less able to find a consistent compromise between prose and the imagistic delicacy he sometimes achieved. The opening line of his description of Chicago, "Hog Butcher for the World," shocked the readers of his first volume of verse, *Chicago Poems* (1916), into an awareness that a new kind of poet had appeared on the scene; and, although he achieved a certain balance in the title poem of *Smoke and Steel* (1920) and broadened his range in *Cornhuskers* (1918) and *Slabs of the Sunburnt West* (1922), he struck no new note until he turned folklorist, folk singer, and imaginative biographer of Abraham Lincoln and incorporated his new interests into a volume of definition and affirmation called *The People, Yes* (1936), which defies literary classification but which contains some of Sandburg's most effective work.

Both Lindsay and Sandburg were protégés of Harriet Monroe and the Chicago *Poetry: A Magazine of Verse*, which was established in 1912 and had the distinction of printing the early poems of Hilda Doolittle, Amy Lowell, William Carlos Williams, John Gould

Fletcher, Wallace Stevens, Edgar Lee Masters, T. S. Eliot, and Marianne Moore as well as those of Robert Frost, Vachel Lindsay, and Carl Sandburg. It also printed in its first issue two poems by Ezra Pound, the Idaho expatriate who became its "foreign correspondent" and proved to be the best informed, most influential, and most sophisticated example of the individual on parade which the "new poetry" movement brought into the limelight. He had the curiosity but not the patience required for graduate work in Romance philology at the University of Pennsylvania, and in 1908, at the age of twenty-three, deserted the academic world for London. By the end of 1912 he had published eight small volumes of original and translated verse which revealed his interest in Latin, Greek, and Provençal poetry, in the work of such modern French poets as Laurent Tailhade, and in the new English "Imagist" movement inspired by T. E. Hulme and F. S. Flint. Pound's interest in medieval France was probably affected by the same sort of academic Romanticism which his fellow admirer of Eleanor of Aquitaine, Cabell, was displaying in the popular American magazines but with the difference that he had seen for himself a harsh reality in Provence which reminded him of the "half-savage country" of his native West and made him feel that with its people, and with the Imperial Romans and the Greek sailors who preceded them, he would have been at home.

So with his heroes from the past he rebelled against what a softer age demanded (and what it was getting in a man like Cabell), and he found in his young English contemporaries men who could appreciate his learning and not only share his rebelliousness but direct it into the productive channel of creating a new poetic style. The style which Hulme demanded would be "cheerful, dry, and sophisticated" in a free-verse pattern which would permit concentration upon the image rather than the metrical line; and although Pound was no model of cheerfulness, despite the implied claims of his "Commission" to his poems, he strove passionately for dryness and sophistication. "Dryness" was the particular aspiration of the Imagist movement whose manifesto in *Some Imagist Poets* (1915) called for concise, clear, hard, exact poetry; but by this time the energetic, self-made but well-heeled poetess, Amy Lowell, had captured the movement for Boston, and Pound was contemptuously referring to it as "Amygism" and fulfilling its aims in his own way. He increased the sophistication of the new poetry by turning, through Ernest Fenellosa, to Chinese and Japanese poetry for new models of imagistic succinctness, by recruiting new talent and ruthlessly editing it (as he edited the manuscript of Eliot's *The Waste Land*), and by beginning his own most ambitious life work in a long series of "Cantos" of which the first three were published in *Poetry* magazine in 1917 and, with revisions, in *Quia Pauper Amavi* in 1919. A year later he abandoned London with severe strictures upon its Victorian traditions and commercialization of literature, in *Hugh Selwyn Mauberley* (1920), and made his way to Paris and eventually to a permanent home in Italy.

Pound's influence upon modern poetry has been so great that it can be treated here only in terms of a manner which is displayed in the early "Cantos" as well as anywhere else. The first, which reads like a free rendering of an Anglo-Saxon adaptation of Homer, bears witness to the eclecticism of Pound's manner—a manner which enabled him to range in allusiveness from the Greeks and Romans, through Dante and the medieval troubadours, to ancient Chinese and modern French poetry while pursuing his general theme of the decay of civilization under the particular influence of usury and in terms of a great variety of personalities ranging from the Italian *condottiere* Sigismondo Malatesta to John Quincy Adams and Henry James. The style is dry in the sense that it is imagistic and colloquial rather than rhetorical, although it reveals a fondness for primitive epithets and often does create the rhetorical effect of deliberate harshness and rudeness. The most striking quality found in the *Cantos* and in Pound's poetry in general, however, is a calculated sophistication achieved by the trick of substituting literature for common human experience as a source for those allusions by which a poet suggests more than he says. Pound's method, then, is the very reverse of that used by such a poet as Frost in that it asks the reader to admire the breadth of his knowledge and take his sensitivity on faith; and it is for that reason that his ultimate influence, by basing poetry on essentially private rather than intensely personal experience, has been to make a substantial body of modern verse academic and erudite rather than popular and simple.

While Pound was avoiding the hackneyed by leading poetry back into the academic environment from which he thought he was revolting, another American expatriate, in Paris, was quietly anticipating and actually achieving the "cheerful, dry, and sophisticated" style which Hulme had set up as the ideal of the Imagists. Gertrude Stein's education had been in psychology at Radcliffe and medicine at the Johns Hopkins University before she went to London in 1902 and then settled permanently in France, where she was to find kindred experimental spirits among the Expressionist painters Pablo Picasso and Henri Matisse, who became her friends, and the many talented young American writers who sat at her feet. Her influence has been greater upon modern prose than upon poetry, but the most interesting of her experimental work has been in what might be called the verses of *Tender Buttons* (1914) and *Portraits and Prayers* (1934). Unlike Pound, who attempted fresh communication through the implications of a vast erudition, Miss Stein attempted to communicate her profound knowledge of people as well as things by means of a calculated simplicity, which is almost always fresh and challenging even when incomprehensible. Her incomprehensibility, however, is the result of her most persistent aim—that of abstracting from her considerable knowledge of a subject the peculiar or "essential" quality of it and attempting to communicate that quality with a minimum of irrelevant associations. When she was experimenting with the communication of peculiar qualities by unconventional means (as in *Tender Buttons* when she undertakes to give the visual image of a moving dog in a rhythmical arrangement of words which literally refer to a monkey and a donkey, or when she gives her opinion of the opera in the rhythmical suggestion of a line drawing of a top hat, cape, and cane), comprehension immediately follows a realization of what she is doing; but when she is dealing with essential qualities, as in her "portraits" of real or typical individuals, comprehension often depends upon the reader's having a sufficiently adequate knowledge of the subject to appreciate the wit and wisdom of what she abstracts as "essential."

Consequently the understanding of Miss Stein's work is likely to be only partially increased by the sort of elaborate annotation which Pound's poetry demands; and readers of her most ambitious novel, *The Making of Americans* (1925), are likely to find some parts of it extraordinarily entertaining and other parts intolerably dull, according to their own background of experience, and turn with greater delight to her first work of fiction, *Three Lives* (1909), and her last, *Brewsie and Willie* (1946), or to the autobiographical works, in which the peculiar directness of her genius can be seen at its comprehensible best. But whether one appreciates the cheerful dryness of her sophistication or not, there was a freshness about her approach to writing which left a good mark on the literature of the twenties and made her one of the most historically important writers of her time. Combining the direct and wholesome wisdom of Frost with the erudite eccentricity of Pound, she joined with them and with the unhappy Robinson and their more flamboyant contemporaries—against the solid background of Henry James—in leading American literature back to the traditional fountain of individual judgment from which it had emerged for its first period of greatness.

This new individualism, however, was different from that of the mid-nineteenth century. For with James and his successors a new consciousness became evident in American literature—a pervading awareness of the conflict between the individual and society. Man was no longer free, as he had been in the mind of Emerson, to vault into his throne and lord it over the creepers and crawlers of the conventional world. He had to assert his individuality, by self-sacrifice, by isolation, by flamboyant rebellion, or by a parade of eccentricity, in order to be sure that he maintained it. The weight of a complex social organization was depressing the confidence of even those who were most determined to declare their independence, and it remained to be seen whether the American tradition would survive as a deep quality of belief or whether it would remain as no more than a symbolic refuge for the maladjustments of second-rate talent.

CHAPTER NINE

Tradition in the Twenties

I

THE consciousness of society was strong in the intoxicating twenties. No period in American history, perhaps, gave greater encouragement to freedom in literary expression, but it was the freedom of iconoclasm rather than that of inspiration. The decade between 1919 and 1929 was an era of rebellion in which writers revolted against the narrowness of their prewar world, against the conventions so dramatically symbolized by the Volstead Act, which made the distribution of alcoholic liquors a crime, and against America itself, as people turned against the idealism of Woodrow Wilson or flocked abroad to take advantage of the favorable rate of exchange which was one of the evidences of their country's new and more powerful position in the world. It was a decade of new writing growing out of the experimental attitudes of the prewar period, of the new psychology of Sigmund Freud, and of a new freedom to do what one wished. It was, in short, a time when the individual walked at large in the liter-

ary scene and wrote as he pleased with the assurance
that some ambitious young publisher would willingly
offer his work to a tolerant and eager public.

The core of the rebellion was against the narrowness
of background—particularly against the small town in
which so many American writers grew up—and, like
most literary manifestations of the twenties, it was foreshadowed by the prewar poetry. In retrospect it can be
seen symbolically anticipated in the first poem of Edna
St. Vincent Millay, *Renascence* (1912), which told of
death and burial, realization that narrowness is of the
spirit, and rebirth to greater awareness of the values of
the world. But the appropriateness of the poem, welcomed more for its youthful freshness than for its
significance, was not appreciated at the time; and the
poetic leader of the revolt from the village was Edgar
Lee Masters, whose *Spoon River Anthology* (1915)
was one of the most popular volumes of verse ever
published in America. Cynical and bitter, Masters used
the form of the free-verse epitaph as a method of revealing the meanness that lay beneath the sanctimonious surface of village life, and his poetry appealed
strongly to young rebels who wanted to get away from
it all and into the freer life of the city. Both poets,
however, proved to be rather sterile. Miss Millay got
to the city and with the gay impertinence of *A Few
Figs from Thistles* (1920) became the poet of
Bohemian Greenwich Village and the idol of a postwar generation of undergraduates; and although she
achieved a fine lyric quality in *Second April* (1921)
and in *The Harp Weaver and Other Poems* (1923) and
grasped at the fringes of greatness in the sonnets col-

lected in *Fatal Interview* (1931), she suffered from the reaction to overpraise and the disillusionment provoked by the socially conscious poems in *Conversation at Midnight* (1937) and *There Are No Islands Anymore* (1940) and has been almost forgotten in the critical devotion to the "new" poetry. Masters, already a Chicago lawyer when he wrote *Spoon River*, continued to imitate himself, in *Domesday Book* (1920) and *The New Spoon River* (1924), in a vain effort to repeat his early success.

The more influential and fruitful leader of the rebellion against the village was Sherwood Anderson, who had written two novels, both expressing a vague dissatisfaction with life, and a volume of poems before he clarified his own point of view in the related stories of *Winesburg, Ohio* (1919)—a book which was to have an extraordinary influence upon the American short story by freeing it from the well-knit formalism of Poe, Bierce, and O. Henry and making it the medium for that perceptive record of a significant moment of experience which was to be perfected by Ernest Hemingway. Anderson's point of view in these stories was like Masters' in that he was interested in the grotesque reality beneath the smug surface of village life but unlike Masters' in that he was sympathetic rather than bitter or cynical toward the "grotesque" or unconventional and nonconforming element in human character. Like Miss Millay, although more inclined to express himself in psychological than in spiritual terms, he was something of a Romantic rebel himself, who found freedom in an irresponsible reaction to conventions; and that attitude provided him with the theme for the best of his novels, *Dark Laughter* (1925). But his finest work was in the short stories of *Winesburg* and of *The Triumph of the Egg* (1921) and *Horses and Men* (1923) which followed, and his literary achievement was that of bringing the reader closer to those queer, frustrated, and sometimes tragic individuals who in Robinson's poems had been appealing characters but who in Anderson's stories became neighbors and friends.

The technique of capturing the reader's entire sensibility and making it—rather than some specialized reaction like sympathy, humor, or respect for the author's quality of mind—a part of his literary response, in fact, became a characteristic of the rebellious realism of the twenties and is nowhere better illustrated than in the novels of Sinclair Lewis. He used it effectively for the first time (after five earlier novels of the American scene) in *Main Street* (1920) and developed it most skillfully in *Babbitt* (1922). The Gopher Prairie in *Main Street*, although located in the Middle West, was everybody's small town, and the characters in it could be identified by practically every small-town resident as his friends and neighbors. The first novel of genuine realism ever to be widely read in America, *Main Street* owed much of its popularity to the accuracy with which Lewis caught the spirit, speech, and mores of small-town life, and also, among intellectuals, to the strong strain of satire which ran through it. But, more than that, it allowed every reader—the satisfied villager, the intellectual who had escaped to the city, or the complacent foreigner—the free play of his own individual consciousness in interpreting what he was enabled to see and hear. Similarly in *Babbitt*, which is a better novel because the central character was more fully conceived and because the small city was more representative of America in transition, every reader was made to feel and rejoice in a secret superiority to the ordinary humanity with which he might, to all appearances, be identified. Even businessmen read the book and began calling themselves Babbitts with a complacency which grew out of a private sense of identity which even so complete an observer as Lewis had not been able to capture and so take from them. Instead of dominating his readers as Howells had done through his style and James through the complexity of his perceptions, Lewis somehow managed at once to open their eyes and give them a feeling of superior vision.

How much Lewis knew about what he was doing is doubtful, for the denial of a spiritual center to his characters is a weakness in a novelist; and it would not have led to popular success in any age other than the twenties, when individualism was rampant and standards of value were more unstable than even Henry Adams might have anticipated. At any rate, it was a sign of increasing maturity when Lewis tried in *Arrowsmith* (1925) to create a character who could rise through a chaos of multiple values and achieve universal respect. He chose a scientist who would move through the academic and medical worlds to a position of eminence and opportunity, only to fail in his great experiment because of a humanizing flaw in his scientific temperament. This plot produced the best of his novels, and it might have been a great one had Lewis chosen to stop at this point and emphasize a tragedy which was genuinely moving because it had been developed in an atmosphere of satire which conquered the chaos of multiple values and made those of Martin Arrowsmith seem real. But a certain intellectual weakness and a strain of sentimentality caused him to lead the reader away from the threat of catharsis and disengage him from the story in its concluding parts; and these qualities affected both of the two other important novels he was to publish during the decade, giving to *Elmer Gantry* (1927) the values of the self-conscious intelligentsia rather than those of the understanding realist and touching *Dodsworth* (1929) with a slight suggestion that he was trying to apologize and make up for the injustice he had done the American businessman in *Babbitt*. With the possible exception of the antifascist hypothetical story *It Can't Happen Here* (1935), Lewis failed in later years to achieve a literary success comparable to his five major novels of the twenties; and these failures perhaps confirm the suspicion that he was peculiarly the representative of the postwar decade—a man whose experience was wide and perceptive but who was so dimly focused within himself that readers in a chaotic age could absorb his experience, bring it to terms with their own inner consciousness, and find satisfaction in the awareness of their own individuality.

Unlike Lewis, the other major novelist stimulated to new artistic achievement by the revolt against small-town life had done some of her best work during the prewar period. Many critics, in fact, consider Willa Cather's early stories of simple people on the Nebraska plains, *O Pioneers!* (1913) and *My Ántonia* (1918), the finest of her novels, and her story of the opera singer who came out of such an environment, *The Song of the Lark* (1915), comparable to them. Certainly her admiration for these immigrant daughters, inured to toil and with the inner strength to rise above adversity, was warm and moving; but the intellectual basis for it was obscure, for she kept them separate in body or in spirit from the social entanglements which tested and revealed the beliefs of Henry James and Edith Wharton. It was not until she undertook the story of a young man who went to and returned from war, in *One of Ours* (1922), that she faced in a full-length novel the problem of a heroic spirit in a frustrating society and found that a feeling for heroism was not enough to sustain the integrity of a realistic story. Her first solution was pessimistic, and in *A Lost Lady* (1923) she produced a compact tragedy of moral and spiritual decay which confirmed the attitude toward village narrowness she had indicated in such early short stories as "The Sculptor's Funeral" and "Paul's Case" (from *The Troll Garden* in 1905) but had generally avoided in her novels. Her next two books, *The Professor's House* (1925) and *My Mortal Enemy* (1926), revealed a continued preoccupation with environmental frustration; but within the first of them was an avenue of escape in the form of an inserted novella called "Tom Outland's Story"—an escape into the American Southwest, which she loved with a passion never felt for Europe however much her early European experiences may have affected her art.

Actually, the theme of the Southwest had been an-

ticipated in *The Song of the Lark* when Thea Kron-
borg, worn out by the pressures of the city and unable
to find the artistic restoration she sought in her native
town, took refuge among the cliff dwellings of "the ancient people," listened to "a voice out of the past, not
very loud, that went on saying a few simple things to
the solitude eternally," and in this communion with the
past found a renewal of strength and character. The
story of the archaeologist Tom Outland and his Blue
Mesa was designed to have the same effect by letting
in a breath of fresh air from the mesa in the form of
Outland's fine disregard for the triviality of "petty ambitions," "quivering jealousies," and "American proprieties" with which Miss Cather had deliberately
made Professor St. Peter's house "stuffy." In these epi-
sodes she was reflecting personal experience and feeling, but it was experience and feeling from which she
was to create a new theory of values which were
environmental but not social and on which the individual could depend for a strength she was not quite
willing to attribute to his Transcendental spirit—a system based upon a few simple things said externally
from the past and thereby uniting the past and present
in one timeless reality.

Miss Cather could have acquired from Henri Bergson or Marcel Proust the ideas that led her into her
recherche du temps perdu in *Death Comes for the
Archbishop* (1927), but her own comments upon the
inspiration of the novel suggest that she was simply following the same sort of sensitivity that caused Hawthorne to become preoccupied with the past prolong-
ing itself into the present as a sort of "gray legendary

mist." In any case, her success in recapturing the legendary quality of the early Santa Fé missionaries, Bishop Latour and Father Vaillant, harmonizing it with the existing atmosphere of the region is one of the finest achievements in American fiction in one of the most secure of modern classics. The fineness of her achievement in interpreting the distinctive atmosphere of a peculiar locality in terms of the past and the few simple things it whispers to the present can be tested by any one who reads her other novel of the same type, *Shadows on the Rock* (1931), set in modern Quebec, where the shadows seem to be more delicately but definitely etched than in New Mexico. But *Death Comes for the Archbishop* is the deeper book, emotionally, in the witness it bears to a sense of the past not as history but as life, and nothing in Miss Cather's later work ever rivaled it.

Comparable to Willa Cather in the opinion of some critics and certainly possessed of more wit if less sensitivity and feeling is Ellen Glasgow, another Virginian by birth but one who remained in her native state and found her literary material almost exclusively there. Miss Glasgow's early ambition was to give in fiction a panorama of Virginia history, but she developed from a historical novelist into a novelist of inbred character and finally, during the twenties, into a witty and sardonic commentator upon contemporary southern life. Born in Richmond rather than in a small town, Miss Glasgow's revolt was against the southern devotion to Romantic illusion, which she so skillfully presented in *The Deliverance* (1904); and she began it early with the realistic story of the Reconstruction period, *The*

Voice of the People (1900), which preceded her Civil War novel *The Battle-Ground* (1902). Her method was that of emphasizing the importance of the lower middle class in southern life in a series of novels culminating with *Barren Ground* (1925), whose heroine, Dorinda Oakley, is comparable to Willa Cather's Alexandra Bergson and Ántonia Shimerda, and of holding up for admiration those people who broke with the southern conventions as did the heroine of *Life and Gabriella* (1916). Under the influence of Cabell, her wit came to full flowering in the three novels of "the Queenborough trilogy," *The Romantic Comedians* (1926), *They Stooped to Folly* (1929), and *The Sheltered Life* (1932), in which she mocked the manners of contemporary Richmond and—in the second and perhaps the best of the three—gave an amusingly ironic representation of the change in attitude toward three generations of lovely ladies who slipped or stepped from the path of virtue.

Miss Glasgow had as deep a feeling for the past as did Miss Cather, but she felt it within a pattern of evolutionary ideas rather than as something from which time selected certain absolute values and incorporated them into the present. To her the past was a cultural heritage which might destroy or preserve, a myth one might live but against which it was better to rebel, a period of selective breeding in a strictly biological sense. It was this last concept which finally prevailed in the most profound of her novels, *Vein of Iron* (1935), in which she paid tribute to the hard firmness of her own Scotch-Irish strain and suggested that the stern cultural heritage of the Presbyterian intellectual was weaker than the inbred qualities of character.

II

The rebellion against conventions, for which Edna St. Vincent Millay wrote the lyrics and H. L. Mencken beat the drum, had the advantage of its own periodical in *The American Mercury,* which Mencken founded in 1923 with the assistance of George Jean Nathan, who had been associated with him in the editorship of *The Smart Set.* Mencken himself had been an aggressive Baltimore individualist for more than two decades, an early admirer of George Bernard Shaw but an outspoken opponent of socialism, a defender of the philosophy of Friedrich Nietzsche, an eclectic critic whose essays had been collected in *A Book of Prefaces* (1917), and a bull in the conventional china shop with *Damn—A Book of Calumny* and *In Defense of Women* (both in 1918). He was also an independent and explosive user, student, and creator of the American language, who had already begun his monumental work of scholarship on that subject with the publication of its first volume in 1919; and he had collaborated with Nathan in an ironic study of *The American Credo: A Contribution toward the Interpretation of the National Mind* (1920). His major literary works of the postwar period consisted of the six-volume series of essays called *Prejudices* (1919–27) which began with a literary emphasis but became increasingly sociological, and with the damning *Notes on Democracy* (1926) and a cynical *Treatise on the Gods* (1930).

His greatest influence was exercised through the *Mercury,* in which he published a quarterly collection of "Americana" gleaned from the country's press and revealing the national life at its sanctimonious worst, denounced the "boobosity" of the country as a whole and especially the service club "wowsers" and the smugness of the "Bible Belt," and defended generously every new or old writer who seemed to be striking at or through the moral or social conventions of which he so vigorously disapproved—Theodore Dreiser, Sinclair Lewis, and especially James Branch Cabell. For the Cabell of Mencken's era had become quite different from the earlier representative of popular if somewhat sophisticated Romanticism. In 1919 he had published in the essays of *Beyond Life* an urbane defense of Romanticism on the grounds that man alone of all animals was able to play the ape to his dreams and that Romantic illusions were necessary if he was to raise himself out of the biological mire. But in the same year he had also published the novel *Jurgen,* which told the story of an old and cynical pawnbroker whose youth was renewed by magic; his renewed youth was devoted to biological activity under the influence of his single remaining illusion. With an intellect entirely too active for the sort of writing he had been doing, Cabell had reached the point of having to decide whether he would develop as a sort of Romantic evolutionist or become a satiric and cynical commentator upon the world as it was. As he approached the threshold of the new era, the choice, in fact, was made for him: he became the latter, writing a companion novel for *Jurgen,* called *Figures of Earth* (1921), in which the hero, Dom

Manuel, followed his own thinking and his own desires under the motto "The world wishes to be deceived," until he achieved every high position the world could offer without ever changing his original simple self.

During these years *Jurgen* was generally suppressed throughout the country on the grounds of indecency, and Cabell busied himself revising all his earlier books in order to bring them into a common pattern. He went so far as to give a new title to the revised version of *The Soul of Melicent* (*Domnei,* in 1920), but most of the revisions were designed to sharpen their cynicism of tone and place them within the mythological framework of his pseudomedieval world of Poictesme, in which Jurgen (as the exponent of the cleverly intellectual way of life which he called "gallantry") and Manuel (representing the simple-minded way of "chivalry") were the two protagonists from whom all his other characters were descended. His whole ingenious plan was charted in *The Lineage of Litchfield* (1922), filled out with the eighteenth-century gallantry (and sexuality) of *The High Place* (1923) and with the chivalric fellowship of *The Silver Stallion* (1926), and rounded off with *Something about Eve* (1927), which is the most sympathetically human of his novels in its representation of the effects of marriage and of a father's transfer of his own dreams to his hopes for a child. Cabell's own greatest illusion, stoutly maintained in the essays of *Straws and Prayerbooks* (1924) at a time when every tendency was in the opposite direction, was that lushness and sophistication were the proper qualities of a good style; and, although critics of a later generation may find in him the stylistic and intellectual ambivalence which has become so attractive in Hawthorne, his immediate successors have ignored him to such a degree that he has become least known of all the major literary figures of the twenties.

Yet Cabell was only one of a considerable group of rebel sophisticates which included the later Joseph Hergesheimer of *Cytherea* (1922) and *Balisand* (1924), the young Thornton Wilder of *The Cabala* (1926) and *The Bridge of San Luis Rey* (1927), and the aging critic James Gibbons Huneker whose privately printed collection of short stories, *Painted Veils* (1920), appeared the year before his death. Huneker's literary successor—and also the successor of Edgar Saltus, whose death in the same year revived an interest in his precious, erotic writings of the previous century—was Carl Van Vechten, music and art critic and devotee of cats, whose novels *Peter Whiffle* (1922), *The Blind Bow-Boy* (1923), and *The Tattooed Countess* (1924) were supposed to contain practically everything a young man should know during the early twenties. Van Vechten's interest in the offbeat aspects of New York life, however, was both genuine and intelligent; and he went on in *Nigger Heaven* (1926) and *Spider Boy* (1928) to explore Harlem and the sporting world with a knowledge which was not to be exceeded in American fiction until Ralph Ellison wrote *Invisible Man* (1952) and Bernard Wolfe *The Late Risers* (1954). But Cabell's closest rival was the short-lived Elinor Wylie, who handled a Romantic style with much more delicacy and taste and produced two minor classics in *Jennifer Lorn* (1923), the story of a young Englishman in the East India Company whose elegant discrimination kept him a year or two in advance of the great minds of his age, and *The Venetian Glass Nephew* (1925), an imaginary episode in the life of Giacomo Casanova told from the point of view of complete innocence. She achieved popular success in *The Orphan Angel* (1926), a Romantic fantasy of Shelley pioneering the American continent, and maintained it to a certain extent in the year of her death with *Mr. Hodge and Mr. Hazard* (1928), a novel which suggestively portrayed in human terms the impact of Victorianism upon the Romantic spirit; but she has been remembered more by a later generation for her poetry (from *Nets to Catch the Wind* in 1921 to *Angels and Earthly Creatures* in 1929), which shares some of the qualities of Edna St. Vincent Millay but is much more clear-cut in style.

While Mencken was encouraging his group of rebels in fiction, George Jean Nathan found his major literary protégé in the person of Eugene O'Neill, who brought to the dreary boards of the American theater a quality of excitement never felt before in serious native drama. O'Neill had got his start with the Provincetown Players on Cape Cod and in the Provincetown Playhouse of New York, and several of his early realistic dramas had been published in *The Smart Set* before he attracted widespread literary attention with the publication of *The Moon of the Caribbees, and Six Other Plays of the Sea* in 1920. O'Neill was primarily a dramatist of frustrations, whose background of realism and whose technical skill, acquired through the early one-act plays, enabled him to be convincing while he made his theme exciting by expressing it in terms of the new theater and the new psychology. *Beyond the Horizon* (1920), the story of a dreamer and would-be wanderer who is held to the farm by a woman's passion while his solid brother is set awandering, was a realistic representation of the basic conflict in most of his plays—a conflict between dreams and desires on the one hand and temperament and practicality on the other. *The Emperor Jones* (1921) translated it into symbolic and psychological terms by making a ruthlessly calculating Caribbean dictator the victim of the little formless fears that arose in his own mind, and *The Hairy Ape* (1922) experimented with its symbolic expression by the use of masks and stereotyped figures. This experimentation was carried in 1926 to its utmost length in *The Great God Brown* (which used masks, not altogether successfully, to stage the conflict in terms of the divided personality of a single character) and in the almost unactable *Lazarus Laughed* of 1927 (in which Lazarus found, through the experience of death, a life beyond desire and a laughter which split the masked personalities of the world to which he returned). In the meantime O'Neill had been developing his more naturalistic means of expression in the unresolved pathos of *Anna Christie* (1922), in the stronger pathos of miscegenation in *All God's Chillun Got Wings* (1924), and in the unadulterated passions of sex and greed in *Desire Under the Elms* (1925), until he was able to bring his realistic and experimental tendencies together in the most ambitious of his dramas—*Strange Interlude* (1928), in which the characters spoke their secret thoughts in motionless pauses between the passages of conventional dialogue.

Much of O'Neill's power seems to have come from the fact that in the infinitely varied twenties he could accept frustration as a way of life and find in that acceptance a source of energy comparable to that which Anderson found in irresponsibility, Lewis in superiority, Cather in the past, Glasgow in inbred character, Mencken in irreverence, and Cabell in cynicism. He was less prolific and less exciting in the more serious decade which followed, when he tried in vain to modernize the Greek tragic spirit in *Mourning Becomes Electra* (1931), was more successful with the nostalgia of youth in *Ah, Wilderness!* (1933), but became lost trying to deal with the religious impulse in *Days Without End* (1934). Positive commitments were not easy for a man who sank into silence for more than a decade before he revealed the essence of his problem in *The Iceman Cometh* (1946): he could neither be content with a drunken dream nor accept the conventional realities of life as sanity. And the reason for his dilemma was to become clear in his revealing posthumous drama, *A Long Day's Journey into Night* (1956). Frustration, violent impulsiveness, and theatric expression were bred in him and formed the tenor of a life which could never quite find ease in irony or really reach the depths of tragedy.

For people who enjoyed the revolt against conventions during the twenties, Mencken, Cabell, and Millay preserve its true flavor; but, for later readers who just missed it, Scott Fitzgerald became the novelist of the great rebellion. Perhaps this is so because Fitzgerald himself did not quite believe the age but played its game with an air of wonder, a double sense of involvement and detachment which made him the immediate historian of an age he was half living and half creating. At any rate, *This Side of Paradise* (1920) was a reminiscent novel at the time he wrote it, drawing upon his experiences as a romantic, Irish-midwestern egoist in prewar Princeton; but it was put together with a postwar feeling that made it a model of emulation for a new generation. Similarly the short stories of *Flappers and Philosophers* (1920), *Tales of the Jazz Age* (1922), and *All the Sad Young Men* (1926) were careful and often fascinated observations of the new era which were widely distributed in popular magazines as examples of a way of life which, as Mencken observed, was "imitated by the flappers of the Bible Belt country clubs" in the weeks that followed. Fitzgerald was more ambitious as a social historian in *The Beautiful and Damned* (1922), a somewhat chaotic portrayal of the attractions and the futility of the New York world to which his success had admitted him; but it was not until *The Great Gatsby* (1926) that he managed to triumph over his early faults of style and achieve a novel which seemed to T. S. Eliot "the first step that American fiction has taken since Henry James." There was, in fact, a Jamesian quality in the book, emphasized by the use of a narrator and the method of presenting the story in scenes, in its conception of flamboyant bootlegger Gatsby as an individual of greater moral sensitivity than the wealthy and well-bred Daisy and Tom; and, although it lacks Jamesian faith inasmuch as Gatsby is killed instead of being allowed to experience some inner triumph, it is this quality which makes it Fitzgerald's most human book rather than another fine example of social history.

Fitzgerald was to preserve this humanity in his next and much later novel, *Tender Is the Night* (1934), by making the reader feel pity rather than respect for the young psychiatrist Dick Diver, whose most successful case was his wife who had no need for him after she was cured. He also carried it over into many of the later short stories collected in *Taps at Reveille* (1935) and into the fragmentary novel, *The Last Tycoon* (1941), which he attempted after his Hollywood experiences and while he was himself going to pieces in the way he so candidly described in *The Crack-up* (1945). But his great achievement was that of capturing, in the person of Gatsby, the major symbol of the rebellion against conventions during the Prohibition era and identifying it with that quality of humanity which Americans traditionally admired.

III

Among the less high-spirited but more pretentious leaders of the rebellious twenties Thomas Stearns Eliot was to have, by far, the greatest literary influence. A native of St. Louis, he had been educated at Harvard and, like Pound but with much better academic training, he had gone abroad to complete his work for the doctorate. There, like Pound, he decided to remain; and at the outbreak of the First World War he settled in England, married, recognized in Pound a poet of kindred interests, and in 1917 published a pamphlet on Pound's metric and poetry and brought out a thin volume of his own verse entitled *Prufrock and Other*

Observations. Some were early satires dating from his Harvard days, a few paid passing allegiance to the Imagist fad, and two of them ("Portrait of a Lady" and "The Love Song of J. Alfred Prufrock") resembled Pound's "Portrait d'une Femme" in suggesting a by-stander's fascination with the world of Henry James. At the end of the war he made a collection of his literary essays in *The Sacred Wood* (1920), prepared for publication a new volume of *Poems* (1920), and, suffering from nervous strain, made a trip to Lausanne, where he composed the first version of *The Waste Land,* which was to be extensively cut and edited by Pound before it was published in 1922. With the publication of *The Waste Land* (which appeared in two periodicals and in book form in the same year) against the background of his *Poems* and his critical essays, Eliot became the most controversial poet of the new era.

Consequently his development during these first postwar years is of unusual interest. Some of it can be traced in the *Poems* and attributed to the influence of Pound, who undoubtedly encouraged him in the greater devotion to the French Symbolists which this volume revealed, who taught him the trick of weaving a poem out of allusions to erudite knowledge, and who set him an example for the sophisticated bad-boy pose, which had been foreshadowed by his early satires and the "Portrait of a Lady" but which became pronounced in "Whispers of Immortality" and "The Hippopota-mus" and in the suggestion of self-identification in "Mr. Eliot's Sunday Morning Service" with a crude character named Sweeney. Pound's influence is also strongly marked in some of the ideas and in the shift away from the Symbolists toward the Dantesque quality of "Gerontion," which led directly to *The Waste Land* in the new quality of its imagery and in the somber seriousness of its tone and attitude. Yet the *Poems* were also a declaration of independence from Pound. For Eliot did not share his friend and mentor's evangelical determination to sacrifice metrical charm to imagistic hardness, and his words sang their way into their readers' consciousness with all the insidiousness of nonsense verse. Much of Eliot's early fame was probably due to this insidiousness and to the prestige given him by intellectuals who partially mastered his erudition and found that achievement created in them a feeling of complacency comparable to that which Sinclair Lewis was creating in the general public; but Eliot had much more to offer, especially in *The Waste Land,* than the charm of Lewis Carroll and intellectual satisfaction for the initiate. He had a theme in the decay of modern civilization which possessed a strong appeal for a generation which was beginning to read Oswald Spengler and was to consider O'Neill a great dramatist, Cabell a man of wisdom, and Fitzgerald a tragic novelist; and his poem had a quality of inner coherence, a suggestion of focus in depth, which was notably lacking in the poetry of Pound.

The search for a point of focus in *The Waste Land,* however, has been confused by the fact that in the critical essays of *The Sacred Wood* Eliot had set forth two quite different theories concerning the relationship of the poet to his work. One (to be found in "Ben Jonson" and "Hamlet" of his *Selected Essays* of 1932) held that the creation of a work of art consisted of the process of transfusing the personality of the author into it and maintained that literary appreciation depended upon understanding the author rather than the "archaeology" of his materials. The answer to the riddle of *Hamlet*, for example, lay in Shakespeare's biography, perhaps on a subconscious level; and the play was an artistic failure because Shakespeare had transfused into his character an emotion too deep and complex to be evoked in the audience by any of the symbols he used to justify it. For "the only way of expressing emotion in the form of art is by finding an 'objective correlative,'" Eliot explained; "in other words, a set of objects, a situation, a chain of events which shall be the formula of that *particular* emotion; such that when the external facts, which must terminate in sensory experience, are given, the emotion is immediately evoked." This was a theory in the tradition of Emerson and James, who thought of art as a selected portion of the external world passed through "the alembic of man." Yet it was almost completely opposed by another theory (found in "Tradition and the Individual Talent") which held that the mind of the poet was merely a catalytic agent that enabled very special or very old feelings to enter into new combinations with a new effectiveness. These feelings would have no necessary reference to the poet himself. For "the more perfect the artist, the more completely separate in him will be the man who suffers and the mind which creates." Consequently "it is not in his personal emotions, the emotions provoked by particular events in his life, that the poet is in any way remarkable or interesting"; and poetry itself "is not a turning loose of emotion but an escape from emotion; it is not the expression of personality, but an escape from personality." Here Eliot was presenting a more subtle and sophisticated version of Poe's "The Philosophy of Composition."

The line which Eliot himself has followed most consistently since has been the second (most emphatically in the lectures *After Strange Gods* of 1934), and it is from this line that there has developed a whole school of "New Critics" in America, who have violated Eliot's notions of "The Function of Criticism" (1923) by falling into the "autotelic" heresy of creative interpretation and have filled university classrooms with creative and catalytic agents rather than instructors. Because of this—and because the author's own notes for *The Waste Land* suggested an anthropological rather than a personal inspiration for the poem—the interpretations of Eliot's most influential work have been in terms of its superficial theme. But if one assumes that his first theory of poetic creation is the more real one—that he was actually writing in the American tradition of insisting that literary materials make sense in terms of his own experience—and if one makes the further assumption that his literary allusions were selected for their genuine allusiveness rather than as bits of arbitrary structural material for an emotional engineer, then the poem itself and Eliot's peculiar power both become more comprehensible.

Under such assumptions, the key to *The Waste Land* might be found in its concluding section, "What the Thunder Said," and especially in the final lines, be-

ginning with the voice of the thunder, which are
introduced by the interwoven imagery of the biblical
journey to Emmaus and the approach to the Castle
Perilous in Jessie Weston's *From Ritual to Romance*.
The associations of this imagery suggest a moment of
time after the Passion and before the Resurrection, a
moment when the Fisher King of the Grail romances
sits waiting for the word which will cause the waters
to flow and restore fertility to the stony places. Then,
out of the author's Harvard studies in Indic philology,
comes the voice of the thunder—"*Da*," which was
variously interpreted, according to fable, as the first
syllable of the words meaning "give," "sympathize,"
and "control." The reflections upon these interpretations seem to be intensely personal in their references
to the gift of "the awful daring of a moment's surrender," to the key of sympathy which had turned in the
door once and once only, and to the control which
would have brought a gay and willing response had it
been exercised upon another's heart; and the implication of personal failure in the last reflection is emphasized in the following lines in which the poet identifies
himself with the Fisher King, sitting with the arid
plain behind him and asking whether he should not at
least set his "lands in order." The ordering is in the
manner of Pound, by a collection of apparently ran-
dom quotations which, however, are highly coherent
in their allusive context. The first conjures up the inevitable association of "my fair lady" with the catchy
words of "London Bridge is falling down," the second
calls to mind the Provençal poet who was being purged
of lust in Dante's Purgatory, the third is a part of a

cry from the violated and mutilated Philomela who wants to be like the swallow and from dumb distress set free, and the fourth recalls a gloomy, widowed, and unconsoled Prince of Aquitaine standing before a ruined tower. "These fragments" of literary feeling from the past, said the poet, "I have shored against my ruins"—in the manner, he implied, of Thomas Kyd's Hieronimo, who escaped from real distraction by pretending madness and agreeing to write a play by which he achieved his rational purpose—and the poem closes with the Sanscrit words of guidance and a benediction inviting an infinitude of peace.

The rights of privacy which any man can claim in his lifetime make it impossible to relate these allusions to a specific experience, but the coherence of its conclusion seems personal enough to invite a reading of the whole poem in such terms and finding in its earlier parts a sustained emotional balance between old dreams and current reality. Cleopatra and Lil, the London of Spenser's "Prothalamion" and that of Mr. Eugenides and the carbuncular clerk, the Thames of Elizabeth and Leicester and that of the cockney boats off Richmond—these represent a balance of opposites which culminates in the foreboding of "Death by Water" and in the resolution of its conclusion. From this point of view it would seem that Eliot's "waste land" is his own emotional waste land and that contemporary civilization is an "objective correlative" which the public, under the guidance of his criticism, has found adequate for its justification. And from this point of view, too, his later and less influential writings may be summarized in terms of a search outside of literature for other means of shoring up his life. He seems to have dwelt in his waste land at least through "The Hollow Men" (1925); made a determined effort to escape in the essays *For Lancelot Andrewes* (1928) when he announced himself a classicist in literature, an Anglo-Catholic in religion, and a royalist in politics; and confirmed himself in the institutional refuge of the church with the poem *Ash Wednesday* (1930) and the poetic drama *Murder in the Cathedral* (1935), while trying, in *Sweeney Agonistes* (1932), to exorcise his bad-boy self along the way. But the indications are that he has not found the institution adequate, and in what appears to be the finest and most mature of his poetical works, the *Four Quartets* (1941–43), he has turned to a past which is neither literary nor institutional but one which whispers "a few simple things" eternally. When he came to the belief that "Time present and time past are both perhaps present in time future, and time future contained in time past," he may have been finding his own personal support in the concept of reality which Willa Cather had tried to capture in *Death Comes for the Archbishop.* Or perhaps his final philosophy represents a return to a subjective concept of time derived from Bergson, under whom he had studied in 1910. At any rate he had explored much and arrived back where he might have started had he been able to know the place the first time.

The basic difference between Eliot and Pound can be expressed, though oversimplified, in terms of the old assumption that a man's wisdom should be tested by the tenor of his own life. Eliot, despite his philosophy of composition, seems to have followed this assumption, whereas Pound has formed his life around the fixed ideas of his early rebelliousness. Of the other participants in what has been called "the melody of chaos" it is more difficult to judge. Among Eliot's younger contemporaries the one most closely linked to him, by reaction rather than by imitation, was Hart Crane, whose first collection of verse (*White Buildings* in 1926) showed a genuine originality in experimenting with the suggestive power of words. But Crane, unlike the troubled Eliot and the eccentric Pound, was using poetry to struggle against a genuine derangement of mind, and the ambitious culmination of his desire to provide a constructive answer to *The Waste Land* took the form of "an epic of modern consciousness," *The Bridge* (1930), which gathered together the myths of American history, literature, and folklore and related them to impressions of contemporary New York but achieved neither epic quality nor inner coherence. E. E. Cummings, whose novel *The Enormous Room* (1922) was one of the most psychologically effective products of the First World War, makes a more lasting impression with his distinctive combination of delicate sensibility and mischievous independence from linguistic conventions; and his volumes with such queer titles as *Is 5* (1926) and *1 x 1* (1945) contain some memorable poems in rather startling arrangements of word forms, grammar, syntax, punctuation, and typography. The most deeply independent minor poet of Eliot's generation, however, was Marianne Moore, who emphasized the objective quality of her work by calling one volume of poems *Observations* (1924) and who has since, by constant revision, stripped her originally stark verses on simple things to the simplicity of skeleton poetry.

Yet among the host of singers in the chaotic twenties there arose only one new voice strong enough, for a while, to rival Eliot's; and that was the voice of the California poet Robinson Jeffers. As well educated as Eliot, though interested in the sciences as well as in the classics, Jeffers had studied abroad and published one volume of rather conventional verse before marrying and settling upon the California coast near Monterey, where he built the stone tower in which he was to live the rest of his life in retirement. His volume of verse, *Californians*, appeared in 1916, but he attracted little attention until rumors of the privately printed *Tamar* began to circulate in 1924 and *Roan Stallion, Tamar, and Other Poems* reached a startled public in 1925. He had been completely untouched by the "new" poetry of Pound and Eliot, but his own was new enough in its own right. His long lines invited comparison with Whitman but were more regular, suggesting at once classical hexameters and the strong beat of Old English verse, and his images had the strength of one who had dedicated himself to absorbing his own wild surroundings. But a greater wildness was in his subjects: *Tamar* was a story of incest and *Roan Stallion* of a woman's frenzied passion for a horse, and both ended in violence. That they owed much to the new psychology was evident, but they possessed a feeling beyond Freud, as though their author was releasing subconscious forces for the purpose of destroying something more than the inhibitions of excessive civilization.

291

Philosophically, *Roan Stallion* suggested as much, for in it Jeffers wrote: "Humanity is the mold to break away from, the crust to break through, the coal to break into fire, the atom to be split." And this proved to be his central theme as successive volumes developed and clarified it, and, though equally violent, modified the impulsiveness of its first statement. In *The Women at Point Sur* (1927) the incest motif became more clearly symbolic of the introversion of society and of Jeffers' belief in its destructive effect; and the poem was also more clearly indicative of his condemnation of man and his civilization, as though the course of evolution had run itself out and it was time for a collapse, as though the decline of the West had actually been speeded up according to the rule of phase, as though the flash in chaos was the light of revelation. Jeffers had found something of his own feeling among the Greek dramatists and in "The Tower beyond Tragedy" (1925) had given Orestes a vision of humanity turning inward upon itself in hate or love and had allowed him to cut himself loose from human passions by falling in love "outward" with the inanimate world. And he too seems to have achieved something like a catharsis through the violence of these poems, for there is pity in *Cawdor* (1928) for the strong man who is betrayed and broken by the primitive egocentricity of a woman and pity in *Dear Judas* (1929) for the betrayer. His own feeling at the end of the decade is perhaps best expressed in this last volume in the best of the shorter poems which reveal both his violence and his philosophy—a succinct version of *The Bacchantes* called "The Humanist's Tragedy." "It is possible for you to break prison of yourselves and enter the nature of things and use the beauty," says King Pentheus. "Wine and lawlessness, art and music, love, self-torture, religion, are means but are not needful, contemplation will do it. Only break human collectedness." A moment later he is torn to pieces by his mother and her frenzied companions, but the "tragic flaw" in the drama appears in the "wild, somewhat too drunken" representatives of humanity rather than in the hero whose "dignity, as a human being, a king and Greek," is maintained and respected. And whether Jeffers would allow himself to be called a humanist or not, his later work, from *Thurso's Landing and Other Poems* (1932) on, seems to be more concerned with violence as an error than with violence as an ideal.

Most of the writers whose spirit was peculiarly that of the twenties wrote in the spirit of *après moi le déluge,* and Jeffers, the introspective recluse, was perhaps no more than an ultimate example of the spirit of an age in which every individual could find a source of energy in his own sense of values, even the values of destruction. At the moment it is probably too soon to say which of the writers of the twenties reflected a "wisdom tested by the tenor of a life" and which represented a mere rebellion against conventional life. Certainly the energy of many appeared to fade with the energy of their decade: their individualism was not rugged enough to survive the stock-market crash of the autumn of 1929 and the economic depression which followed. The symbol of the American tradition had flourished, gaudily enough for a while, but the real test of its power was to be made in the sterner years to come when a new generation of writers arose and a few older ones continued to mature.

EPILOGUE

The Test
1930—

CHAPTER TEN

Power and the Past

I

THE most radical effect of the economic depression upon the American consciousness was to make the old attitude of *laissez faire* impossible. From the most conservative stockbroker who turned his face to avoid buying an apple from a former colleague on the streets of New York to the most ardent socialist who welcomed the New Deal in politics as "a step in the right direction," people were forced into an awareness that individuals did not stand alone in the complex society they had created. Many, of course, did not want to stand alone. Even the twenties had been marked by a gradual decrease in enthusiasm for the new freedom, a lessened willingness to live in the present, a noticeable tendency toward second thoughts in literature. But these signs were in older writers who may have been simply losing their energy, and so it required a newcomer on the literary scene, a young man with an apparently inexhaustible gusto, to show that this change in attitude was a sign of the times rather than an evidence of individual exhaustion.

This newcomer was Thomas Wolfe, whose first rich and crowded novel, *Look Homeward, Angel* (1929), was a product of the twenties with all its exuberance but with a pervading suggestion that its author felt lost in the chaotic world his older contemporaries had created and enjoyed. Significantly, it was the one major novel of the decade that was wholly autobiographical in design, re-creating the places and persons of Wolfe's North Carolina background with a quantity of detail that suggested total recall but that was actually memory engaged in interpreting the environment from which Wolfe was glad to escape but for which he had found no satisfactory substitute. His next novel, *Of Time and the River* (1935), was equally autobiographical, dealing with the larger world of Harvard, New York, and Europe, and equally suggestive of the lost "hapless youth" to which the title of the first had referred; but by this time he was trying to find a meaning in his wanderings in terms of the mythological figures to whom he referred in the subdivisions of the book. As he caught up with his own actual experiences in his writing, he planned a vast historical panorama dealing with his ancestral background; but the impulse to re-create his own personal past in terms of its current emotional meaning seems to have been primary with him, and the last years of his short life were devoted to a more mature and disciplined re-ordering of his early experience, with the introduction for the first time of wholly fictitious characters, in *The Web and the Rock* (1939), *You Can't Go Home Again* (1940), and the fragmentary *The Hills Beyond* (1941)

—all posthumous publications which contain sections rejected from his two earlier books but which suggest the struggle of a man of enormous literary energy who could neither accept the values of the decade in which he reached manhood or that into which he survived.

If Wolfe is the best representative of the emotional attitude of the transition period, John Dos Passos was the best representative of its intellectual state of mind. A Harvard esthete of the generation after Eliot's, Dos Passos had gone to war and given his impressions of the experience in two novels, *One Man's Initiation* (1920) and *Three Soldiers* (1921), reported on his postwar European wanderings in several travel books, and attracted wide attention as an experimenter with the technique of fiction by *Manhattan Transfer* (1925) —a novel which succeeded in capturing the peculiar quality of New York life much better than Howells had done (in the house-hunting introduction to *A Hazard of New Fortunes*), by the device of using many apparently unrelated scenes and incidents and gradually pyramiding them into a relationship which produced a story. After other travels and travel books he began his ambitious trilogy of twentieth-century America which was eventually to appear under the title *U.S.A.: The 42nd Parallel* (1930), *1919* (1932), and *The Big Money* (1936). His method was impressionistic, consisting of the episodic pursuit of a variety of representative characters and the use of three extraordinary devices for the purpose of transmitting a timely background of impressions to the reader—"the camera eye" of a sensitive and perceptive observer's stream of consciousness, a "newsreel" of headlines and fragments of news stories and of bits from popular songs, and impressionistic biographies of historical figures who were related to the fictitious action. The whole was aimed at an unfocused portrayal of the American cultural scene during the first quarter of the twentieth century, when its economic center was moving westward along the forty-second parallel and the moral energies of its people were collapsing into the postwar search for "the big money."

Time alone will tell whether the technical ingenuity of Dos Passos gave him a new means of vivifying the novel of social history or whether it merely served as a successful mnemonic device for readers of his own generation. But his critical attitude toward the United States in which he developed is both clear and representative of the early thirties: he considered it a moral chaos in which malefactors of great wealth were more powerful than the leaders of labor and in which little men were the victims of social ideals that were largely mercenary. Such constructive implications as it contained were socialistic, and, although Dos Passos was to attempt to modify and correct these implications in *The Ground We Stand On* (1941) and other later works of history and fiction, the attitude revealed in *U.S.A.* was the attitude which controlled the search for new values by most of the writers who came to maturity in the thirties.

The writer who developed most during the decade was John Steinbeck, whose considerable versatility was displayed in the early books through which he sought those values which would give assurance to his creative powers. His first, *Cup of Gold* (1929), was a romance based upon the buccaneer Henry Morgan; his second, *The Pastures of Heaven* (1932), a collection of fine and sympathetic short stories about the ordinary people of a "happy valley" in California; and his third, *To a God Unknown* (1933), a novel packed with religious and sexual feeling so intense that it could pass for mysticism. The relative quality of these early volumes suggests that he had found what he was seeking in the second; and Steinbeck may have felt so himself, for his next book, *Tortilla Flat* (1935), was another collection of stories about simple people, *paisanos* of Mexican descent, which was unified by Quixotic humor and the suggestion of Arthurian fellowship. Sympathetic and happy-go-lucky in tone, it was the best of his early books and the first to achieve, though slowly, a wide popular success. Before its qualities were recognized, however, it was followed by *In Dubious Battle* (1936), a novel of class warfare in the California farm lands, which in effect announced Steinbeck's conversion to the new proletarian movement in American fiction—a movement represented ideologically by Mary Heaton Vorse's *Strike: A Novel of Gastonia* (1930), Robert Cantwell's *Laugh and Lie Down* (1931) and *The Land of Plenty* (1934), Grace Lumpkin's *To Make My Bread* (1932), and Jack Conroy's *The Disinherited* (1934) and *World to Win* (1935). Without more research than has yet been done, however, it is difficult to estimate any writer's affiliation with the proletarians, for even so anti-Marxian an author as Pearl Buck showed a strong sympathy for the poorer classes in *The Good Earth* (1931) and her other novels of Chinese peasants. In any event, the power of Steinbeck's new book suggested that he had found in the proletarian movement the strength lacking in his short stories and necessary for his development as a major novelist.

But Steinbeck hesitated. Although *Of Mice and Men* (1937) identified his human sympathies with the itinerant worker on at least two levels of interpretation, *The Red Pony* of the same year marked a return to his more spontaneous sympathies, and it was not until 1939 that he was able to produce a really fine novel of social consciousness in *The Grapes of Wrath,* which has properly been called "the epic of the great depression." The story of the Joad family, who had been driven off their farm in the Oklahoma dust bowl by a combination of natural and economic circumstances, it follows them in their transcontinental migration to the promised land of California, capturing the atmosphere of the time with a discreet use of impressionistic devices borrowed from Dos Passos but telling a genuinely human story of frailty, endurance, and disillusionment. It was not, however, an orthodox proletarian novel; and although the book was praised by the Marxian critics, it marked the end of Steinbeck's association with the movement. The good and evil in the book were not completely separated by class lines; and, although Tom Joad certainly was allowed to acquire strength from his radical social philosophy, the strongest personality in the book was Ma Joad, whose strength came from character and her determination to hold the family together. Steinbeck's sympathy for individual human beings had enabled him to avoid the rigid demands of Marxism, but his difficulty seems to have been that he did not have much to escape to. An insistence that "people are people" was not enough, as he discovered when he tried to apply that principle to the Nazi invaders of Norway in *The Moon Is Down* (1942). What was left was emotion—physical, as he tried to give depth to his interest in the *paisanos* in *Cannery Row* (1945), and almost mystically sexual in *The Wayward Bus* (1947)—and with it he has maintained his public but not his literary power.

What would have happened had Steinbeck been able to hold firmly to the sense of values he undoubtedly gained for a while from the proletarian movement? The question is of course entirely speculative, but it suggests an approach to Erskine Caldwell, who is one of the most widely read American authors abroad and who shared many of Steinbeck's characteristics. Caldwell began with a theme of sensational violence and degeneracy in *The Bastard* (1930) and attracted widespread attention when his novel *Tobacco Road* (1932) was made into a play which ran for seven years in New York. Although it was also concerned with violence and degeneracy, *Tobacco Road* revealed a grotesque humor which was developed in *God's Little Acre* (1933) to the point of making the latter book a spontaneously amusing story of the realities and eccentricities of southern poor whites. Both books displayed, too, a deeper quality in their indication of a sympathetic understanding of a peasant-like attachment to the soil which was the last sign of stability among mean people who were being uprooted by industrialism and fascinated by its products.

Furthermore there was a Steinbeck-like quality of emotionalism in both books which developed into the intensely erotic religiosity of *Journeyman* (1935). These were the qualities recruited to the proletarian cause and devoted to it, with a minimum of humor, in the grim tragedies of *Kneel to the Rising Sun* (1935), the title story of which is especially powerful in its treatment of racial injustice and of the inability of human attachments to survive racial consciousness and class pressures.

Although never brought into balance in a single book, there was a Gogol-like quality in Caldwell's writing which held remarkable promise at the time he became primarily interested in reporting (with the photographs of Margaret Bourke-White) the human effects of the American depression, the atmosphere of central Europe, and the Russian battle front. For this reason his announcement of a major novel dealing with the Russian popular resistance to the German invasion of the Ukraine was of unusual interest at a time when Nikolai Gogol's Russians were doing the resisting but Leo Tolstoi's *War and Peace* was a best seller in the United States. Yet when the book, *All Night Long* (1942), actually appeared, it was not only a disappointment to literary expectation but a swan song for the proletarian impulse in American fiction. The Germans and their collaborators were beasts. The communists and the peasants of the resistance were martyrs. The passion and the violence, the eccentricity and high spirits, the humor and the sympathy, and the basic love of the land—qualities which had appeared in Gogol's portrayal of the Russians in *Taras Bulba* and Caldwell's portrayal of the meanest of Georgia crackers—these were nowhere. Caldwell held the line as Steinbeck did not when each got his great chance, and the Marxian line disciplined him out of all contact with his material and with his readers.

James T. Farrell, the third major new novelist to mature in the proletarian atmosphere of the thirties, was saved from Caldwell's fate by the rugged Dreiserian honesty which pervaded all his work and by his Wolfeian tendency to engage in a constant re-evaluation and reinterpretation of material derived from his own early background. In his Studs Lonigan trilogy—*Young Lonigan* (1932), *The Young Manhood of Studs Lonigan* (1934), and *Judgment Day* (1935) —he was an effective recruit to the proletarian cause, writing of the vicious social environment of Chicago's South Side and its destructive effect upon a member of the *petite bourgeoisie* in a naturalistic way which refrained from preaching but used the symbol of a communist parade to suggest a better way than that followed by Studs. But in the year the trilogy was completed Farrell quarreled with the communist bureaucrats who dominated the American Writers' Congress, prepared *A Note on Literary Criticism* (1936) which came out strongly against the application of political directives to the creative process, and began the Danny O'Neill tetralogy—*A World I Never Made* (1936), *No Star Is Lost* (1938), *Father and Son* (1940), and *My Days of Anger* (1943)—which was more personal in its representation of the O'Neill and O'Flaherty families and more autobiographical in its account of a sensitive hero who set out to get an education and fight in his own way for the betterment of society. Farrell's own way was one of stubborn independence amidst the many shifts of opinion, and when the reaction against radicalism set in he reasserted his freedom in *The League of Frightened Philistines* (1945) and began a new series of novels—*Bernard Clare* (1946), *The Road Between* (1949), and *Yet Other Waters* (1952)—in which the progress of his hero (who was renamed Bernard Carr after a lawsuit over the first volume) marked his own break with the Communist party but maintained the socialistic ideals he asserted in *Literature and Morality* (1947) at a time when so many of his former intellectual associates were recanting their radicalism or taking refuge in silence.

There was more vitality in the Studs Lonigan and the first of the Danny O'Neill books than in the later novels, for Farrell, like Wolfe, was at his best when his material was fresh; and there is no doubt that he and his contemporaries found genuine strength in the values of the new social consciousness of the early thirties. But it was the strength of shock, anger, and impulsive rationalization rather than the strength of an ideology, for creative power survived only in its resistance to the strangling effects of Marxian orthodoxy. Calverton, at the beginning of his reaction, was to blame the ineffectiveness of orthodox proletarian writing upon a compulsion to view America through Russian eyes. But he was only partially right. The writers of the thirties had to learn the larger lesson that so many of their American predecessors had learned before them—that their material had to make sense in terms of their own experience if their writings were to earn the lasting respect of their readers. Farrell alone knew this almost instinctively, and he would have been the great novelist of the era had he been less prolific and more patient in making sense of his experience before transmuting it into fiction.

I I

However much the novelists of the thirties may have failed to find trustworthy and durable values in the social consciousness of the period, they nevertheless exhibited greater vitality than the writers in any other form. The lack of vitality was particularly ironic in the drama, for the Federal Theatre Project during the depression offered American dramatists for the first time a nationwide opportunity for expression and also offered the theater as a whole the chance to recapture the audiences it had been losing to the rapidly developing sound films. Furthermore, the American drama itself, which had for so long lacked any considerable literary character, had taken on a new quality during the twenties with the success of O'Neill and with the exploration of new forms and materials in such plays as George Kaufman's *Beggar on Horseback* (1924), Elmer Rice's *The Adding Machine* (1923), the psychological dramas of Sidney Howard and George Kelly, and the folk plays of Hatcher Hughes and Paul Green. There were also actors' groups prepared to take advantage of the noncommercial theater and at least one able dramatist and dramatic theorist, John Howard Lawson, capable of guiding younger playwrights into the proletarian camp.

The best of Lawson's early plays, *Processional* (1926), had drawn sharp class distinctions, and *The International* (1927) had celebrated the labor movement throughout the world; and after his Marxism became more clearly defined in *Gentlewoman* (1934) he was to write a practical handbook for the proletarian dramatist in *The Theory and Technique of Playwriting* (1936), illustrating it with the spectacular tribute to strikers, *Marching Song* (1937), which was voted the best play of the year by the second American Writers' Congress. Lawson's formula for a successful drama was that of achieving "revolutionary clarity" in an action which embodied "both conscious will and social necessity." He believed that the essential quality of drama was social conflict, but not a conflict of mechanistic or fatalistic forces so much as a conflict of wills directed toward specific aims which brought the action to a state of crisis and, regardless of the outcome, contributed to social progress by creating a new awareness of environment. Lawson's own comparative failure and that of most of his followers seem to have been the result of a greater concern for "revolutionary clarity" than for the presentation of a convincing conflict of wills and social necessities, and the most capable of his younger associates, Clifford Odets, was at his best when he was closer to Lawson's precepts than to his practices.

Although Odets achieved a certain spectacular success with his audience-participation play, *Waiting for Lefty* (1935), he proved himself a dramatist with *Awake and Sing* (1935), in which interest was centered upon the characters, and explicit revolutionary implications were left for the final scene and actually presented as only one means of escape from environmental pressures. The compulsion toward revolutionary clarity, however, pushed him away from realism in *Golden Boy* (1937) and revealed how difficult it was for a genuinely talented American dramatist to compose a tragedy along party lines. For Joe Bonaparte is the victim of his own weakness rather than of "the system," and his death is symbolic and theatrical rather than a social necessity.

But the best illustration of the devitalizing effects of the thirties can be seen in the work of Maxwell Anderson, who has come nearest to being O'Neill's successor in the field of literary drama. An extraordinarily versatile craftsman, he achieved his first success with a realistic war play, *What Price Glory* (1924), in collaboration with Laurence Stallings; mastered the light comedy with *Saturday's Children* (1927); gave expression to his social consciousness (with the collaboration of Harold Hickerson) by indignant comments on the Sacco-Vanzetti Case in *Gods of the Lightning* (1928); and boldly turned to historical verse tragedy in *Elizabeth the Queen* (1930), *Mary of Scotland* (1933), and *Valley Forge* (1934). He was also one of the most serious dramatists of the time who had reached the opinion in "the godless twenties," as he was to say later, that "the theatre is a religious institution devoted entirely to the exaltation of the spirit of man." The message of tragedy was "simply that men are better than they think they are," and it was delivered through an action which included the discovery of some element in the soul or environment of the hero which enabled him to face death or life with "a new vision." Like Lawson's formula for the proletarian drama, it was a good theory if it could be put into practice; and Anderson's major shortcoming as a tragic dramatist was that he could not find anything in the human soul or environment, during the thirties, which made death noble or life worth while.

The result was a tendency to identify the tragic spirit with a compulsion toward martyrdom which had neither a sound psychological or social justification—an arbitrary expression of "faith" in human nobility so far removed from real belief that it might almost be founded on the notion, expressed in *Elizabeth the Queen*, that the noble, the valiant, and the admirable are always destroyed in their prime while "the rats inherit the earth." This was particularly evident in *Winterset* (1935), his first effort to adapt verse tragedy to the treatment of contemporary problems. Based upon the same material used for *Gods of the Lightning*, it was primarily concerned with the effects of injustice rather than with injustice itself, especially upon a son who is anxious to clear his father's name and upon the judge who (like the Captain Vere of Melville's *Billy Budd*) had sent an innocent man to his death on the theory that "the common good" was worth more than "one small injustice." But Anderson did not set up the clear conflict between individual and social morality that Melville did, for Judge Gaunt's notion of the common good is as false as the judgment of guilt he had once directed. Nor does Anderson set up a conflict between truth and falsehood, for Mio Romagna makes only the most implausible of efforts to avoid the death he chooses in order to avoid revealing the truth he had sought so long. The whole implication is not that he dies because he is noble but is noble because he dies and allows the rats of the Estrella gang to inherit the earth. The "tragedy" of *Winterset,* like that of *Key Largo* (1939) afterward, is one which finds virtue in neither struggle nor sacrifice but simply in giving up.

In such a negative atmosphere as this—to which Robert E. Sherwood's *The Petrified Forest* (1935) also bears witness—there was no more breath for the comic than for the tragic spirit; and the instability of Philip Barry and the thinness of S. N. Behrman reveal the difficulty that even the wittiest of playwrights had in finding a solid basis from which to view the world around them. Only in the fresh, uninhibited whimsicality of William Saroyan's *My Heart's in the Highlands* (1939) and *The Time of Your Life* (1939) at the end of the decade did there appear a really positive affirmation of values, even though they seem to be the values of the pure animal spirits reflected in Saroyan's earlier short stories and so well suggested by the title of his first volume, *The Daring Young Man on the Flying Trapeze* (1934). There may have been little more than this, set forth with much more sophistication and greater pretensions to profundity, in Thornton Wilder's celebration of the eternal "something" within man which made the stark simplicity of *Our Town* (1938) so impressive, but in this play and in his affirmation of the constructive impulse in his comic allegory of survival, *The Skin of Our Teeth* (1942), the drama escaped from the false values of proletarian ideology and romantic pessimism and acquired a new vitality.

The vitality of American verse during this period is more difficult to estimate, for the age was one of considerable poetic activity and talent and of even more active criticism, which brought about many changes in poetic reputations and perhaps sustained some of them beyond their deserts. Certainly one of the most influential men of the time was John Crowe Ransom, whose three early volumes of verses—*Poems about God* (1919), *Chills and Fever* (1924), and *Two Gentlemen in Bonds* (1927)—revealed the irony and delicacy of a fine though minor poet but whose greatest influence was exercised through his leadership of the self-designated "fugitives" of Nashville, Tennessee, and through the criticism to which he turned in *God without Thunder* (1930) and reviewed in *The New Criticism* (1941). His attitude and that of his followers, as revealed in the collection of essays *I'll Take My Stand* (1930), was conservative if not reactionary in its retreat from the modern world of science and industry into an agrarian regionalism. During the thirties the members of the group became rather widely dispersed in academic circles, where they found kindred spirits who shared their self-conscious intellectuality and the tendency toward dogmatism which was so characteristic of the decade, and their influence remained strong in American universities long after the dogmatic proletarians became unfashionable.

The result has been a peculiarly academic type of poetry which has as its distinguishing characteristics a more intimate relevance to learning than to life and a ready susceptibility to critical exposition. The most important literary influence upon it has been that of

Eliot, especially through his theories concerning the poet's detachment from his work and his use of the "objective correlative" to express emotion; but Eliot's poetic mannerisms have also been extensively imitated, and even the best of the younger members of the original "fugitive" group, Allen Tate, has not been able to avoid frequent echoes of the master's cadences and a haunted recollection of the animal symbols in "Gerontion" and *The Waste Land*. The more productive Robert Penn Warren has tried to escape the excessively intellectual metaphysical quality of his early poems by a greater use of folk material; but the essentially academic nature of his imagination is revealed in the most widely read of his novels, *All the King's Men* (1946), where the reader of William Faulkner's *The Sound and the Fury, Absalom, Absalom!*, and *The Wild Palms*, and of Dashiell Hammett's *The Glass Key* will find a hero who is as recognizable as he is perhaps unconsciously composite. The dangers of an excessive literary consciousness and too great an ideological awareness, however, can be nowhere better illustrated than in the career of Archibald MacLeish, who had been writing poetry for nearly a decade before becoming a follower of Eliot in the early twenties and to a certain extent of Pound in *Conquistador* (1932)—a historical poem even more ambitious than Stephen Vincent Benét's spirited narrative of the Civil War, *John Brown's Body* (1928), of a few years before. For MacLeish, though genuinely talented and perhaps the most adaptable poet of the century, has been so sensitive to the climate of opinion that he seems to have no sensitivity from within; and the incoherence of his work as a whole shows how difficult it is for an American writer to achieve a firm position in literature by taking his stand on intellectual grounds as shifting as those of the twentieth century.

The writer's dilemma after the exuberant twenties, in short, has been that of finding a relationship to the world which would permit his creative energy to develop and mature; and this relationship was not found in proletarian dogmatism, romantic pessimism, or academic self-consciousness. Consequently it is perhaps not insignificant that the two poets who seem to have grown most in importance as they approached the mid-century were both men who had persistently sought to solve this problem in their own individual ways but in ways which were also within an older American tradition. The younger of them, William Carlos Williams, was old enough to have been in the University of Pennsylvania with Ezra Pound, to have brought out his first volume of poems in 1909, to have been one of the original contributors to *Poetry* magazine, and to have been an active participant in the literary excitement of the twenties with novels and essays as well as with poems—all composed while the author was engaged in the busy life of a successful physician. During these years he passed from a conventional lyricism through the influences of Imagism into a distinctive style of his own, based upon colloquial language and unpredictable in such transitions from seriousness to mockery and humor as may be found in his poem on "The Sea-Elephant." Yet there was a stubborn objectivity in his manner (for, as he observed in one complete poem, "so much depends upon a red wheel barrow glazed

314

with rain water beside the white chickens") which
kept him concerned with the external world and convinced that there was nothing in it which could not be
brought to life and meaning by the force of imagination. His own imagination, especially when affected by
the social consciousness of the thirties, was sometimes
grotesquely sentimental (as may be seen by comparing his poem "The Yachts" with William Vaughn
Moody's "Gloucester Moors") and sometimes aggres-
sively nonsentimental as he moved toward a philosophy of accepting the world, which gives him a firmer
place in the Whitman tradition than is occupied by
such earlier professed followers of Whitman as Carl
Sandburg and James Oppenheim.

Although he has been one of the most genuinely independent poets of the century, Williams has accepted, by following the Whitman tradition, some of
the limitations of Whitman—especially those involved
in committing himself to independence as a principle
or symbol with the consequent risk of unevenness or
affectation in his determination to accept everything as
material for poetry. And this unevenness is evident in
the first four volumes of *Paterson* (1946–51), the ambitious work undertaken at the age of sixty in an effort
to make a small New Jersey city—its history, its aspirations, and its beauty and sordidness as a physician,
after years of practice, had come to know it—the emblem of his acceptance of the whole of life as something which could be lifted out of the commonplace
and made exciting by the vitality of the poetic imagination.

Wallace Stevens, although four years older than

Williams, was much slower to come before the public —perhaps because he was inclined by temperament to place himself in a quite different sort of relationship to the world, finding in poetry a retreat rather than a form of acceptance. Although he had been intensely active in undergraduate literary circles at Harvard at the beginning of the century and a leading contributor to the new *Poetry* magazine, he did not publish his first volume of verse, *Harmonium* (1923), until he had reached the age of forty-four. By this time he was a successful lawyer and insurance executive, completely separated by age and experience and by his matter-of-fact life in Hartford, Connecticut, from the flamboyant individualism of the self-consciously "lost" generation of the twenties. Yet the volume showed that he was at heart, in his disciplined way, as flamboyant and as individual as any of his younger contemporaries. Two of its poems are especially interesting as revelations of their author's point of view and methods of expression. The earliest, "Sunday Morning" (1915), revealed a basic but thoughtful and highly sophisticated hedonism—a renunciation of belief in the supernatural and a conviction that "the blood of paradise" courses through the heart of any mortal human being who is capable of seeking enjoyment in the sensations of daily life, of feeling the power of "enduring love," and of realizing that "death is the mother of beauty" which would become insipid if it were imperishable. The second was a short funeral poem which mocked the traditional majesty of imperial death in sonorous lines which at once presented a drab picture of the reality and reduced pretentiousness to nonsense with the high-sounding refrain "The only emperor is the emperor of ice-cream." In some respects it resembles the poetry of Williams, but it is much more coherent in its use of a precise balance of music, visual imagery, and intellectual content in order to communicate a meaning which could not be achieved in the unbalanced art of such a poet as Vachel Lindsay who shared Stevens' belief in "the essential gaudiness of poetry."

But Stevens' gaudiness was accompanied by a rare elegance; and both became incidental, during his prolific period in the thirties, to a pursuit of more serious values in poetry. His *Ideas of Order* (1935)—"the order," as he was to say later, "of a man's right to be as he is"—had direct reference to the Marxian "panorama of despair"; and the poems in the volume reaffirmed the power of the imagination to master darkness by its own creative force. But it should not be an imagination based upon tradition or directed by reason, he felt when he wrote *Owl's Clover* (1936) at a time when the literary world seemed to be divided between the traditionalists and the proletarians. It was "enough to live incessantly in change"—a change caused by an unchangeable "subman," who exists below the thinking level in every man and corrects the errors of logic by his irrational consciousness. This was not a return to the popular Freudianism of the twenties, however, for Stevens was being impelled by the times to find a more serious substitute for religion than the hedonism of his early "Sunday Morning." In *The Man with the Blue Guitar* (1937) he had clearly found it in poetry, and much of his considerable literary activity during the remaining eighteen years of his life was devoted to an attempt to define poetry in terms of a disciplined perceptiveness. "Poetry is the statement of a relationship between a man and the world," was one of his *Adagia,* and it was a relationship of intuitive creativeness, based upon observation but opposed to formal reasoning. "For a poem is a nature," he said, echoing Emerson, "created by the poet"; and it was in this older tradition of finding reality within himself rather than in the world about him that he stood opposed to Williams and found both a refuge from his times and a strength which made the last two decades of his long life his most creative.

III

Detached though Wallace Stevens was from the professional world of literature, his development begins to appear symptomatic when we turn to the two writers of fiction, William Faulkner and Ernest Hemingway, who emerged after the First World War and proved to be the only two who survived the time spirit of a particular era and continued to grow in stature for more than three decades. Faulkner's first two novels, *Soldiers' Pay* (1926) and *Mosquitoes* (1927), reflected the spirit and life of the twenties in a small Georgia college town and the region around New Orleans, and it was not until *Sartoris* and *The Sound and the Fury* (both published in 1929) that he discovered his vital source of literary material in his native Mississippi where he created the microcosm of Yoknapatawpha County in which his imagination has largely dwelt ever since. *Sartoris,* in fact, provides the geographical and social frame of reference for the greater part of his later writing. The small town of Jefferson, haunted by traditions, is situated on the edge of the red-hill country, where tradition has no meaning, and within driving distance of the lowlands, where remnants of the Chickasaw Indian hunting culture still survive. The aristocrats of Jefferson, the Sartorises and the Compsons, are never quite free from the past, in which they live or against which they react in accord with standards of behavior set on the plantations before the Civil War, by the lost cause of the war itself, and during the speculative period which followed the Reconstruction era. The poor whites, represented by the Snopes family, are free from all inhibitions and are subject to the driving forces of greed and perverse meanness. Between the two classes, culturally, are the Negroes—free from all traditions except the tradition of service, and free also from greed and meanness—and a few solid white men who trade and hunt with no feeling of class responsibility. Out of these people Faulkner created his literary world.

The Sound and the Fury made it a world in depth as Faulkner used the extraordinary device of the stream of consciousness of an idiot named Benjy to unify a period of thirty years in the history of the Compson family and show the quality of love which the unreasoning child could attract while his calculating brother Jason descended to all the meanness of the poor whites and his sensitive brother Quentin, torn between family pride and sentiment on the one hand and an awareness of family degeneracy on the other, committed suicide. But the story was not complete, as

Faulkner was to indicate seven years later in *Absalom, Absalom!* (1936) when he associated its psychological depth with a depth in time by identifying Quentin's emotional stresses with his knowledge of the wild story of Thomas Sutpen, who had tried to establish a plantation and found a family in the early days when cotton was king and the future aristocrats of Mississippi were all pioneers. In the meantime he had ranged widely in his own approach to fiction, writing in the stream-of-consciousness method a grimly powerful novel of a hill family's epic attempt to deliver a corpse to the family burying ground in Jefferson in *As I Lay Dying* (1930), shocking the public and attracting wide attention with the story of a degenerate gangster and a group of moral weaklings in *Sanctuary* (1931), seriously considering some of the social and racial problems of the South in *Light in August* (1932), and returning to his early theme of postwar recklessness in *Pylon* (1935). He was a great storyteller whose tales were sometimes as tall as any that grew out of the frontier tradition, but he was finding it difficult to achieve a firm medium of communication with a public which was puzzled by his rhetoric and experimental techniques and impressed (during a period of proletarian solemnity) more by his preoccupation with violence and degeneracy than by his pervasive humor.

Actually he was finding his medium and stabilizing himself in the short stories he published in various magazines before collecting them in book form. Some of them, like those in *Doctor Martino and Other Stories* (1934), were simply good tales; others, like the ingeniously heroic adventures of a grandmother and two small boys during the Civil War in *The Unvan-quished* (1938) and the chronological account of the Snopes invasion in *The Hamlet* (1940), were coherent enough to form novels; but the most significant group were those in *Go Down, Moses, and Other Stories* (1942), which revealed the strong attraction held for Faulkner by the primitive values of the hunt—values which made "The Bear," within the context of the collection, perhaps the most positive ethical statement its author had made in fiction up to this date. By this time and with the assistance of the two contrasting stories woven together into a single novel, *The Wild Palms* (1939), Faulkner's prevailing attitudes were becoming reasonably clear. He possessed a stronger and more consistent sense of the past than did any other American writer, but he did not find in it the source of strength that Willa Cather and T. S. Eliot attributed to it. Instead, he saw it as a cultural tradition, often romanticized, which sapped the energies and eventually destroyed (through rhetoric, alcohol, or a subconscious death wish) the people who were affected by it. On the other hand, the rapacious, unprincipled, materialistic, and mean impulses of people like the Snopes threatened all values and society itself. What remained to form the basis of any hope for humanity was the blind courage and enduring spirit which could be found in even the meanest of mankind (witness the Bundrens of *As I Lay Dying* and the convict in "The Old Man" story in *The Wild Palms*) and which acquired a simple ethical pattern in the wilderness stories of *Go Down, Moses*.

The qualities of blind courage and persistence were

attributed alike to the sophisticated and garrulous lawyer, the old maid, the boy, and the Negro Lucas in
Intruder in the Dust (1948); and this first novel after
nearly a decade, though widely misunderstood by
critics preoccupied with racial relationships, prepared
the way for the Nobel Prize speech of 1950, in which
Faulkner surprised the many critics who admired the
myth of southern degeneracy more than they admired
his books by his positive affirmation of those values he
had always recognized and had come to believe in. "I
decline to accept the end of man," he said from his
"pinnacle." "I believe that man will not merely endure:
he will prevail. He is immortal . . . because he has a
soul, a spirit capable of compassion and sacrifice and
endurance. The poet's and writer's duty is to write
about these things. It is his privilege to help man endure by lifting his heart, by reminding him of the
courage and honor and hope and pride and pity and
sacrifice which have been the glory of his past. The
poet's voice need not merely be the record of man, it
can be one of the props, the pillars to help him endure and prevail." The speech was Faulkner's declaration of independence from the fears of the atomic age,
designed to encourage younger writers to cast off the
bondage of fear, and it is not hard to see in it the pattern of thought and the attitude of mind incorporated
in the political Declaration of nearly two centuries before: in the course of human events it had become
necessary to take a stand and declare a few self-evident
truths agreeable to reason only if its observations are
guided by an intellectual light within. Since then, in
Requiem for a Nun (1951) and *A Fable* (1954), he

has asserted these truths somewhat more positively in his fiction; and in *The Town* (1956) he has even attributed to the Snopes an inclination toward respectability which may lift them to the level of humanity before their story is finished.

Ernest Hemingway, in most respects, seems to be as far removed from Faulkner as any contemporary could be. A native of the Middle West, he remained in Europe as an expatriate after the First World War, brought out a volume of *Three Stories and Ten Poems* (1923) in Dijon and a collection of short stories and sketches called *In Our Time* (1924), and for reasons of his own published in America a burlesque novel *The Torrents of Spring* (1926) before becoming the leader of the self-conscious members of the "lost generation" with *The Sun Also Rises* (1926) and the short stories in *Men Without Women* (1927). Since then the little part of his life that he has spent in the United States has been lived in such out-of-the-way places as Montana and Key West, and he has made his permanent home in Cuba. He has written of these places and of France, Spain, Italy, and Africa with no implications of a regional microcosm and has written in the style of a laconic observer who stands generally outside his characters and at the opposite pole from Faulkner's rhetorical stream of consciousness. His immediate success was that of becoming Scott Fitzgerald's successor as the spokesman for the period's bored sophisticates and of speaking in an idiom which was at once more striking and more convincing than Fitzgerald's, and his lasting success came from the artistic discipline by which he achieved this idiom and kept his materials within its power of expression.

In its origin the Hemingway style was not new, for the best known of his earliest stories, "My Old Man," and the Nick Adams stories of *In Our Time* are suggestive of *Huckleberry Finn* and the first half of Melville's *Redburn* in that they are told from the point of view of a boy who can see, hear, and feel acutely but has little capacity for analyzing or interpreting his feelings and no desire to explain or do anything more than co-ordinate what he sees and hears. It is only when an adult becomes the narrator in *The Sun Also Rises* and adopts this point of view as his own—acting as noncommittal as an adolescent about the emotions aroused by a bullfight or a fishing trip or the peculiar complications of the relationship between himself and Lady Brett—that he becomes the representative of a generation which prided itself on an ability to accept any experience without judgment. The success of this technique depends primarily upon the accuracy and restraint with which the author presents material which will allow the reader to draw inferences beyond the adolescent power of expression; but it could not be achieved without such stylistic devices as an extensive use of dialogue and of a grammatical tone derived from the spoken language, a simplification of the narrative diction to a level below that of the dialogue, and a syntax which avoids the sort of judgments which are implied by subordination. *The Sun Also Rises* and many of Hemingway's early short stories were pitched on an emotional level so low that his deliberate simplification would have been ridiculous (and it was, in fact, often ridiculed) had it not been new and extraordinarily representative of people who actually were filled with a sense of futility and who would admit few emotions stronger than the desire to escape boredom. Had his work remained on this level it would have been no more than an interesting manifestation of the twenties, and it was not until he began his constant and prolonged effort to increase the emotional content of his writing without violating the fundamental principles of his style that he proved himself the most serious artist in twentieth-century American prose.

As with Faulkner, much of Hemingway's development was through his short stories; but the milestones of his progress may be found, much more readily than with Faulkner, in his novels. *A Farewell to Arms* (1929) advanced to the emotional level of romantic love, but it was love free from all social implications; and it provides an interesting illustration of the dominance of style over plot in that Hemingway was forced to kill off his heroine at the end, not because he wanted to follow the hackneyed plot of the sentimental novel, he explained, but because numerous efforts at a different conclusion had shown him that he could not handle his subject outside the restricted environment of a hospital. During the early thirties he refrained from any prolonged attempts at fiction, publishing *Death in the Afternoon* (a serious study of bullfighting, with some excellent and revealing literary comments) in 1932, a new collection of short stories called *Winner Take Nothing* in 1933, and the *Green Hills of Africa* (a book about hunting, with some rather petulant literary comments) in 1935. But the social consciousness of the new decade was having its effect upon him; and, after becoming actively interested in the Spanish Civil War, he published a novel of the depression, *To Have and Have Not* (1937), in which the cynicism of his first novel and the romantic love of his second was supplemented by a proletarian emotion toward the decadent rich and an evident sympathy for his hero's despairing belief that "a man alone doesn't have a . . . chance."

For a while the tone of this novel and of his dispatches from Spain suggested that Hemingway was adopting the ideological line of his major literary associate in the Loyalist cause (the André Malraux of *Man's Hope*) which his American contemporaries were already finding so unproductive; and his antifascist play, *The Fifth Column* (1938), was so intellectually undetermined that an extraordinary interest centered around the publication of his Spanish novel, *For Whom the Bell Tolls*, in 1940. The most ambitious and richest of his literary works, it presented a greater variety of characters than any other and went into more individual minds, and it added to the emotional ingredients of the other books a new sense of humanity and of sacrifice. But this new sense had no ideological support. On the contrary, Hemingway was embittered by the "isms" of the war and attributed to his hero, Robert Jordan, only a simple impulsiveness—almost Transcendental in quality—toward the general welfare of mankind. What he might have added to this had he completed his promised novel of the Second World War is uncertain, for the only book to come out of it was *Across the River and into the Trees* (1950), in which his own anticipation of death seems to have thrown him off balance and caused him to forget the heroism he had admired in his journalistic coverage of the Royal Air Force during the Battle of Britain and of the *maquis* of the French resistance. What was left was a celebration of good wine and good food, love, companionship, and good hunting, and a hatred of high brass and of mutilation, bound together with an emotion that only his style kept from appearing maudlin. His more natural development in a world of increasing emotional complexity was displayed, very simply, in *The Old Man and the Sea* (1954)—the basic individual human qualities of compassion, courage, and endurance which Faulkner had affirmed in his Nobel Prize speech and which seems also to be Hemingway's ultimate concept of value.

The difficulty of looking into the future makes it impossible to say what significance there is in the attraction of two such different writers toward a common standard of values which had become traditional in American literature—an attitude of mind which had developed in the past and from which they derived a power not given to their contemporaries as they gradually realized it in terms of their own experiences. Yet it is possible to find it in the types of popular literature which are most distinctively American. The spirit of courage and endurance and compassion, incorporated in a single individual, has been basic in the western novel from Owen Wister's *The Virginian* (1902) to Jack Schaefer's *Shane* (1949), despite the efforts of some recent writers to get away from it as a convention and make the Western more "realistic" and psychological. The same ideal was carried over into the peculiarly American hard-boiled detective story by Dashiell Hammett, who perfected its technique in a style that rivaled the early Hemingway's until either his capitalistic resources or his Marxian principles (for Hollywood served as a double agent during the thirties) caused him to quit writing. But his successor in the mastery of this genre, Raymond Chandler, has persuasively defended the American type of detective story as the last refuge for these values in popular literature. Yet they are beginning to emerge in the newly fashionable science fiction, and David Karp in *One* (1953) has looked into a future more skillfully regimented than that imagined by George Orwell in *1984* and expressed his faith in the ability of the individual human spirit to survive influences far more diabolical than those which made the hero of the English novel love the dictatorial symbol of "Big Brother."

Of the more serious writers of fiction it is less easy to judge, for the economics of postwar publishing tend to divide the literary scene between the occasional writers of "quality" short stories—such as Katherine Anne Porter, Eudora Welty, and Truman Capote—and the heavyweight novelists like Norman Mailer, James Jones, and Herman Wouk, whose experiences provide them with a single best seller rather than with the sustenance for growth. The highly competent professional, like James Gould Cozzens, who can do a variety of jobs in the fashion of the moment seems to have a more than ordinary advantage today over the writer who persists in his individual view of the world until his persistence gives it the validity of his own being. Yet it is interesting to note that among those who have persisted through a half score of novels, with more critical acclaim than sales, Wright Morris—in a final passage dealing with the queer psychologist and his even queerer patient in *The Field of Vision* (1956)—has come in his own way of sardonic understatement to express the same belief that was romantically expressed by Wallace Stevens, rhetorically by William Faulkner, and inferentially by Ernest Hemingway. It is a belief in the creative power of the human spirit to endure and prevail and to exist in the meanest and queerest of individuals.

This is the belief which budded beneath Puritan orthodoxy, found its way through eighteenth-century reason to a declaration of independence, transformed the symbols of European literature into something new, and became established as an American tradition which could survive the impact of an almost overwhelming materialism, the disillusionment of false hopes, and the charms of new dogmatisms. Tacit rather than rational in its pervasiveness, its expression has been shaped by so many intellectual contexts that it refuses to become a part of any system or orthodoxy and exists only as a sort of intangible national quality in American literature and an under-the-surface source of that power which contemporary literature—and perhaps America itself—derives from the past.

Index

NOTE: The American authors discussed or referred to in the text may be identified by the birth and death dates given in the Index. References by adjectives derived from authors' names are indexed under the proper names (e.g., Cartesian and Platonic under Descartes and Plato).